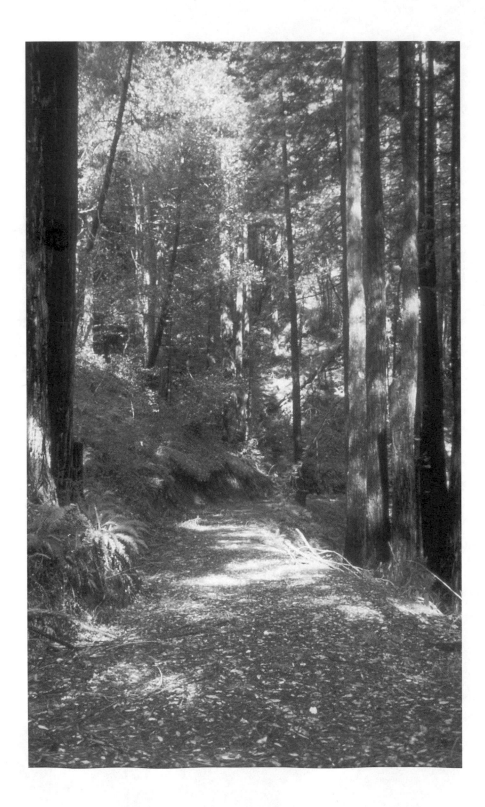

PENINSULA
TRAILS

HIKING & BIKING TRAILS ON THE SAN FRANCISCO PENINSULA

Jean Rusmore

with Betsy Crowder, Frances Spangle, and Sue LaTourrette

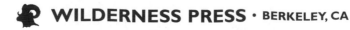 **WILDERNESS PRESS** · BERKELEY, CA

Peninsula Trails: Hiking & Biking Trails on the San Francisco Peninsula

1st EDITION January 1982
2nd EDITION January 1989
3rd EDITION May 1997
4th EDITION January 2005
Copyright © 2005 by Jean Rusmore, Frances Spangle, and Betsy Crowder

Front cover photo copyright © 2005 by David Weintraub
Interior photos, except where noted, by Jean Rusmore
Color photos, except where noted, by David Weintraub
Cover design: Lisa Pletka
Book design: Margaret Copeland—Terragraphics

ISBN 0-89997-366-3
UPC 7-19609-97366-9

Manufactured in the United States of America

Published by: **Wilderness Press**
              1200 5th Street
              Berkeley, CA 94710
              (800) 443-7227; FAX (510) 558-1696
              info@wildernesspress.com
              www.wildernesspress.com

Visit our website for a complete listing of our books and for ordering information.

Cover photo: *The Spring Ridge Trail connects Windy Hill with Portola Valley*
Frontispiece: *Portola Redwoods State Park*

Dedication

To the memory of Betsy Crowder

Acknowledgments

During the period of exploring new trails, revisiting familiar ones, and writing this fourth edition of *Peninsula Trails*, I have enjoyed the cooperation and help of many people. I especially thank Sue LaTourrette for accompanying me on the scouting hikes and for proofreading the text. Her sense of adventure and good humor made each trip a treat. To Peter LaTourrette for donating his bird photos and sharing his extensive knowledge of avian species, many thanks. To the many family members and friends who joined me on the trail, to Marilyn Walter, an outstanding trail advocate ready to hike and explore on short notice, to Joane and Ross Anderson who scouted several new trail routes, to my colleagues on the former San Mateo County Trails Advisory Committee, and to my delightful friends in the Walkie-Talkies women's hiking group, I extend my thanks.

The directors, rangers, and staffs of the public agencies through which these trails wind have been most helpful. In addition to their individual help, their maps, internet sites, and brochures have been indispensable. I thank all the dedicated people who plan, protect and care for the beautiful parks, preserves, watersheds, baylands, and beaches that grace the San Francisco Peninsula—Golden Gate National Recreation Area, State of California Parks and Recreation Department, California Coastal Commission, Midpeninsula Regional Open Space District, San Mateo County Parks and Recreation Department, Santa Clara County Parks Department, the Bay Area Ridge Trail, the San Francisco Bay Trail, the Juan Bautista de Anza Trail, and the many city parks and beaches. Two nonprofit organizations that secure land for future parks and open spaces deserve special mention—Sempervirens Fund and the Peninsula Open Space Trust. Their longtime efforts to save magnificent redwood groves, ridgeline forests and meadows, and coastal properties continue to add lands for preservation and passive recreation on the San Francisco Peninsula.

Frances Spangle and I authored the first two editions of *Peninsula Trails* and *South Bay Trails*; when Frances moved away, Betsy Crowder joined me for the third edition. Unfortunately, an accident took her life on September 29, 2000. Sue LaTourrette joins me in dedicating this fourth edition of *Peninsula Trails* to Betsy.

Jean Rusmore
November 2004

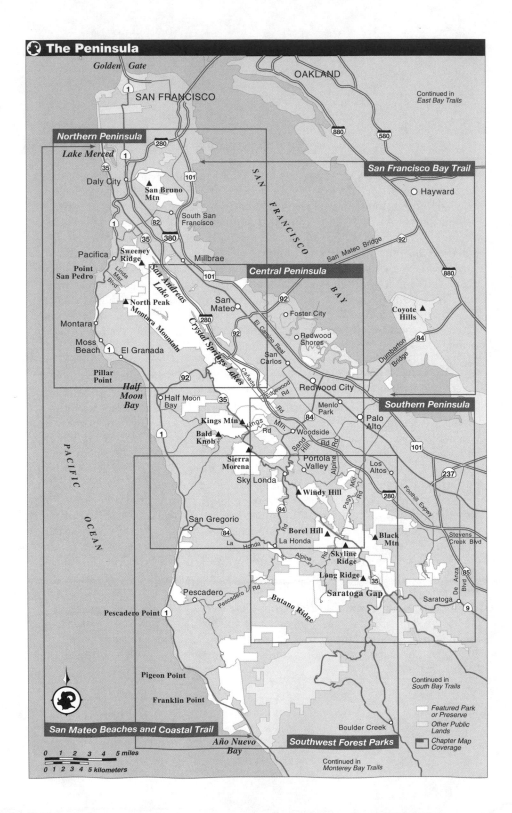

The Peninsula

OAKLAND

Continued in
East Bay Trails

Northern Peninsula

Golden Gate

SAN FRANCISCO

Lake Merced

Daly City

San Bruno
Mtn

South San
Francisco

San Francisco Bay Trail

○ Hayward

Pacifica

Sweeney
Ridge

Millbrae

San Mateo Bridge

Point
San Pedro

Linda
Mar
Blvd

▲ North Peak

San
Mateo

Central Peninsula

○ Foster City

S A N

F R A N C I S C O

B A Y

Coyote ▲
Hills

Montara

Moss
Beach

El Granada

San Andreas Lake

Crystal Springs Lakes

Montara Mountain

Redwood
Shores

San
Carlos

Dumbarton
Bridge

Pillar
Point

*Half
Moon
Bay*

Half Moon
Bay

Redwood City

Southern Peninsula

Menlo
Park

Palo
Alto

Kings Mtn ▲

Bald ▲
Knob

Kings
Rd

Woodside

Sand Hill Rd

Portola
Valley

Los
Altos

P A C I F I C

Sierra
Morena ▲

Sky Londa

Windy Hill ▲

Page Mill Rd

Alpine Rd

San Gregorio

Borel Hill ▲

La Honda

Black ▲
Mtn

Stevens
Creek Blvd

O C E A N

La Honda Rd

Skyline ▲
Ridge

Alpine Rd

Long Ridge ▲

Saratoga Gap

Saratoga

Pescadero

Pescadero Rd

Butano Ridge

Pescadero Point

Pigeon Point

Franklin Point

Continued in
South Bay Trails

■ Featured Park
or Preserve

■ Other Public
Lands

▢ Chapter Map
Coverage

San Mateo Beaches and Coastal Trail

Southwest Forest Parks

Boulder Creek

*Año Nuevo
Bay*

Continued in
Monterey Bay Trails

0 1 2 3 4 5 miles

0 1 2 3 4 5 kilometers

Table of Contents

Preface

Since the publication of the first edition of *Peninsula Trails* in 1982, the number of parks, preserves and open spaces and the miles of trails increased more than twofold. In the last two years Sue LaTourrette and I visited all the parks covered in the 3rd edition and hiked every new trail in each new park, preserve, beach or bayside. We marveled at the beauty and accessibility of the San Francisco Peninsula—from the San Francisco county line to Saratoga Gap and from San Francisco Bay to the Pacific Ocean. Therein is a magnificent treasury of open space for all to enjoy. Described here are 19 open space preserves, 2 watersheds, 11 lakes, 4 Golden Gate National Recreation sites, 5 state parks, 16 county parks, 11 state beaches, and 9 Coastal Access points.

We hope this book will help you, the reader, find these open spaces—the tiny coves and broad sandy beaches along the San Mateo Coast, the miles of paved Bayside trails, the route of the Juan Bautista de Anza Trail or the Bay Area Ridge Trail, the newest park or preserve, or the summit route to one of several 2400′+ peaks on the Skyline ridge. Awaiting you is the pleasure of seeing a tiny wildflower brightening the trailside in spring, the discovery of a shaded dell beside a rushing stream, a picnic lunch in a new park, and the sense of wonder when gazing at the vast Pacific from a bluff recently designated Coastal Access.

Jean Rusmore and Sue LaTourrette

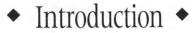

✦ Introduction ✦

The Peninsula Bayside, Mountain, and Coastside Setting

Geography

The Santa Cruz Mountains are part of the Coast Ranges of California. They run northwest to southeast, extending from Montara Mountain near San Francisco to Mt. Madonna near Watsonville. A natural divide splits the range into two parts at the Highway 17 pass between Los Gatos and Santa Cruz. The Spaniards called the southern section the Sierra Azul ("blue mountains") and the northern part, the Sierra Morena (brown or dark mountains). The area covered by this guide centers on the Sierra Morena and includes land from the San Francisco Bay on the east to the Pacific Ocean on the west. The highest mountain in the Sierra Morena, at 2800 feet, is appropriately called Black Mountain.

The east side of the Santa Cruz Mountains, steeper than the west, is cut into deep canyons by streams that empty into San Francisco Bay. The upper reaches of these creeks, which still flow more or less untrammeled down through the mountains and the foothills, are some of the main delights of the mountainside parks. Where these creeks meandered across the Bay plain, they were once the dominant features of the landscape, bordered by huge oaks, bays, alders, and sycamores. Now they have all but disappeared from sight in the flatlands, being mostly confined to concrete ditches and culverts and bordered by chain-link fences. Two happy exceptions are the lower reaches of Los Trancos and San Francisquito creeks, which still retain their parklike tree borders as they wind through Portola Valley and the undeveloped lands of Stanford University. They are the sites of popular creekside trails.

The western slopes of the Santa Cruz Mountains are a different world from the eastern side. Very few roads cross the summit; those that do usually follow old Indian trails or Spanish routes or are remnants of former logging roads. Originally thickly forested, the canyons and ridges now support a second or third growth of redwoods and Douglas firs, interspersed with live oak, black oak, tan oak, bay laurel, and smaller shrubs and trees. Some groves of giant redwoods were spared the axe and saw. Toward the Coastside some areas formerly ranched are still open grassland.

Westflowing creeks are generally larger and longer than Bayside streams, due to the heavier rainfall on the Coastside and the greater distance from the mountains to the sea. Present-day trails follow major creeks flowing through state and county parks to the ocean along routes trod by early settlers.

Geology

The Santa Cruz Mountains were formed over the millennia by the uplifting, folding, and faulting of rocks. Frequent earthquakes in the area tell us that forces

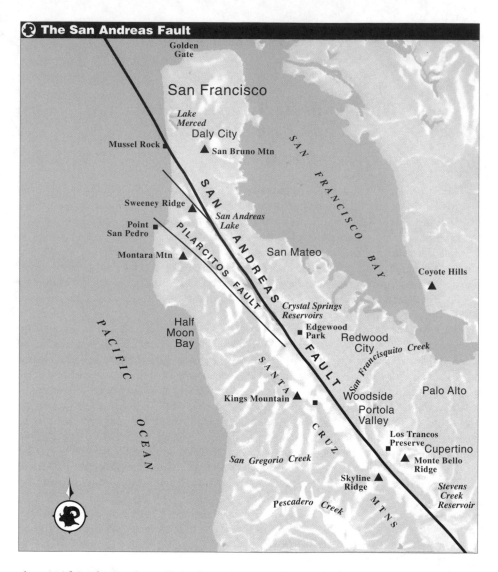

The San Andreas Fault

deep within the earth continue to reshape the land. The San Andreas Fault, which spans the length of California, is the most influential feature of the Peninsula land-scape. It runs northwest-southeast roughly parallel to the main and highest ridge of the Santa Cruz Mountains, popularly known as The Skyline.

In the 1890s Andrew Lawson, a noted California geologist, recognized the rift valley running south toward Loma Prieta and Mt. Umunhum and north up the Crystal Springs Valley as far as San Andreas Lake, about 25 miles in each direction. He named the fault for the northernmost of the rift-valley lakes. The great earth-quake of 1906, centered a few miles offshore and west of San Francisco's Lake Merced, made the San Andreas Fault famous around the world. A dramatic van-tage point from which to view this fault is the top of Los Trancos Open Space Preserve on a fault saddle between the Skyline ridge and Monte Bello Ridge.

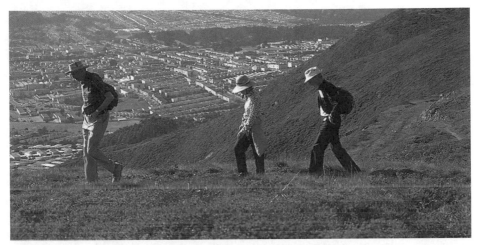

Hikers mind their footing on the trail to San Bruno Mountain's summit.

The Santa Cruz Mountains are very young geologically. The oldest exposed rocks on the Peninsula were formed only 150 million years ago, whereas the oldest known rocks on earth are four billion years old. In spite of its youth, Peninsula geology is extremely complex because the area lies at the boundary between the Pacific and the North American plates. These plates have been (and still are) moving very slowly past each other for the last several million years at an average rate of 1 to 2 inches per year. As a result of movements along the fault, granitic rocks originally formed about 90 million years ago in the area now occupied by Southern California lie deep under most of the land west of the San Andreas fault, and are exposed on Montara Mountain.

From the concept of plate tectonics, and the kind of bedrock formation found in the Santa Cruz Mountains, the following geologic history can be inferred. Between 150 and 65 million years ago, massive quantities of lava flows, red ooze, sand, and mud accumulated in complex layers on the Pacific Plate in a location west of what is now the California coast. These deposits on the ocean floor were hardened to rock, partly crushed and thoroughly mixed as the edge of the Pacific Plate was pushed under the North American continent, thus moving what is called the Franciscan Complex to its present location on the east side of the Pilarcitos and San Andreas faults. This complex is composed of shale, siltstone, limestone, sandstone, chert, and greenstone. Outcrops of these rocks occur on Sweeney and Sawyer ridges, San Bruno Mountain, Belmont Hill, and Monte Bello Ridge.

Serpentine, the California state rock, occurs in outcrops along Sawyer Camp Trail, in road cuts along I–280 from Woodside north, in Edgewood Park, and in scattered locations on Monte Bello Ridge. The linear fault valleys of the Peninsula exist because rock broken by fault movements erodes more rapidly than rock farther from the fault. You can see other and more recent signs of faulting on the Peninsula. Where the fault crosses the ridge at the top of Los Trancos Open Space Preserve, the crushed rock has eroded to form a fault saddle. Sag ponds at the preserve result from horizontal fault displacements that shifted hill slopes, blocked ravines, and created undrained depressions. Earthquake movements have changed stream courses along upper Stevens Creek Canyon. Landslides occur frequently in the steep Santa Cruz Mountains; many were triggered by the 1906 and 1989 quakes and their prehistoric counterparts.

The San Gregorio Fault runs northwest-southeast inland from the coast on the west side of the Santa Cruz Mountains. Its effects are seen in the shifts of creek directions near Butano State Park, at Fitzgerald Marine Reserve, and near Mussel Rock.

Plant and Animal Life

In this guide we mention some of the trees, flowers and creatures you may encounter, but we can touch only briefly on a few of the many species. Following are brief descriptions of the major plant communities. Fortunately for those whose curiosity is aroused, there are many excellent publications that focus on the plants and wildlife of the Bay Area and California. See Appendix II.

More than 1700 species grow in the Santa Cruz Mountains and on their western and eastern flanks, categorized into what are known as plant communities—a group of plants with similar tolerances and similar adaptations to environmental conditions.

On the east side of the Skyline ridge there are four main plant communities:

1. Mixed woodlands—characterized by the rounded forms of the oaks, madrones, bays, and buckeyes that cover much of our hillsides.

2. Open, rolling grasslands—a noticeably different community of mountainside meadows and foothill pasturelands. Mostly imported annual grasses, they are green in winter, dry and golden in summer, and characteristic of California and other Mediterranean climates, distinguished by winter rains and summer drought.

3. Conifer forests of firs and redwoods—tall, evergreen trees that cover thousands of acres in the Skyline ridge watersheds, parks, and sheltered canyons. Although the redwoods were cut over in the 19th century, extensive stands have grown again.

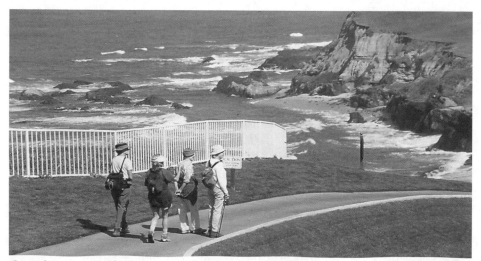

Coastal Trail south of Miramontes Point

4. Chaparral—a dense growth of shrubs and trees specially adapted to winter rains and long, dry summers that thrive on hot dry slopes. Their leathery or waxy evergreen leaves, sometimes curled inward, conserve moisture, and their long taproots reach water deep below the surface. These plants form a scratchy thicket, unfriendly to the hiker but home to many species of wildlife. The Spaniards are said to have named the vegetation "chaparral" after a Spanish evergreen oak, the chaparro.

On the west side of the Santa Cruz Mountains, heavy winter rainfall and summer fog nurture a thick forest in the canyons and on the upper slopes. Up to 60 inches of rain falls in wet years, about 45 inches in normal years. Summer fog is formed when cold water beside the coast upwells to the surface and chills the moisture-laden air above, causing condensation. The rising hot air inland creates a partial vacuum, into which foggy air flows.

The west side has three main plant communities:

1. Giant coast redwood trees—the moisture encourages lush growth in southern San Mateo County and nurtures associated Douglas firs; tan oak and bay laurel trees grow among these conifers until they are shaded out by the taller redwoods.

2. Grasslands—found on exposed west- and south-facing ridges, making sunny pockets scattered along the trails. They are either native grasses or introduced species.

3. Coastal scrub—a softer version of chaparral found on the coast itself, where the winds are strong and the salt spray pervasive, covering consists of some native grasses and introduced species that cover most of the coastal terraces and bluffs.

Fauna—You will also see and hear numerous birds, and if you look closely you will notice lizards, salamanders and the myriad spiders and insects of the earth. You may see a squirrel in the trees or an occasional rabbit in the brush. Larger animals, once so plentiful, are now seldom seen, though you may have the pleasure of catching sight of a deer in the woods or an occasional coyote in the grasslands. Mammal predators such as gray foxes, coyotes, bobcats, and even an occasional mountain lion live in the wild areas.

Footprints in the wet earth by a stream or in the dust on a sunny trail will tell you there is still animal life nearby. Small holes in the ground and tunnels underfoot are probably all you will see of the many burrowers, such as badgers, voles, field mice, and gophers. In thick woodlands you may find the three-foot-high piles of sticks that are the homes of woodrats. Along the San Francisco Bay Trail there are a few places where small populations of the burrowing owl are still extant.

The Peninsula's and Coastside's Past

Although humans have lived on the Peninsula for at least 3000 years, it is only in the past 200 years that they have significantly changed the natural landscape. Spanish newcomers in the 18th century hunted game with their guns, brought herds that grazed the hills, and introduced annual grasses that supplanted the native bunchgrass. By the mid-19th century, Anglos from the East were changing the face of the Peninsula, logging over the forests and farming the valleys and foothills.

But it was not until the mid-20th century that the settlements scattered down the length of the Peninsula suddenly spread over the valley, reshaped the hills, and replaced woodlands and orchards with houses, roads, and shopping centers.

However, the Bayside, which four decades ago was seemingly about to be engulfed in buildings, is now witnessing renewed efforts toward containing its urban spread. Public and private groups are setting aside parks, preserves, and trail corridors that complement the increasingly dense settlement patterns of the Bayside. An expanding system of public greenbelts now gives us the opportunity to walk through the lovely foothill landscape, follow a stream, or climb a trail up our steep mountains to thousands of acres of forest on both sides of the Skyline ridge. Public beaches and a coastal trail offer access to the length of the San Mateo County Coast. A walking and bicycling trail on the Bay's shore extends from the San Francisco to Palo Alto with only a few gaps. The total size of public parklands in the area covered by this book is more than 60,000 acres. Peninsula and Bay Area residents are fortunate that foresighted citizens urged the state and counties to buy so much beautiful, unspoiled land for public parks. It is the goal of this guide book to help the reader explore all the wonderful parks and preserves lying on both sides of the Skyline ridge from the San Francisco County line to roughly the area north of Highways 85 and 9.

Earliest Inhabitants

The first people to walk these hills were the Ohlones, a tribe of hunter-gatherers who lived along the Bay and Pacific shores and in the foothills between San Francisco and Monterey. When the first European explorers came to the Peninsula, they found their way crisscrossed by trails worn by these Native Americans as they went from their creekside villages to the shores of the Bay, into the hills, and across the mountains to the coast. Before the Spanish era the Peninsula supported one of the densest Native American populations in the country. Nearly 10,000 Ohlones lived between San Francisco and Monterey.

The Ohlones lived well without cultivating the land. They thrived on the incredible bounty of Peninsula woodlands, streams, and shores. Elk, deer, antelope, coyote, fox, bear, and mountain lion roamed the hills, along with plentiful small game. Birds, particularly waterfowl, filled the air in sky-darkening numbers. Acorns, the staple of the Ohlones' diet, were gathered from the thick stands of oak in the hills and on the valley floors. Families returned to ancestral groves year after year to harvest. Welcome seasonal additions to their diet were the plentiful grass and flower seeds, roots, fruits, and berries. They also used the bountiful supply of fish and shellfish from the Bay, the creeks, and the ocean. Indeed, when early explorers were offered gifts of food, they commented that native fare was palatable, even tasty.

Although the tribelets traveled between Bay and foothills most of the year to gather food, they did not stray far from the small territories they considered their own. A few groups made longer expeditions to trade with others for beads, salt, pine nuts, obsidian, abalone shells, and wood for bows. Regular trade routes crossed the hills between Bay and ocean.

The Ohlones were able to provide well for their people and lived in relative peace with their neighbors and in harmony with the land. Save for the periodic burning of the native bunchgrasses and underbrush in the meadows to keep them open for better hunting and acorn-gathering, and the paths worn by centuries of their footprints, these peoples had little impact on the land or the animals around them. Early Europeans reported that the natives moved among the wildlife and small game without arousing their fears. As Malcolm Margolin states in *The Ohlone Way*, animals and humans inhabited the very same world, and the distance between them was not very great."

The coming of the European, with guns, horses, and cattle, changed all this. The antelope, elk, and bear soon disappeared, and other animals retreated from sight. Changes in the land were profound. Cattle grazing and the inadvertent introduction of European oat grass nearly eliminated the native perennial grasses. For the native peoples, change was swift and complete with the advent of the Spanish missions.

The Spanish-Mexican Period

Two centuries after Europeans first explored the California coast by ship, the overland expedition of Gaspar de Portolá discovered San Francisco Bay in 1769. This event paved the way for permanent Spanish settlement. Mission Dolores and the Presidio of San Francisco, as well as Mission Santa Clara, were founded in 1776. A year later, the Pueblo of Guadalupe in San José was built. Mission Santa Cruz on the Coastside was founded in 1791.

After the founding of these missions and their supporting ranches and outposts, most of the natives had been moved from their villages to missions and ranches, their families broken up, their old ways lost. In just over half a century the stable culture that had changed little over thousands of years disappeared. In the final tragedy, the native people succumbed by the thousands to imported diseases to which they had little or no resistance.

In the brief period of Mexican rule the missions and their supporting farms were secularized, and the ensuing disruptions of mission life further demoralized the remaining natives. Then, with the Gold Rush came land-hungry Easterners,

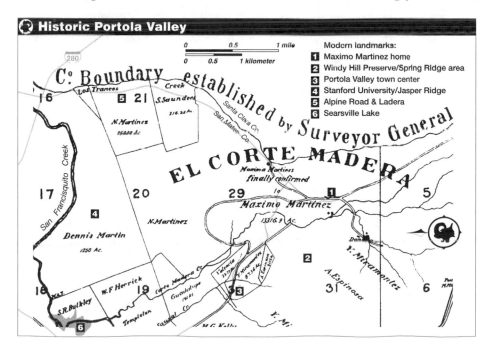

who gained title to the few remaining lands occupied by the native peoples, displacing these first Americans who had lived in harmony on the Peninsula for so long. The United States census of 1860 listed only 62 persons on the Peninsula as Native Americans.

In the early Spanish days the entire Peninsula was divided into a few vast supporting ranches for the missions and Presidio. Herds of cattle and sheep grazed over the hills. Grains, vegetables, and fruits from the ranches on the Bayside near San Mateo and from the coast north of Santa Cruz supplied these Spanish outposts.

When Mexico gained independence from Spain in 1821, the government secularized the missions and their ranches. To encourage settlement of the land the Mexican governors of California made grants of land to individuals. They divided the Peninsula into huge ranchos, as large as the 35,000-acre Rancho de las Pulgas. (East of the Skyline ridge in the area covered by this guide were the Ranchos Guadalupe, BuriBuri, Feliz, Raimundo de las Pulgas, Martinez, Corte de Madera, Purissima de Concepción, and San Antonio. To the west were the Ranchos San Pedro, Corral de Tierra, Miramontes, Cañada Verde y Arroyo de la Purisima, San Gregorio, Pescadero, Butano, and Punta del Año Nuevo.)

The brief flowering of these Mexican ranchos ended in 1848 when the American flag was raised over California. The Treaty of Guadalupe Hidalgo, intended to protect the titles of Mexican land grants, failed to do so. Hordes of Americans from the east, eager for land after the discovery of gold, poured into northern California. The great ranchos were soon divided and sold or even usurped by squatters.

On the San Mateo Coastside, American settlers took over the lands from the Mexican rancheros by fair means or foul. By 1853, Andrew Johnston, having come by wagon over the mountains from San Mateo, had settled in a large house (still standing) near present-day Half Moon Bay. In 1855 a toll road was built on this mountain alignment, making it easier to send farm produce to the Bayside towns. Other settlers moved north from Santa Cruz—the Moore family established a homestead in Pescadero and the Steele brothers started a dairy near Punta Año

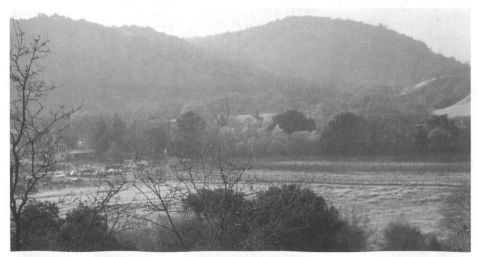

Webb Ranch nestled at the base of the Portola Valley foothills

Nuevo. Butter and cheese, shingles, and tanbark were shipped from a variety of rather precarious wharves and chutes.

Eventually tourists discovered the Coastside, and by 1907 the Ocean Shore Railroad was built south from San Francisco, reaching as far as Tunitas Creek. Another railroad worked north from Santa Cruz, but the two never met. The gap between Tunitas and Swanton (present-day Davenport) was crossed by Stanley Steamer. In 1920, storms washed out parts of the Ocean Shore Railroad and it never was reconstructed.

When modern-day roads were built along the alignments of the earlier railroad tracks, the Coastside settlements grew apace, mainly as "bedroom communities" for Bayside workers. Half Moon Bay is the only incorporated city on the Coastside, but the communities of Montara, Moss Beach, El Granada, and Pescadero are expanding as fast as their limited water supplies allow.

Logging

The Spanish had dealt lightly with the forested Peninsula hills. They felled by ax the redwoods cut to build their missions. In fact, they later expressed concern over unrestrained logging by the Anglos. The greatly increased demand for lumber to build Gold Rush San Francisco brought the first major change to the Sierra Morena, particularly to that part known as the Pulgas Redwoods—the forest above present-day Portola Valley and Woodside. The new owners of these lands logged them heavily with whipsaws. They built sawmills powered first by water, then by steam engines. As many as 50 sawmills operated in these forests, turning out lumber to build San Francisco and then rebuild it after its fires. By 1870 the huge trees, some 10 feet or more in diameter, were gone. Hardly a redwood tree remained standing east of the Skyline, but logging continued in the vast forests on the western slopes. Most of the original giant trees were cut by 1900, but redwoods are fast-growing in this climate, and second-growth trees of marketable size still are being harvested on private lands.

Farming and Ranching

With the redwoods gone in eastern San Mateo County, some of the lower slopes of the mountains were planted with orchards and vineyards. Dairy farms and large estates covered the foothills. During the late 1800s in northern Santa Clara County, ranchers planted vineyards and orchards of plums, apricots, peaches, pears, and cherries on the valley floor and in the lower foothills. This area became one of the most productive fruit-growing areas in the world. The scent of blossoming trees filled the air every spring. Ripening fruits on the trees and trays of apricots, peaches, and prunes drying in the fields made summers colorful in the peaceful orchard country. On western slopes open land became livestock and dairy farms. Later, row crops of artichokes and brussels sprouts were grown in large acreages and greenhouses containing flowers proliferated.

Urbanization and Public Open Space

In eastern San Mateo County, a century of settlement saw the gradual break-up of large estates and the burgeoning of towns. By 1863, tracks for the San Francisco and San Jose Railroad had been laid as far as Palo Alto and soon they extended to

San Jose. By 1900, a string of suburban towns had grown up along the railroad, which shaped the growth of the Peninsula until the coming of the automobile.

The Santa Clara Valley orchards survived until the middle years of the 20th century, when people poured into the Peninsula after World War II. Industry expanded in the valley, and orchard after orchard gave way to housing tracts. Towns grew until their borders touched to form the present unbroken urban band along the Bay.

Although houses had been built on the gentler slopes of the eastern foothills, the steeper hillsides, where road building was too difficult, remained wild. By the mid-1950s there were still many undeveloped hillsides, forested slopes, and canyons in a relatively natural state. As the concept of public open space evolved, the precipitous canyons and oak-covered hills were seen as welcome breaks between subdivisions. These are the lands that have become parks and open space preserves where miles of trails beckon hikers, equestrians, and bicyclists today. By the 1980s many forests and ranchlands west of the Skyline were acquired for parks and preserves.

In the 1990s and early in this century on the Coastside, the Peninsula Open Space Trust purchased farm lands and resold them to farmers who signed conservation easements that permanently reserved the land for agriculture. POST bought the 5638-acre Cloverdale Coastal Ranch in the late '90s and later gave 905 acres to enlarge Butano State Park. Also on the Coastside, Sempervirens Fund purchased an undivided one-half interest in 1800 forested acres along Gazos Creek south of Butano State Park. In 2004 the State of California park system bought some of these acres to add to Butano State Park.

In addition, several private citizens gave sizeable properties to POST, one of which, the Thysen Bald Knob piece, is now part of Purisima Creek Redwoods Open Space Preserve. More recently, the Mike and Margaret O'Neill family gave 482 acres adjacent to Rancho Corral de Tierra's southern boundary. Eventually this property will provide an exceptional link to the already vast public lands in the northwest corner of San Mateo County.

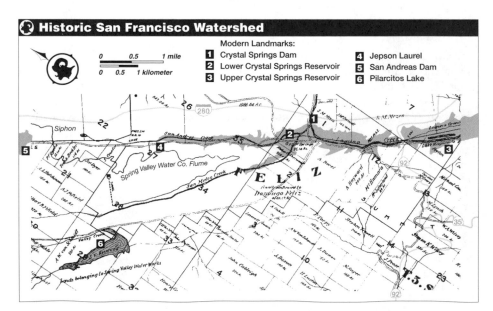

Historic San Francisco Watershed

Modern Landmarks:
1 Crystal Springs Dam
2 Lower Crystal Springs Reservoir
3 Upper Crystal Springs Reservoir
4 Jepson Laurel
5 San Andreas Dam
6 Pilarcitos Lake

San Francisco Watershed Lands

The vast city of San Francisco Watershed lands in the heart of San Mateo County have remained relatively wild since early logging ceased here, their hills spared from development and their reservoirs forming a sparkling chain of lakes. Its 23,000 acres lie between the wooded northern Santa Cruz Mountains and the lower hills to the east. It drains into upper San Mateo Creek, which was dammed in the 1890s. The resultant Crystal Springs Lakes and San Andreas Lake to the north are now water-supply reservoirs for San Francisco and much of the Peninsula.

When San Francisco needed more water than local wells could supply, the city's Spring Valley Water Company began buying up lands in the Watershed and building reservoirs. In 1862 they dammed Pilarcitos Lake in the northwest part of the Watershed, bringing water by gravity to San Francisco along a 32-mile wooden flume. Next they built the San Andreas Dam and the two Crystal Springs dams. The last of these dams, built across the gorge of San Mateo Creek, was completed in 1896, the engineering feat of its time. Although it is only 1200 feet from the San Andreas Fault rupture of 1906, it withstood the earthquake. Today a road and a trail cross this dam.

When San Francisco's needs were again outpacing its water supply, the city acquired the private Spring Valley Water Company and started the ambitious project of bringing water from the Sierra Nevada. In 1934 the O'Shaughnessy Dam at Hetch Hetchy was completed and a pipeline was built across the San Joaquin Valley. Sierra waters flowed into the Crystal Springs lakes through the Pulgas Water Temple, built to celebrate this event. This large water system now provides water to San Francisco, and parts of San Mateo, Santa Clara, and Alameda counties.

Trail Planning

History

As the Peninsula became more urban, opportunities for walking, riding, and picnicking diminished. Then NO TRESPASSING signs and houses appeared where once you could climb a fence to walk or picnic. The counties began to recognize the recreational value of some of the steep canyons, hillsides, and once-cut-over lands.

In 1924 Santa Clara County acquired lower Stevens Creek Canyon, its first county park, which has been a favorite place for hiking and riding ever since. Also in 1924 the Spring Valley Water Company laid out 10 miles of equestrian trails near Lake Merced adjacent to northern San Mateo County, probably the earliest formal trails built on the Peninsula. According to a bulletin of the Spring Valley Water Company, "These trails were planned to give riders as great a diversity of scenery as possible while at the same time minimizing the danger of trespassing on Lake Merced, the golf courses and vegetable gardens." To this day these concerns remain for trail planners as they seek routes through the countryside that will not conflict with the interests of farmers and property owners.

San Mateo County in the mid-1930s began requiring dedication of riding-trail easements as a part of land subdivisions to prevent loss of pre-existing trail links when land was subdivided.

The continued interest in trails, particularly for riding, was manifested in the late 1940s and early 1950s in a grand plan for a statewide California Riding and Hiking Trail system. In San Mateo County, with the support of horsemen's associations and hikers and with some funding by the state, trails were laid out over easements through private property along the Skyline ridge, through the San Francisco and Bear Gulch watersheds, and along the right-of-way of Skyline Boulevard and Cañada Road. The California Riding and Hiking Trail was marked by posts with gold symbols of horseshoes and hiking boots. Regrettably, in time, a number of easements through private property lapsed and freeway building obliterated parts of the trail. But many miles of the trail survived, and San Mateo County's trail from north of San Andreas Lake to Wunderlich Park and SkyLonda uses much of this same route.

The 1940s saw the acquisition of Huddart Park and the development of riding and hiking trails there. San Mateo County, with trail-club cooperation, laid out still more hiking and riding trails on road rights-of-way along Cañada, Whiskey Hill, and Portola roads through the present-day towns of Woodside and Portola Valley.

In a burst of trail-planning activity in the 1950s and 1960s, San Mateo County mapped over 400 miles of trails in the City/County Regional Plan for Parks and Open Space, adopted in 1968. Unfortunately, at that time neither the funding nor the support for trails was sufficient to bring these trails into being.

However, with funding from a federal pilot project to encourage trails in urban areas, three important trails were built in 1969—the Waterdog Lake and Sheep Camp trails from Belmont to Cañada Road and the Alpine Road Hiking, Riding and Bicycle Trail.

In the 1970s, with renewed appreciation for the remarkable potential for hiking and riding trails in the Peninsula mountains and foothills, conservation, hiking, and riding organizations pressed for specific programs and funding for trails. Voters in San Mateo County adopted a Charter for Parks establishing a special tax for park purposes, and Santa Clara County voters passed a park bond issue. In 1974 a gift of Wunderlich Park's 942 acres of conifer forest and meadows provided hikers with many more miles of trails. The city of Palo Alto bought 1400 acres of hillside woodland, which have become the much prized Foothills Park. Other cities reserved canyons, streamsides, and hillsides for public use.

But the citizens of the Peninsula, still concerned with the rapid disappearance of open space and the slow pace of park acquisition, proposed by initiative a Midpeninsula Regional Park District. Northern Santa Clara County voters formed this district in 1972 and were joined by voters in southern San Mateo County in 1976, after which the name was changed to Midpeninsula Regional Open Space District (MROSD).

The District's major purpose is to acquire and preserve foothill and Bayland open space to protect it from development, and to open it to public use consistent with protection of the environment. These lands provide protection for natural vegetation, wildlife, and areas of scenic beauty. The District's goal is to help preserve a greenbelt of open space linking District lands with state and county lands. By 2004 the District had acquired almost 49,000 acres in San Mateo and northern Santa Clara counties and a corner of Santa Cruz County. This greenbelt is creating a system of regional trails with outstanding opportunities for hiking, riding, bicycling and running. This large aggregation of open space lands creates important wildlife corridors.

In 2004, the District voted to expand its boundaries to the edge of the Pacific, an area of 220 square miles in San Mateo County (its current district encompasses 330 square miles in northwestern Santa Clara and southwestern San Mateo County). Shortly a group circulated a petition to repeal the action. The petitioners needed 4071 signatures to qualify a ballot measure, but the elections office certified fewer than 3450. On September 3, 2004, Judge Carl W. Holm issued a three-page ruling that rejected annexation opponents' claim that they had gathered enough qualifying votes. He also lifted a temporary restraining order, dated July 13, that halted the annexation process launched in April.

This coastside protection program, endorsed by farmers, conservationists, and business leaders, is designed to protect the region's unique rural and agricultural heritage. The MROSD gave up its right to eminent domain in this area and agreed only to buy from willing sellers. The District will soon conduct workshops and develop a process needed for democratic representaton of Coastside residents in the open space district.

In 1994, the voters in southern Santa Clara County formed the Santa Clara County Open Space Authority (SCCOSA), a special district with a purpose similar to that of MROSD. It has purchased several parcels, one of which is open to the public—the Boccardo Open Space.

The Peninsula Open Space Trust, a nonprofit land conservancy, takes another approach to open-space acquisition. The Trust is dedicated to private and public preservation of open space in San Mateo and Santa Clara counties. Organized in 1977, the Trust has protected over 55,000 acres through purchase, gift and provision of local, private matching funds for public projects.

In 1995 the Santa Clara County Board of Supervisors adopted a Trails Master Plan, which was the product of several years' work by citizens' committees and commissions. This plan identifies 522 miles of trails and trail corridors that in the future will link the county's urban areas and parks and connect with trails in adjoining counties.

San Mateo County's Trails Plan was adopted by the Board of Supervisors in March 1990; a revision was drafted in 1995 and approved and made part of the County's General Plan in 2002. This plan proposes a system of trails that would link county parks to other public parklands in this county and in adjacent counties.

Pressure for trails sparked state legislation for funding major trails to link state and county parks. Growing interest in regional trails led to bold programs initiated in 1987 for two Bay Area trail systems—the San Francisco Bay Trail and the Bay Area Ridge Trail. Statewide citizen action has spearheaded planning for the Coastal Trail and the Anza Trail.

Hostels and Overnight Camping

As long-distance trails take shape, more camping and hostel facilities will be needed. In the area covered by this guide, camping by reservation is possible at many county and state parks in the mountains and at the beaches in the western part of the county. See Appendix I for a complete list and Appendix III for addresses and phone numbers. Backpack camps on Black Mountain in Monte Bello Open

Space Preserve and in Butano State Park are available by reservation. Some camp-sites are reachable by long trails from the Bayside, such as the Hickory Oaks/Ward Road Trail from Long Ridge OSP to Portola Redwoods State Park. The Hikers' Hut in Sam McDonald County Park and the Jack Brook Horse Camp in Sam McDonald Park are also available to groups by reservation with San Mateo County Parks Department.

Hidden Villa Hostel at the base of Black Mountain in Los Altos Hills, the first and oldest hostel in the West, is open September through May, but closes in sum-mer to accommodate a youth camp. Welch-hurst Hostel in Sanborn-Skyline Park and the Montara and Pigeon Point Lighthouse hostels provide accommodations for travelers year-round. Be aware that most hostels close from 9:30 A.M. to 4 P.M. daily. Hidden Villa Hostel closes from 11 A.M. to 4 P.M.

Trail Building and Maintenance

The success of trail programs depends to a great extent on careful operation, good maintenance and citizen cooperation. Various organizations, including the Santa Cruz Mountains Trail Association, Scouts, Sierra Club, the Trail Center, school groups, MROSD Preserve Partners, and San Mateo County volunteers, are making valuable contributions in trail building and clean-up projects. They also perform an important role in disseminating trail information and promoting a sense of stewardship for public land and respect for private property. See Appendix III.

Long Distance Trails

Four long Bay Area trails include segments in the area covered by this guide-book. With the completion of more than 267 miles of the proposed 400-mile Bay Area Ridge Trail and 251 miles of the San Francisco Bay Trail, users already have an unparalleled opportunity to explore our region at its highest elevations on the ridgetops and at sea level along the San Francisco Bay. Local pathways, like spokes of a wheel, will eventually connect our communities with both these encircling trail systems.

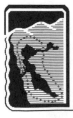
The **Bay Area Ridge Trail** is being developed by the Bay Area Ridge Trail Council working with the National Park Service, state and local park departments, regional open-space districts, and water agencies, and has completed 267 miles. In the area covered by this guide, it will link Peninsula trails from the Golden Gate National Recreation Area in San Francisco through San Mateo County's moun-tainside parks to Saratoga Gap. Already more than 44 miles of trail in this corridor are completed; only a few gaps remain.

The **San Francisco Bay Trail** is being implemented by the
Association of Bay Area Governments, the Metropolitan Transportation Commission, and the nonprofit San Francisco Bay Trail Project. At the time of this guide's publication, 251 miles of trail are in place, 43 miles of which are in San Mateo County.

The **Coastal Trail** along the San Mateo County Coastside, part of a Pacific Coast Trail from Canada to Mexico, is being implemented by federal, state and local juris-dictions. Local citizens assist in planning, implementation and trail maintenance.

Many sections are completed and are described in the San Mateo Coast Beaches section of this book. At this writing there are 42 miles of trail completed.

The **Anza Trail**, a National Historic Trail, follows the path of Captain Juan Bautista de Anza on his quest to find a land route from Mexico to San Francisco in 1776. Now local agencies, under the auspices of the National Park Service, are marking this trail. Handsome signs along Highway 85 indicate that the trail goes somewhere nearby.

For more information on these ongoing projects, see Appendix III.

Information for Trail Users

The main purpose of this guide is to describe trips through our parks and preserves, giving a detailed account of each trail and information on elevation change, terrain, orientation, trip distance, and hiking time. The authors have drawn on their own experience of hiking on all the trails in this guide. Their enthusiasms are, of course, subjective, but directions, trail distances, and details of natural features are intended to be objective and concise.

Travel times are based on a moderate hiking pace, which averages about two miles an hour, taking into account the difficulty of the terrain and the elevation gain. Trip distances are stated as one way, loop, or round trip. Trip times are those required to complete the trips as described. Of course, time for bicyclists or equestrians will differ from that for hikers.

Figures for *elevation change* tell the vertical footage gained or lost from the start to the highest or lowest point of the trip. These figures do not include minor elevation changes along the way. When the outward leg of a loop or a round trip is uphill, the elevation change is given as a gain; then, of course, the return leg will be an elevation loss. Conversely, when the outward leg is downhill, the elevation change is given as a loss.

To estimate the time required for a trip where the cumulative gain is more than 1000 feet or where there are steep climbs within a short distance, the authors used an old hiking rule: for every 1000 vertical feet gain, add ½ hour to the time that would be required on level ground.

Trails for Different Seasons and Reasons in Appendix I groups trails for a variety of purposes and situations, from long hikes and steep mountain climbs in large parks and preserves to strolls on gentle paths past tidal marshes and ocean beaches. These suggestions may help those unfamiliar with the Peninsula and its Coastside to find a suitable trail or perhaps inspire seasoned hikers to try new trails in our parks and open-space preserves. It is not an exhaustive list. Users can add their favorites.

Every effort has been made to make this guide up-to-date, but new parks and preserves opening in the future undoubtedly will provide new trails.

Maps

On the *Map of Peninsula Trails* in the beginning of this book, the general locations of parks, preserves, and watersheds are shown keyed to three sections that correspond with the table of contents—Northern, Central, and Southern

Peninsula—as delineated by the three major roads crossing from Bay to Coast. An enlarged map precedes each of these three sections in the text., and a map also accompanies each park or preserve. Separate maps of the San Francisco Bay Trail and the Coastal Trail in San Mateo County precede those sections of the book and are presented from north to south.

Individual maps of all the parks and preserves, specially prepared for this book, show trail routes and entry points, main natural features, elevations, park facilities, and parking areas for cars and horse trailers. These maps are a valuable reference for hikers, runners, bicyclists, and equestrians, as well as for those who wish to picnic or just relax in public recreation sites. Although many parks and preserves offer trails maps, these are not always available. To secure more information, leaflets, and maps, and free docent-led walks and tours in MROSD preserves, federal, state, and county parks, write, phone or visit the agency's website listed in Appendix III.

Map Legend

Paved Multi-Use Trail	Freeway
Multi-Use Trail	Road
Hiking & Equestrian Trail	Minor Road
Hiking Only Trail	Rail Transit/Station
Disabilities Access	
Bay Area Ridge Trail	Major Stream
	Seasonal Stream
Publlic Transit Stop	Lake/Pond/Bay/Ocean
Trailhead Parking	Marsh/Swamp
Limited Parking	
Equestrian Parking	Peak
Picnic	
Camping	Featured Park or Preserve
Rest Room	
Visitor Center/Museum	Adjacent Park or Preserve
Ranger Station	Private Land
Building	
Gate/Number — WH02	
Point of Interest	
Bridge/Tunnel	True North

In addition to these public agencies, the Trail Center is a volunteer organization that serves as a source of information about local trails and trail activities. Among publications available are a four-county parks map and a trail map of the southern Peninsula, now available through Wilderness Press.

Excellent topographic maps are available from the United States Geological Survey headquarters and from many sporting-goods stores. The western district headquarters of the USGS is at 345 Middlefield Road, Menlo Park. The map sales and information office, Building 3, a fascinating place worth a trip in itself, is open from 8 A.M. to 4 P.M. USGS maps are published in a 7.5-minute series. Some local trails are shown on these maps, but it is the topographic information that is of particular interest to the trail user—contours and natural features, such as wooded areas, clearings, creeks, lakes, and mountains. Although topo maps are not necessary for using the trails in this guide, they can add to your understanding of the terrain. After you have learned to read the contour lines, you can visualize the shape and elevation of the land they represent. Then you can tell by the spacing of the contour lines whether the grade on the trail will be steep or gentle.

The area of this guide is covered by quadrangles of the 7.5-minute series, listed here from north to south: *San Francisco South, Montara Mountain, San Mateo, Half Moon Bay, Woodside, Pigeon Point, Palo Alto, Mindego Hill, Cupertino, La Honda, San Gregorio, Big Basin, Franklin Point,* and *Año Nuevo.*

At some sports shops, one can print parts of or full-size topo maps on waterproof paper for a price somewhat higher than the USGS charges.

Trail Rules, Etiquette, and Safety

Park and open-space preserve regulations are few, but they are important. Based on common sense, they are necessary for your own safety, the protection of the parklands, and to preserve the beauty of the natural setting.

- All plants, animals, and natural features are protected. Leave them undisturbed for others to enjoy.
- Stay on the trail. Shortcuts across trail switchbacks break the trail edge and accelerate erosion.
- Don't smoke on the trail, and build no fires except where permitted in established fireplaces.
- Firearms and bows and arrows are prohibited.
- Hours: generally open 8 A.M. to dusk; MROSD preserves open dawn to dusk.
- Fees for some state and county parks; subject to change.
- Trail closures: in wet weather trails often are closed to bicyclists and equestrians. Newly constructed trails are temporarily closed until treads harden.
- Dogs: prohibited in all San Mateo County parks. In Santa Clara County dogs are prohibited except in some parks that permit dogs on a short leash in picnic areas, but never on trails. Midpeninsula Regional Open Space District permits dogs on leash in some preserves; call for information. State parks allow dogs on leash in campgrounds but not on trails.
- Hikers and runners: yield to equestrians.

- Bicyclists: ride on designated trails only. Observe closure signs. Helmets required in all parks and preserves. Speed limit in MROSD preserves and Santa Clara County parks is 15 m.p.h.; 5 m.p.h. when passing. Yield to equestrians and hikers.

- Equestrians: observe closure signs. Indicate to other users when it is safe to pass.

- Safety: travel with a companion rather than alone. See list of organizations offering group trips in Appendix III.

Some Hazards For Trail Users

Poison Oak: This plant, *Toxicodendron diversilobum*, is widespread through most of the Peninsula hiking country. You don't need to remember its Latin name, but you should learn to recognize this ubiquitous plant with its three-lobed leaves. A pretty cream-colored flower cluster is followed by white berries. It looks different according to the season and the environment where it is growing. In spring its gray branches send out reddish buds, then shiny, young, light-green leaves. In autumn it has rosy red leaves that are brilliant in the woods and along the roadsides. To touch the twigs or leaves is to court the outbreak of an uncomfortable, itchy, blistering, long-lasting rash.

Avoid it! Wear long sleeves and long pants for protection; bathe with cool water and soap when you get home. If you have unavoidably brushed against some poison oak, wash the area in the nearest stream or even use water from your canteen. Investigate new pharmaceutical products designed to prevent contamination and others to remove its effects.

Rattlesnakes: Another, and far less common, hazard is the rattlesnake. It has a triangular head, diamond markings or dark blotches on its back, and from one to ten or more rattles (segments) on its tail—it adds a new rattle each time it sheds its skin. It is the only poisonous snake native to our hills; it inhabits many hillside parks, though it is rarely seen. The rattlesnake will avoid you if it possibly can. Just watch where you put your feet and hands, and stay on the trails.

Lyme Disease: A potentially serious illness can result from the bite of the Western Black-Legged tick, a ¼-inch-diameter insect. Ticks brush off onto you from grasses and trailside bushes. Wear long pants, tucked into boots or socks, and a long-sleeved shirt.

Mountain Lions: Sightings of these shy, native residents of wild lands have become more frequent due to increased use of their habitat by people. A mountain lion is about the size of a small German shepherd, with a thick tail as long as its body. It is recommended that trail users stand facing any mountain lion they encounter, make loud noises while waving their arms, and not run away.

Bobcats: Although generally shy, if aroused they can be treacherous. They are about twice the size of a house cat with 6-inch-long tails.

Feral Pigs: Imported from Europe, these animals interbred with domestic pigs and have spread over many acres of wild lands since their introduction for hunting in the 19th century. While generally not dangerous to humans, they can be fierce when cornered. If you see large areas of meadows and open forest that appear to have been tilled, you are proably seeing the work of these animals.

Coyotes: Their numbers are increasing; frequently sighted in open grasslands; seem curious about humans and have been known to attack humans.

Remember, wild animals normally avoid humans, if possible. Trail users must be careful not to entice them closer by giving them food, as they may lose their natural fear and cause problems.

Weather

The vagaries and variety of our local weather require some flexibility in planning hikes. Summer weather can vary from day to day, even from hour to hour where coastal fogs and winds influence the temperature. The Coastside, Skyline ridge and the northern Peninsula are often windy and dripping with fog in summer while the rest of the Peninsula is mild and sunny. In other seasons the mountains can be drenched in rain when the Bayside cities are merely cloudy. Fall, winter, and spring are best on the Coastside, when fresh breezes bring clean air and crystal visibility.

Summer and fall bring sunny, hot days to the southern Peninsula. Midday hiking is best then in the cool, forested canyons. In any season, south- and west-facing slopes are the warmest. A winter hike on such slopes is delightful on a sunny day.

What To Wear

Walking is surely the prime low-cost sport. The rewards are unrelated to the outlay for equipment.

The only essential is comfortable, sturdy footgear. The many available walking and running shoes with good treads are fine for Peninsula trails. Some hikers still prefer boots for the protection they give on rough terrain and on wet trails.

Clothing—dress like an onion, so you can peel off layers as needed:

- sweater and windbreaker
- long-sleeved shirt and long pants for protection from sun and poison oak
- hat for shade in summer and a scarf or warm cap for cold and windy days.
- all-purpose bandana or scarf

Water—an essential; no drinking fountains on trails; stream water is unsafe to drink

- snack or lunch
- this guidebook
- day pack—for extra clothing, lunch, and water

And, if weight is not a problem:

- binoculars for birds
- magnifying glass for flowers, lichen, and insects
- flower or bird guide

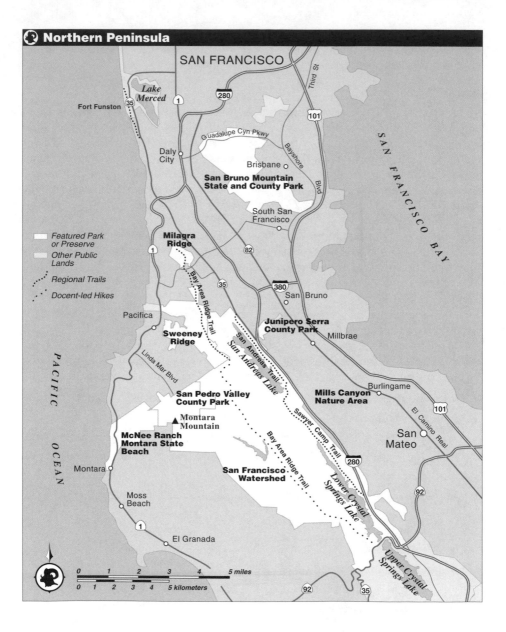

Northern Peninsula

◆ Northern Peninsula ◆

From the San Francisco County Line to Highway 92

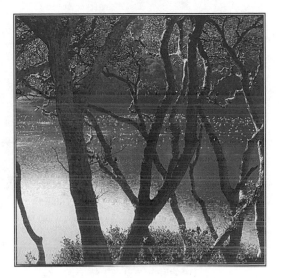

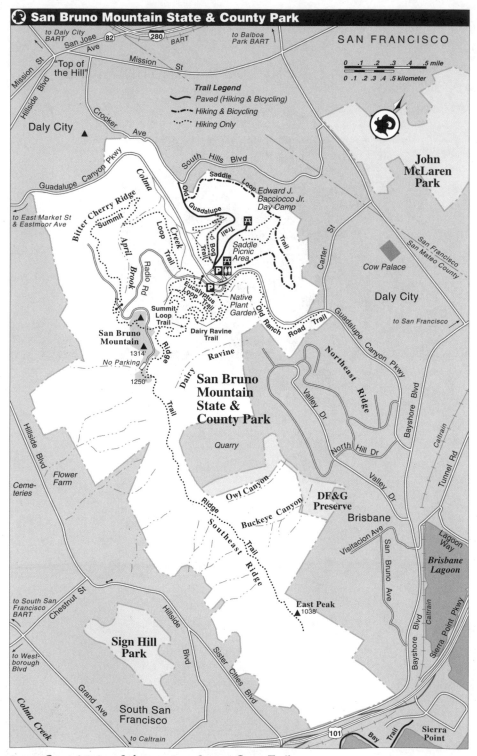

San Bruno Mountain State & County Park

to Daly City
BART
San Jose
to Balboa
Park BART
82   280   BART

SAN FRANCISCO

Mission St

Hillside Blvd

Mission St

"Top of
the Hill"

Crocker   Ave

Daly City

Guadalupe Canyon Pkwy

Colma

to East Market St
& Eastmoor Ave

Trail Legend

Paved (Hiking & Bicycling)

Hiking & Bicycling

Hiking Only

0   .1 .2 .3 .4   .5 mile
0 .1 .2 .3 .4 .5 kilometer

**John
McLaren
Park**

South Hills Blvd

Saddle   Loop

Old   Guadalupe   Trail

Edward J.
Bacciocco Jr.
Day Camp

Bitter Cherry Ridge

Summit

April   Brook

Creek   Loop   Trail

Bog   Trail

Saddle
Picnic
Area

Carter   St

San Francisco
San Mateo County

Cow Palace

Daly City

Radio   Rd

Eucalyptus
Loop   Trail

Native
Plant
Garden

Old   Ranch   Road   Trail

Guadalupe Canyon Pkwy

to San Francisco

**San Bruno
Mountain**
1314'
No Parking

Summit
Loop
Trail

Dairy Ravine
Trail

1250'

Ridge

Dairy   Ravine

Trail

**San Bruno
Mountain
State &
County Park**

Quarry

**Northeast
Ridge**

Valley   Dr

North Hill Dr

Bayshore   Blvd

Caltrain

Hillside Blvd

Ceme-
teries

Flower
Farm

Ridge

Owl Canyon

Buckeye Canyon

Southeast   Ridge   Trail

**DF&G
Preserve**

Brisbane

Valley   Dr

Visitacion Ave

San Bruno Ave

Lagoon
Way

*Brisbane
Lagoon*

to South San
Francisco
BART

Chestnut   St

to West-
borough
Blvd

Hillside   Blvd

**Sign Hill
Park**

Sister Cities Blvd

East Peak
1038'

Tunnel Rd

Bayshore   Blvd

Caltrain

Sierra Point Pkwy

Colma Creek

Grand   Ave

**South San
Francisco**

to Caltrain

101

Bay   Trail

**Sierra
Point**

Lower Crystal Spings Lake seen from Sawyer Camp Trail.

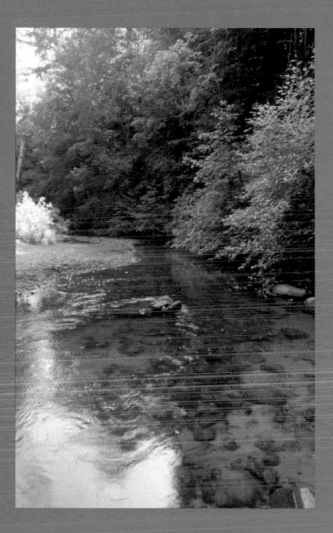

PENINSULA TRAILS
Photo Exploration

All photos by David Weintraub unless otherwise noted

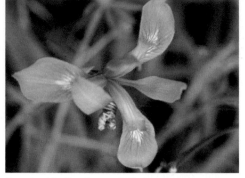

Douglas iris, Bay Area wildflower

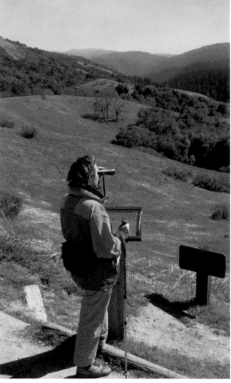

Peter LaTourette

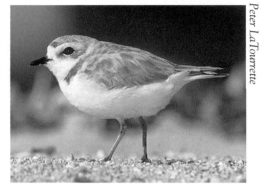

Snowy Plover

Stevens Creek Nature Trail

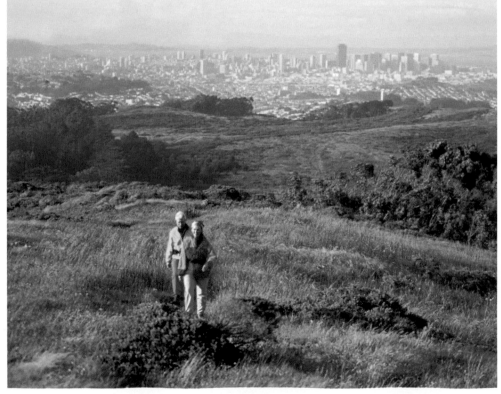

Summit Trail, on the north side of San Bruno Mountain

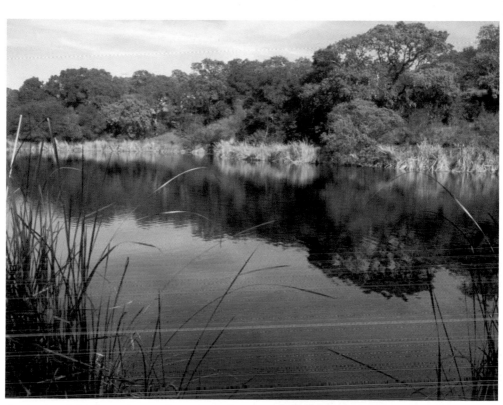

Arastradero Lake, formerly a ranch stock pond

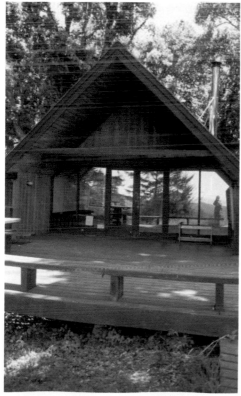

Hikers Hut, Sam McDonald County Park

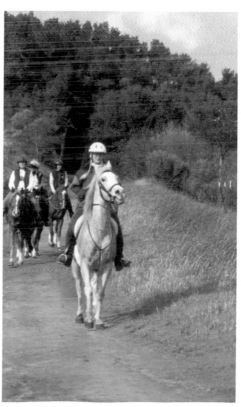

Equestrians ascend the Spring Ridge Trail

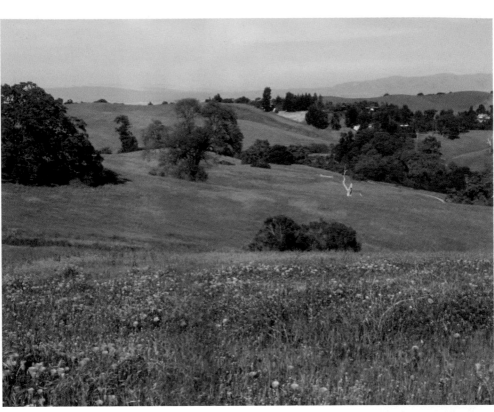

Arastradero Preserve

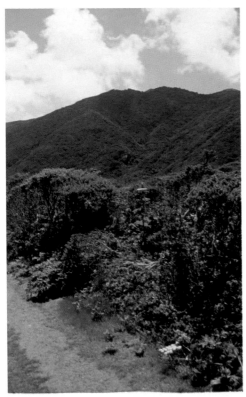

Montara Mountain Trail

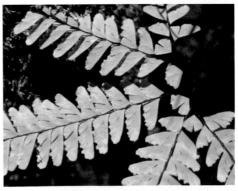

Fivefinger fern in a coast redwood forest

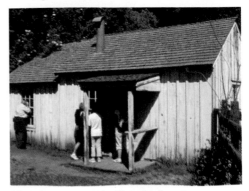

Historic Grant Cabin, Deer Hollow Farm

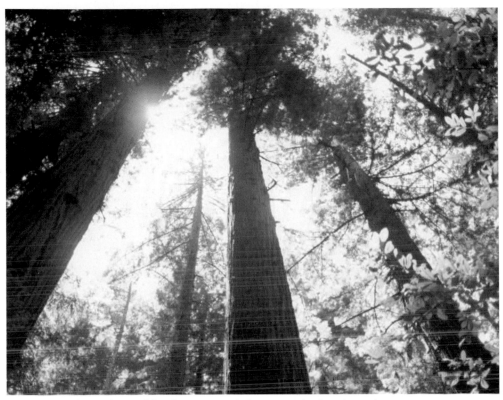

Coast redwoods are the world's tallest trees and also among the fastest growing.

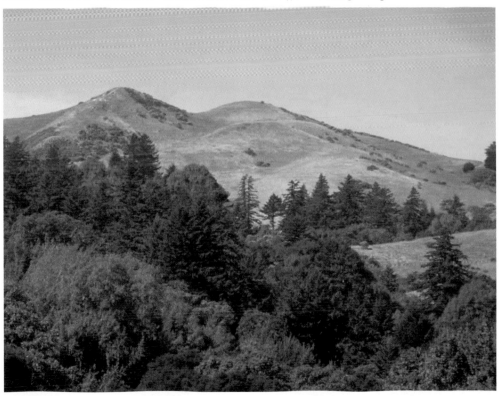

Windy Hill's twin summits, from the junction of the Lost and Hamms Gulch trails

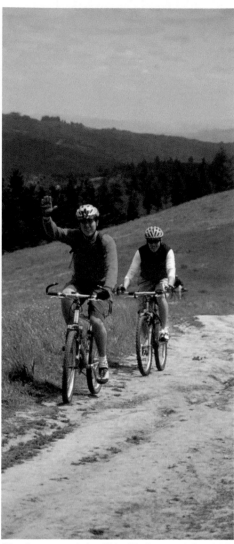

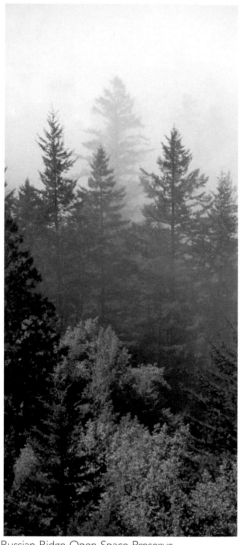

Bicyclists ascend the Ridge Trail toward Borel Hill

Russian Ridge Open Space Preserve

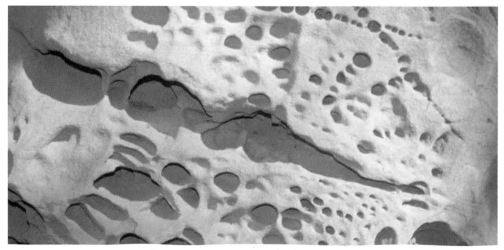

Erosion by acidic rain creates fantastic sandstone formations called tafoni.

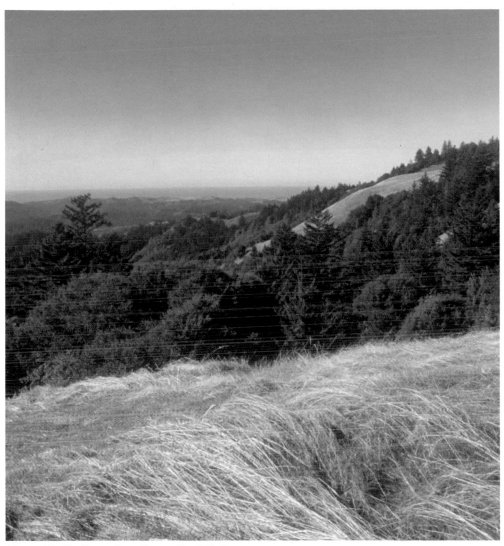

View of Pacific Ocean from Peters Creek Trail

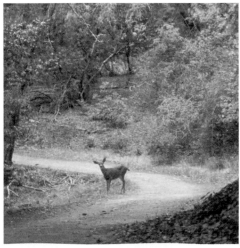

Deer on the Alambique Trail

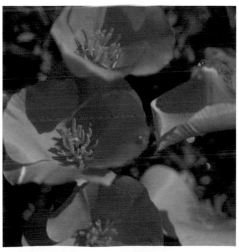

California poppies, the state flower

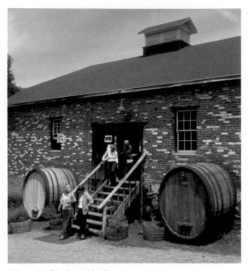

Historic Picchetti Winery

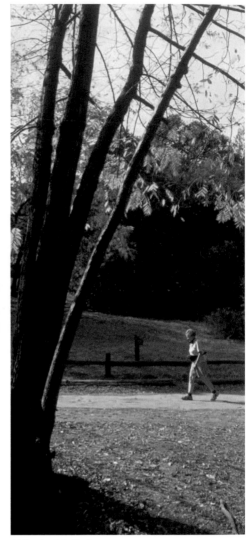

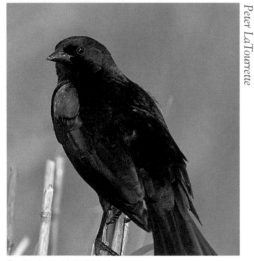

Red-winged blackbird

Wunderlich Park

Peter LaTourrette

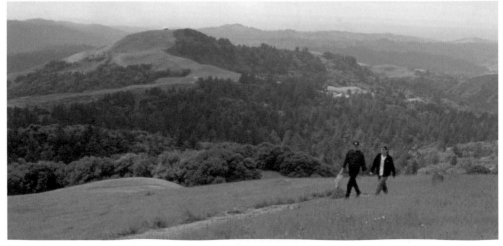

Views from the Ridge Trail near Borel Hill extend westward to the Pacific Ocean.

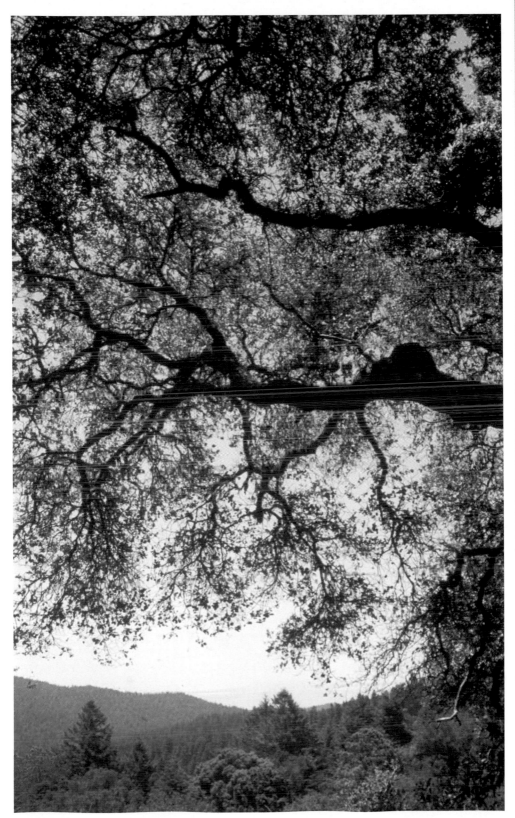

Pescadero Creek County Park

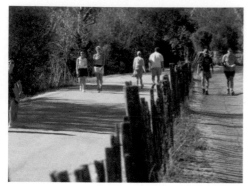

Rancho San Antonio

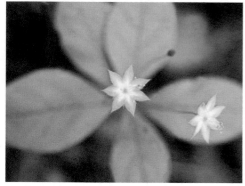

Starflower, found on shady forest floors

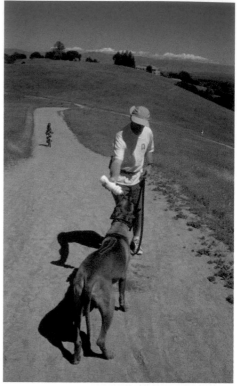

Fremont Older Open Space Preserve

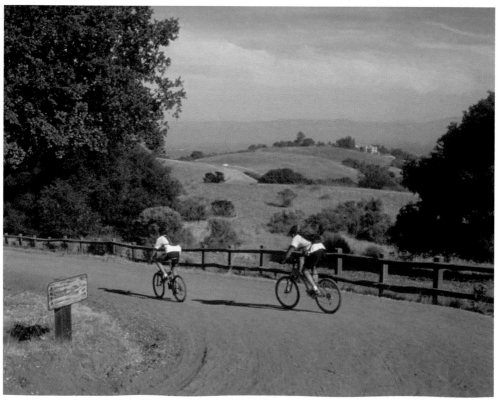

Fremont Older Open Space Preserve

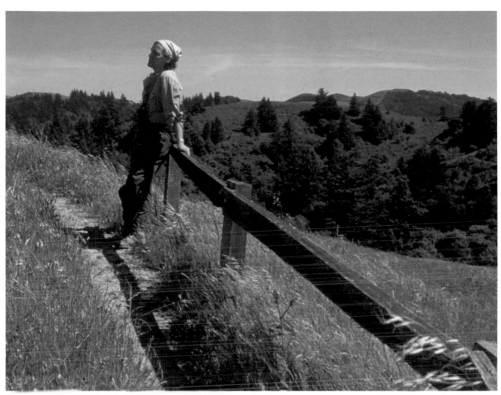

Anniversary Trail, toward Windy Hill summit

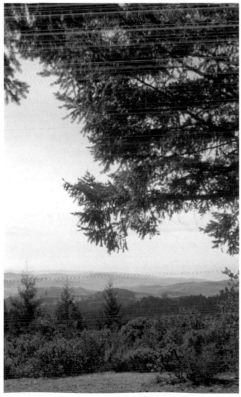

El Corte de Madera Open Space Preserve

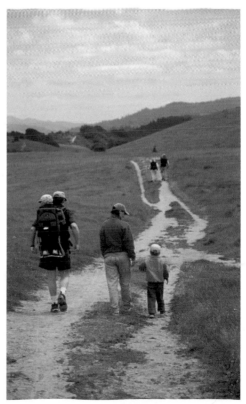

Russian Ridge Open Space Preserve

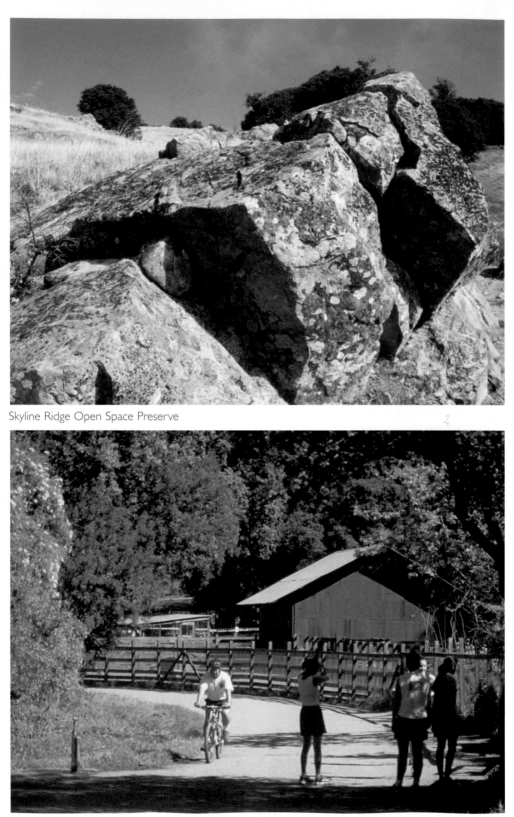

Skyline Ridge Open Space Preserve

Deer Hollow Farm

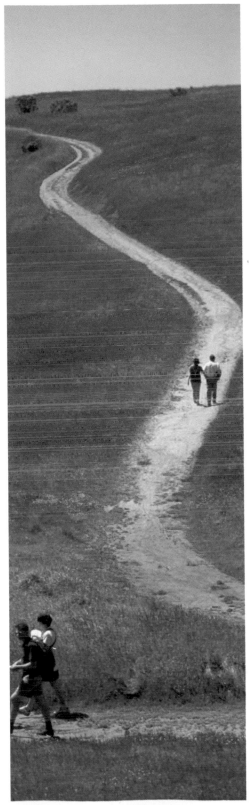

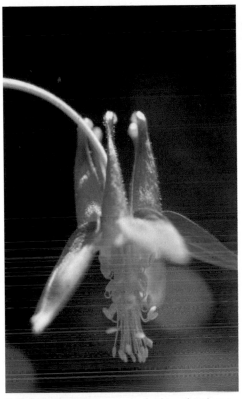

Crimson columbine grows in shady, moist places.

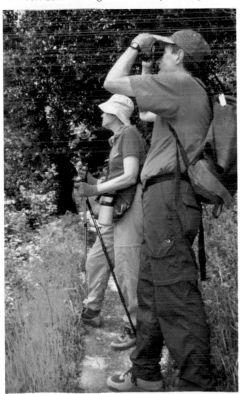

Russian Ridge Open Space Preserve

Purisima Creek Redwoods

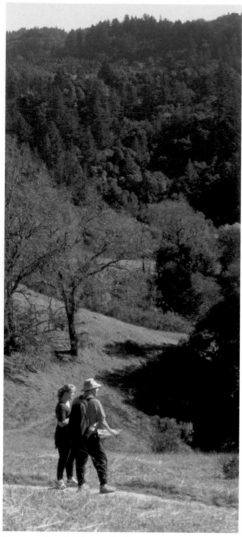

Stevens Creek Nature Trail

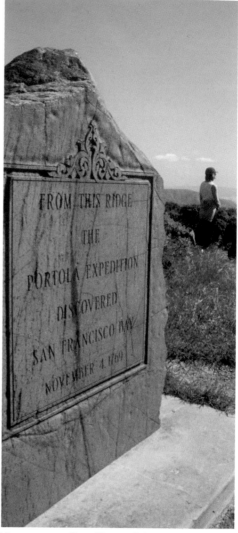

Monument to Portolá expedition

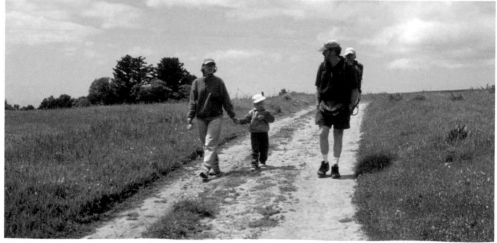

The Ridge Trail, Russian Ridge Open Spacde Preserve

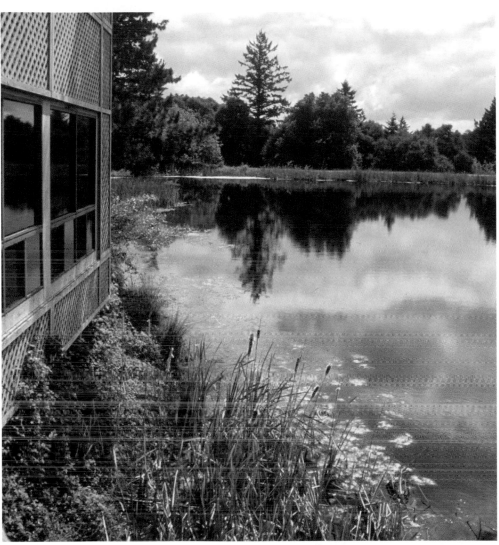

The Daniels Nature Center on Alpine Pond, Skyline Ridge Open Space Preserve

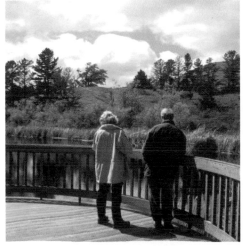

Looking out on Alpine Pond

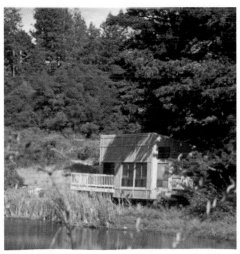

View of Daniels Nature Center

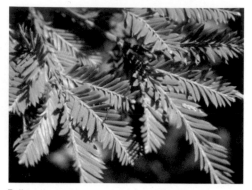

Foliage on young coast redwood

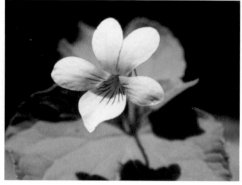

Redwood violet

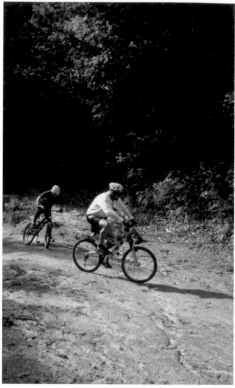

Biking on the Methuselah Trail

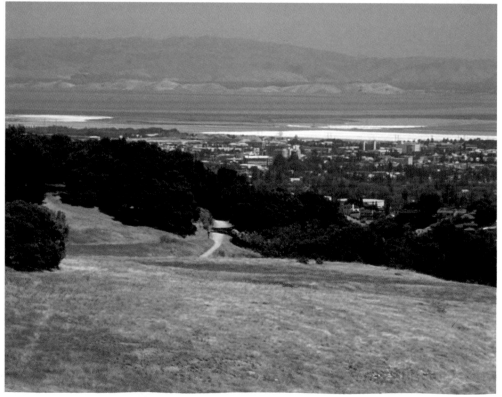

Edgewood County Park and Preserve

◆ San Bruno Mountain State and County Park ◆

San Bruno Mountain rises starkly from the Bay to an elevation of 1314 feet, dominating the northern Peninsula landscape, its bare, steep flanks creased by narrow ravines and a few wooded canyons. The cities of San Francisco, Brisbane, South San Francisco, Colma, and Daly City surround the mountain.

From the top of this seemingly barren mountain rising above the cities encircling it, you see the other Bay Area landmark mountains, the Pacific Ocean, San Francisco's skyscrapers, and the ships on its great Bay.

In 1978 the mountain became San Bruno Mountain Park with the purchase by the State of California and San Mateo County of 1500 acres and the gift of 500 acres by the property owner. Later additions brought the park's total to 2266 acres, which are managed by San Mateo County.

Guadalupe Canyon Parkway, running generally east-west across the park, leads to the park entrance. North of the parkway is a relatively level area known as the Saddle, where visitors find beautiful views and attractive picnic areas screened by Monterey cypress and sheltering low walls. A day camp nestles in the center of the Saddle and trails loop around the perimeter.

South of the parkway, trails ascend the mountain's steep sides and a road to the summit leads to trails along its high ridges. Superb views from this mountaintop make it a fine place to take visitors for an orientation to the Bay Area, all laid out before you.

More than 11 miles of trails take the visitor over the mountain's varied terrain: short, easy nature trails accessible for the physically limited, moderate loop hikes, and longer trips up the mountain. Although the ridges of the mountain are exposed to the prevailing winds and fog from the ocean, and buffeted by the storms of winter, the ravines in the lee of the main ridgeline are often sunny and relatively warm. After winter rains clear, the superb 360° views are worth a trip to the mountain with windbreaker, binoculars, and camera. Even in blustery weather, the hiking is good if you are prepared with proper clothing.

Considered an outlier of the Santa Cruz Mountains, San Bruno Mountain geologically is an elevated fault block composed largely of a dark gray Franciscan rock with the catchy name of graywacke (three syllables). You can see jumbled outcroppings of this rock above Guadalupe Canyon Parkway as you come up the canyon from the west.

History

Some evidence of Indian habitation has been found in Buckeye Canyon and shell mounds are known along the edge of the Bay below. A few years after the Portolá expedition discovered San Francisco Bay in 1769, Captain Fernando Rivera, the principal officer of Father Francisco Palou's exploring party, climbed the mountain with four of his men to watch the sunrise. Humans have since greatly altered the land they saw around them, but the mountain itself remains very little changed. It is believed that the mountain was named for the patron saint of Captain Bruno Heceta, who commanded an inland party mapping the Bay and the surrounding lands.

From Spanish times the mountain was considered good pasture, and from those times until World War II cattle grazed these grassy slopes. During these war years the army set up a small camp in today's Saddle area where they used searchlights for anti-aircraft maneuvers. The buildings are gone but some traces of its former use remain.

In one of the early grants of the Mexican regime, in 1836 Governor Luis Arguello bestowed on Jacob Lesse, a naturalized Mexican citizen, the Rancho Cañada de Guadalupe, Concepción y Rodeo Viejo. The ranch took in the whole mountain, Visitacion Valley and the old rodeo grounds near the Bay. Over the years the ranch changed hands many times as it was traded, sold and divided, until 1872 when the Visitation Land Company secured the largest holding. In 1884 H. W. Crocker acquired the company's 3814 acres. This large holding remained for nearly a century in the Crocker Estate, until the establishment of the park.

However, in 1964 a huge development scheme had proposed slicing off the top of the mountain to fill the Bay from Hunters Point to Coyote Point, after which houses would cover the mountaintop and the Bay fill. Fortunately, the scheme did not come to fruition, although a later development plan did gain approval for some housing. The Saddle area was saved along with all the land south of the parkway up to the summit and on its southern slopes.

The Mountain's Special Flora

The mountain, so dun-colored from a distance after its grasses dry up, is at close view colorful and lively with a great variety of plants, lichen-covered rocks, and fern-lined canyons. In spite of over a century of grazing, San Bruno Mountain is a botanical island with vegetation typical of that which once covered the San Francisco hills. A great number of native species of plants grow on the mountain— 384 have been counted, including some rare and endangered species and a few unique to this special environment. E.O. Wilson wrote in the Diversity of Life that San Bruno Mountain is one of the world's best examples of biodiversity.

Nearly 50 varieties of grasses grow here, half of them native, including many of California's perennial bunchgrasses. In the grasslands from February on, you can see impressive displays of wildflowers—sheets of pearly everlasting, colonies of goldfields, clumps of Johnny jump-up, slopes covered with Douglas and coast iris- es, and steep hillsides of brilliant, showy, scarlet, orange, and yellow Indian paint- brushes. The mountain's most extensive and varied displays of annual flowers are found on some 150 acres of the April Brook slopes known as the Flower Garden.

Four rare butterflies, among them the endangered Mission blue, the San Francisco silverspot, and the San Bruno elfin, live and feed on the plants of San Bruno Mountain.

Habitat Conservation Plan

Long years of concern over potential effects of construction on the mountain's flora and its rare and endangered species led to a landmark decision in 1982. Known as the Habitat Conservation Plan, it granted developers a 30-year permit to build on some of the endangered species' habitat in return for their funding pro- grams to enhance the species' chances of survival on the park lands.

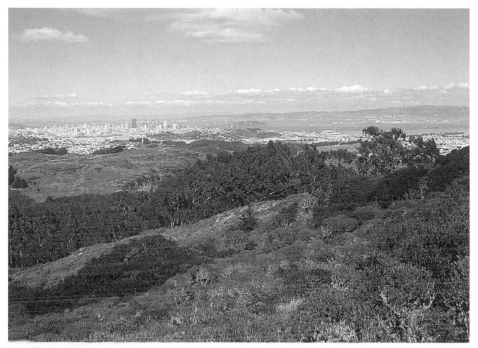

San Bruno Mountain, open space surrounded by urban development

This plan sets up an annual fund, the San Bruno Mountain Habitat Conservation Trust Fund, which will be used to eliminate invasive gorse and eucalyptus and to seed host plants, such as lupine and violas, for food and refuge for the endangered species of butterfly.

Gorse elimination projects are ongoing; 1995 saw the beginning of eucalyptus removal. Time will tell how well these fragile native species can survive in limited space and in close contact with urban development. In the meantime, building moves right up to the boundaries of the park.

Jurisdiction: State of California and San Mateo County: 650-363-4020

Facilities: Trails for hikers, one for bicyclists and another for physically limited; picnic areas; barbecues; meadow play area; restrooms; day camp

Rules: Open 8 A.M to sunset; no dogs allowed in park; bicycles allowed on Old Guadalupe Trail and Saddle Loop Trail only

Maps: San Mateo County *San Bruno Mountain Park* and USGS topo *San Francisco South*

How to Get There: From I-280: (1) Southbound—Take Eastmoor Ave. exit and turn left on Sullivan Ave., which parallels freeway. At first street on left, turn left onto San Pedro Rd., which goes over freeway. Across Mission St, San Pedro Rd. becomes East Market St, which becomes Guadalupe Canyon Pkwy. Park entrance is on north side of parkway. (2) Northbound—Take Mission St exit. At first stop signal, turn left onto Junipero Serra Blvd., then right on San Pedro Rd. and follow directions above. From Hwy 101: Take Bayshore Blvd., turn west on Guadalupe Canyon Pkwy and go 1.5 miles to park entrance on right.

SADDLE LOOP TRAIL

SEE MAP
ON PAGE
22

*Circling the northern Saddle area of the park, this is an invigorating hike
when fresh breezes sweep in from the Pacific. Views stretch beyond San
Francisco to its dramatic setting of Bay and mountains.*

Distance: 2.9-mile loop

Time: ½ hour

Elevation Gain: 150′

Marked off in 0.5-mile segments, this loop is a longtime favorite of joggers. Now
open to bicyclists too, it is becoming an even more popular trail. Starting on the
Old Guadalupe Trail on the west side of the north parking area, follow this former
ranch road lined with eucalyptus and Monterey cypress. It traverses the side of a
ravine, where moisture-loving plants grow by the path. On foggy days the aroma
of eucalyptus leaves is intensified when they are crushed underfoot.

In 0.8 mile veer right past new subdivisions crowding the park boundary, to
climb into open grasslands where you have long views out to the Pacific Ocean and
Point Reyes. If the day is very clear, the Farallon Islands seem closer than their
31-mile distance.

The trail arcs right, staying close to the boundary of the park, with flowers
brightening the way at most any season. Particularly brilliant in spring with goldfields, lupines, and some rare species, this path even in summer is dotted with
magenta farewell-to-spring and white yarrow.

Downtown San Francisco high-rises puncture the skyline, and the Bay Bridge
stretches across to Oakland. As your trail continues to its highest point, the view
spreads toward the South Bay shoreline. From about the halfway point of this loop,
a service road cuts straight back to the park entrance, passing the pleasant Edward
J. Bacciocco, Jr. Day Camp area en route. As you continue around the Saddle Loop,

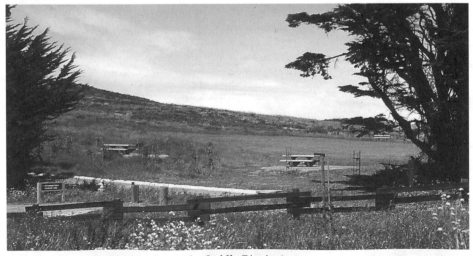

Old Monterey cypress trees frame the Saddle Picnic Area

the view changes to take in the full height and breadth of San Bruno Mountain. It beckons the hiker to cross the parkway and climb its trails to even wider views of the entire Bay Area.

Heading back to the parking area, you pass the gorse elimination projects. European gorse has taken over large areas of this saddle, threatening to wipe out the host plants for the rare and endangered butterflies. Because gorse seeds can live up to 25 years, gorse is very difficult to eradicate.

In small ravines coastal scrub harbors many bird species. You may recognize the quail's warning call and see wren-tits and song sparrows flitting from shrub to shrub. These birds and the rare plants and butterflies of the mountain are now protected through the establishment of San Bruno Mountain Park.

BOG TRAIL

A short nature trail aligned on a gentle grade and having a stable surface skirts a little swale west of the park entrance. A bridge over an intermittent stream leads from it to the Old Guadalupe Trail. This 0.4-mile trail, accessible to the physically limited, offers an opportunity for all nature lovers to enjoy the riparian environment.

The Bog Trail, together with a section of the Old Guadalupe Trail (the first leg of the Saddle Loop Trip), makes a loop of less than a mile. Try this before sitting down to lunch at one of the picnic sites just beyond the old cypress trees at the park entrance.

EUCALYPTUS LOOP TRAIL

A relatively easy trail samples the lower slopes of the mountain with views up to its long ridgetop.

Distance: 1.08-mile loop

Time: ½ hour

Elevation Change: 170' gain

This trip is just right for a brisk walk before lunch. Before you set off, pause to learn about the natural wonders of the mountain from the exhibits on the display board by the trailhead at the south-side parking area. Here too, you can see the botanical garden, funded by the Habitat Conservation Trust Fund and planted and maintained by the volunteer group, Friends of San Bruno Mountain. At present three of the five plant communities found on San Bruno Mountain are represented—grassland, coastal dune scrub, and wetland. The remaining two will be added later.

Then take the left hand trail to begin this loop trip. When past the eucalyptus removal area and the botanical garden, you see the deeply furrowed sides of the mountain, dark green against the sky. Water rushes down the mountain in winter, carving still deeper furrows in the mountain's side. After a few bends in the trail, turn right at the first junction. Your way straightens out above the former eucalyptus grove to cross Dairy Ravine. High above, the long spine of the park extends for more than 2 miles southeast. Up close, the mountain has a magnificent profusion of poppies and goldfields glowing golden in spring and early summer.

A right turn at the next junction takes you into the trees and thence back to the trailhead. For lunch you can take the footpath through the underpass to the north-side picnic area by the old Monterey cypresses that mark the north entrance to the park.

DAIRY RAVINE LOOP

Climbing higher on the mountain, this trip zigzags up and down the sides of Dairy Ravine past trailside gardens of remarkable beauty.

Distance: 1.75-mile loop

Time: 1 hour

Elevation Change: 325′ gain

In return for the extra elevation gain and extra mileage, this loop offers the delights of coming upon a different rock garden at every turn. Lichen-covered rocks shelter gray-green sedums, their tall flower stalks bearing coral and yellow blossoms.

Starting from the trailhead on the south side of Guadalupe Canyon Parkway, take the left branch of the Eucalyptus Loop Trail (see Saddle Loop Trail, above) and at the first junction bear left onto the Dairy Ravine Trail. This 0.5-mile-long trail climbs the east side of Dairy Ravine in wide switchbacks to meet the Summit Loop Trail at the head of Dairy Ravine. When you meet the Summit Loop Trail, veer right on it, and see the San Francisco skyline looming in the distance. Below are the old cypress trees in Dairy Ravine. The name and these trees are all that remain of the dairy farm that once operated at the foot of the ravine.

The trail crosses over and makes a switchback above the steep east side of Cable Ravine, then descends quickly through waist-high cream bush, coffee berry, and snowberry to meet the Eucalyptus Loop Trail. Here you take a left turn to return to the south-side parking area.

SUMMIT LOOP TRAIL

This mountaintop climb takes you past the Flower Garden of April Brook Ravine, along the west ridge for its views, and down the steep north face below the summit.

Distance: 3.1-mile loop

Time: 2 hours

Elevation Change: 725′ gain

Although you can complete this trip in less than two hours, you may want to linger longer in spring to enjoy the views and the flowers at every step of the way. From the trailhead on the south side of Guadalupe Canyon Parkway, take the path to the right through the eucalyptus grove.

After crossing the road, you soon come out into dense, waist-high growth—tall cow parsnip with its flat clusters of white blossoms, pink-flowered honeysuckle, and California bee plant with its small, dull red flowers. Along the way you come across the many wet places in the trail where even in summer water is seeping from springs above.

You are soon at the ravine where April Brook flows into willow-bordered Colma Creek. It's a protected little swale that catches the noontime sun. The brook is heavily lined with sword ferns and big clumps of coastal iris edge the trail. In winter, you can distinguish the coastal iris from the Douglas iris, also found on the mountain, by the former's straplike leaves that are green on both sides; in contrast, Douglas iris leaves are shiny green on top and dull-grayish green below. Come back in April and May to see the long-petaled flowers in shades of blue.

But even in winter you can see the promise of spring in the emerging foliage of California poppies, lupines, and other annual flowers. Stone outcrops by the trail form rock gardens of such satisfying design as to serve as models for our domestic landscaping efforts. Needlepoint-textured, orange and gray lichen cover the rocks; pink-hued succulents, small polypody ferns, and thick-leaved daisies fill the crevices.

The trail crosses April Brook Ravine and ascends via switchbacks to Bitter Cherry Ridge, where the skyscrapers of San Francisco and the blocks of Daly City homes come into view. East of April Brook in the sloping meadow below Radio Road is the Flower Garden, a carpet of color from early March through May.

At the very top of the ridge the trail joins a paved road, which you cross and look for the continuation of the trail on the south side. Keep to the narrow trail going uphill and avoid an old jeep road that contours around to a lower destination. Southwest and far below are the cemeteries of Colma, with lawns, lakes, and headstones.

The first stretch of the trip on the south side goes through a brilliant summer garden of knee-high golden yarrow, contrasted with purple pennyroyal, crimson pitcher sage, white yarrow, and pink owl's clover. If you look back over this sea of blooms, you will see up the coast all the way to Point Reyes. A few steps farther around the east side of the hill, low, pink-edged succulents and gray-leaved, lemon-yellow-blossomed Indian paintbrush encrust the stony stairs. Below the next bend in the trail the saucer of a telephone relay rises like a giant white bloom from this stony garden.

A switchback in the trail takes you up to Radio Road, where above you rises a spindly forest of antennas springing from the commercial communications installations in an enclave of private property. Cross the road and start north down the mountain in wide switchbacks with ever-changing vistas and a succession of trailside gardens as varied as the views. Just 400 feet down the Summit Loop Trail you pass the Ridge Trail going east. You could turn here and walk out to the East Ridge and back, thus extending your trip by 5 miles.

Continuing down the Summit Loop Trail, you pass a rocky promontory where rare varieties of huckleberry and manzanita form ground-hugging mats. This species of manzanita, found only on San Bruno Mountain, is now sold in nurseries as a drought-resistant ground cover. From the promontory you can see down the flank of the mountain to the Bay. After a hairpin turn you look east to Blue Blossom Hill, mantled with deep-blue wild lilac blossoms in early spring.

At the next trail junction you can choose the east or the west ridge above Dairy Ravine. Both have fine views and remarkable flower displays long after the spectacular spring show. To stay on the Summit Loop Trail bear left (west). On this long traverse you pass a series of little gardens in a sheltered spot. Low-growing pink daisies are blooming along with blue brodiaeas, accented with crimson sage, and a patch of pennyroyal is splashed with some scarlet paintbrush. Here and there are clumps of iris edged with monkey flower.

At the next trail junction, veer left and follow the Eucalyptus Loop Trail around a big bend down to the parking area.

SEE MAP ON PAGE 22

RIDGE TRAIL TO EAST PEAK VISTA

An invigorating hike goes out to East Ridge for commanding views of the Bay Area and far out over the Pacific Ocean.

Distance: 8 miles round trip from lower, south-side trailhead

Time: 4½ hours from lower trailhead

Elevation Change: 725' gain from lower trailhead

The summit parking area is now closed to cars, but hikers who want to do this challenging 8-mile hike start at the lower, south-side parking area and take the Summit Loop Trail up to the Ridge Trail, which is on the northeast side of the summit. Then follow the Ridge Trail, contouring east below the mountaintop, to join the trail to the East Ridge. This trip calls for windbreakers against the usual mountaintop winds and sturdy shoes for the often rocky Ridge Trail.

Only 0.25 mile out on the trail you can begin to take in the wonderful panorama. You stand with the San Francisco skyline in view in one direction, the Bay in front of you, and over your shoulder the blue Pacific Ocean. Right at your feet is the mountain, its grassy slopes flowering in early spring. You can see down into the steep ravines, the first to the southwest, Sage Ravine, grayed with artemisia. The northeast slopes tend to be brush-covered or wooded. Past the quarry, rock outcroppings, tall chaparral, and trees cover Buckeye Ravine.

On either side hawks ride the updrafts. You may see one make its swift glide for a ground squirrel in the grass below. If it has a wing spread of 4 feet or more and a tail that shows reddish orange against the sky, it is a red-tailed hawk, the most common kind on the mountain.

By late February wildflowers begin to bloom through the grass, earlier here than elsewhere on the Peninsula. Clumps of California poppies and ground-hugging Johnny jump-ups color the ridgetop. Creamy yellow wallflowers blow in the

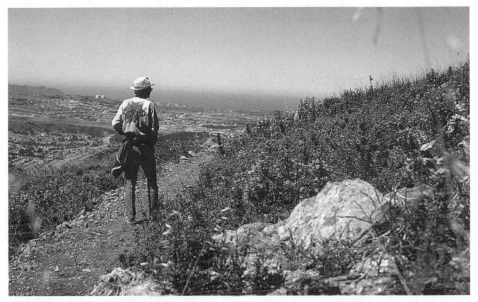

Graywacke rocks and wildflowers crowd San Bruno Mountain trails

breeze on ten-inch stems, and blossoms of white milkmaids are sprinkled down the shadier northeast slopes.

When you reach the transmission towers, note that the ridge falls off rapidly just beyond. This makes for a very steep climb back. As you return to the summit, the ocean is before you; on a clear day you can see Point Reyes on the northwest horizon.

A TRAIL TO NEARBY OFFICES

The **Old Ranch Road Trail** leaves the south side parking area and meanders downhill through the trees and shrubs beside the parkway to a crossing to the Carter Street business park complex. Those who work there can enjoy a lunchtime walk to the park on this trail.

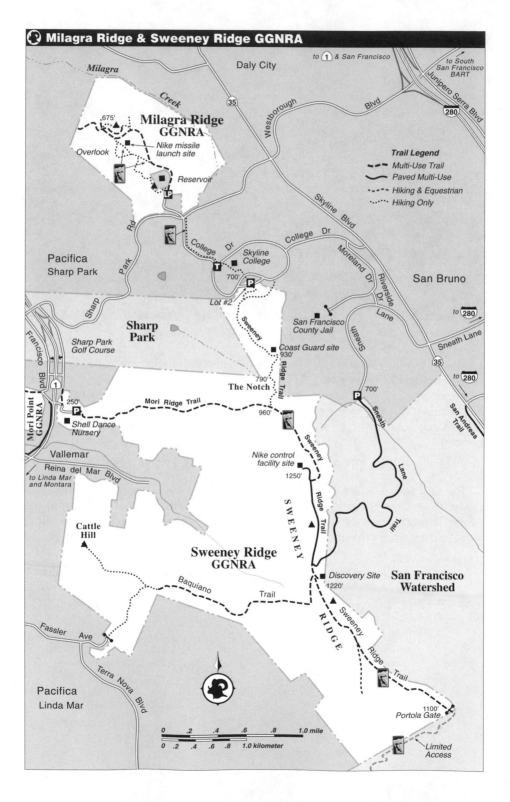

Milagra Ridge & Sweeney Ridge GGNRA

✦ Milagra Ridge ✦

Several years after World War II, the Army closed this hilltop site, a former Nike installation. They temporarily placed it under the wing of the San Mateo County Parks. When the Golden Gate National Recreation Area took over the land, they began a concerted drive to remove invasive plants, particularly the fields of pampas grass. While removing the exotic plants, they protected the native species, particularly the lupine that is the host plant for the Mission Blue Butterfly, an endangered species.

Today new lupines and native grasses are thriving, the piles of rubbish are gone, eroded hillsides are filled and protected with straw and a new trail reaches two view sites overlooking the Pacific. This trail is a segment of the Bay Area Ridge Trail that extends south through Skyline College to GGNRA's Sweeney Ridge.

Jurisdiction: Golden Gate National Recreation Area

Rules: Trails for hikers only; open 8 A.M. to dusk; bicycles on roads; dogs on leash

SEE MAP ON PAGE 32

LOOP TRAIL TO THE NIKE SITE

Try this on a clear day when you can see for miles north, south, and seaward.

Distance: 1.5 mile

Time: ¾ hour

Elevation Change: 690' gain

After going around the preserve gate at the end of College Drive North, bear left on the trail that climbs a few steps and then meanders northwest. This trail for hikers only is about 6 feet wide, demarcated by ropes strung between sturdy wooden posts, and laid out on a comfortable grade. It passes a reservoir, goes up and down the low hills beside bush lupines, native grasses, and low-growing shrubs, punctuated by wildflowers in season. In early spring the authors saw the blue blossoms of silver-leaved lupine just emerging.

After the reservoir there is a wide meadow, from which you can get your first glimpse of the sparkling sea (on a day without fog). You can watch the breakers crashing against the rocks at Mori Point and scan the horizon from Pedro Point to the Marin Headlands. On very clear days you can see the Farallons.

Continuing on the trail northwest, you come to a gravel road, which you take for a short distance to the left, then climb the steps on your right to reach a fenced platform. Here was a battery of six-inch guns set on a retractable mount. Today you can admire the peaceful view out over the surrounding GGNRA lands—Mori Point, Sweeney Ridge, and north to Fort Funston and the San Francisco shoreline.

From this platform you can descend a different set of stairs and follow the preserve road beside the sloping grasslands to the east. Pass a trail junction on your right and in less than a mile, you are back at the preserve gate.

This trail is marked as a segment of the Bay Area Ridge Trail.

◆ Sweeney Ridge ◆

The Sweeney Ridge addition to the Golden Gate National Recreation Area takes in the high ridge just north of Montara Mountain. Its grassy hilltop commands sweeping views of ocean and Bay. From this site Gaspar de Portolá's scouts first saw the expanse of water now known as San Francisco Bay.

In 1980 the Golden Gate National Recreation Area expanded its jurisdiction south from Marin County and San Francisco to include more than 27,000 acres of land within San Mateo County. Much of this land was already in public ownership, though not some thousand acres along Sweeney Ridge. The GGNRA purchased this land in 1982 to "preserve the natural, cultural and recreation values of the ridge." Included in this acquisition was the Portolá Discovery Site, already owned by the city of Pacifica and San Mateo County. In 1987 the GGNRA assumed jurisdiction of San Mateo County's adjacent Sweeney Ridge Skyline Preserve and Milagra Ridge Preserve less than a mile north.

In addition to their place in history as the spot from which Europeans first saw San Francisco, these wind-swept, foggy heights were grazing lands for Spanish ranches. By 1875 the enterprising Richard Sneath, for whom the lane is named, acquired these lands, ideal for dairy farming. He operated his dairy here until well into the 1920s. His barns were on Sneath Lane at El Camino Real.

From the rounded ridgetop, steep slopes and narrow, brush-filled canyons descend. At the northwest end of the preserve Mori Ridge reaches beyond Highway 1 to Mori Point, also in the GGNRA, see page 300. Sweeney Ridge's hogback is flanked east and south by San Francisco Watershed lands; west is the city of Pacifica. Only a few thousand feet west from the southern boundary of the preserve is San Pedro Valley County Park.

Described here are three trips, one from each of the present access routes to the preserve. The quickest and most direct for those living on the Bayside is the approach from Skyline Boulevard on Sneath Lane. From the north there is a direct route from Skyline College to the ridgetop. The third trail leaves Highway 1 in Pacifica just north of Vallemar and climbs Mori Ridge to join the Sweeney Ridge Trail. The County's Trail Plan calls for a new trail to reach the ridge from the existing San Andreas Trail north of San Andreas Lake.

Sweeney Ridge is a key segment of the San Francisco Bay Area Ridge Trail, which extends from the Portola Gate on the southern Sweeney Ridge boundary with the San Francisco Watershed north through the Skyline College campus and on through Milagra Ridge. As of 2004 the Bay Area Ridge Trail route through the San Francisco Watershed connects to Sweeney Ridge from the south at Highway 92, subject to reservations on docent-led trips, see website: http://sfwater.org.

Jurisdiction: Golden Gate National Recreation Area: 415-561-4700, 415-556-8642, 415-239-2366

Facilities: Trails for hikers, equestrians, and bicyclists; portable toilet near old Nike site

Maps: See map on page 32; GGNRA *Sweeney Ridge*, USGS topo *Montara Mountain*

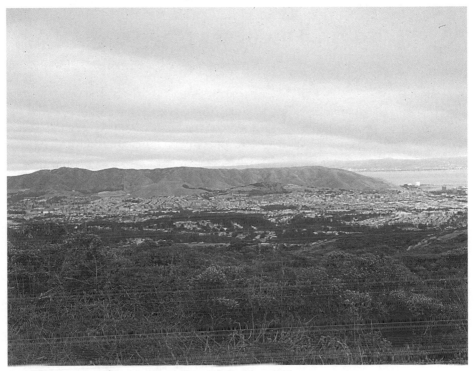

Sun Bruno Mountain seen from Nike site, Sweeney Ridge

Rules: Open from 8 A.M. to dusk; dogs on leash only; bicyclists on Sneath Lane, Mori Ridge Trail, and trail to Portola Gate only; equestrians use trail from Pacifica to Portola Gate and Mori Ridge Trail junction only

How to Get There: There are 5 access points: (1) Sneath Lane trailhead—From Skyline Blvd. (Hwy 35) in San Bruno go 2 miles west on Sneath Lane to off-street parking at gate; (2) Mori Ridge trailhead—Going north on Hwy 1 in Pacifica, pass Reina del Mar Ave., turn abruptly right into Shell Dance Nursery and continue past nursery buildings to parking at end of dirt road; going south on Hwy 1 in Pacifica, make a U-turn at Reina del Mar Ave. and go north, following directions above; (3) Skyline College—From Skyline Blvd. in San Bruno go west on College Dr., turn left at college entrance and proceed to parking lot 2 (several spaces reserved for GGNRA trail use); (4) South entrance, Bay Area Ridge Trail from Highway 92 to Portola Gate—(5) Milagra Ridge—From Hwy 1 or from Skyline Blvd., take Sharp Park Rd., turn north on College Dr. Extension N. and continue to roadside parking at Milagra Ridge gate. SamTrans buses reach Skyline College from Pacifica, Daly City BART, and Serramonte-Tanforan.

FROM SNEATH LANE
TO THE DISCOVERY SITE

A bracing hike with superb views to an historic site and the trail's southern terminus.

Distance: 1.8 miles one way from Sneath Lane parking area to Discovery Site, and a 2.4-mile loop from Discovery Site to south end of preserve and back, altogether a 6-mile round trip

Time: 3¼ hours round trip

Elevation Change: 700′ gain

From the Sneath Lane trailhead, access point (1), enter through the stile to the paved service road through the San Francisco Watershed lands and descend by a willow-bordered watercourse that flows into San Andreas Lake. (Close by is the proposed junction with the San Andreas Trail extension.) The road soon starts its rise in and out of ravines that furrow the eastern slopes. From the outer bends of the road you catch glimpses of San Andreas Lake below. The grade is easy and the only traffic is an occasional official vehicle or a few bicycles.

Partway up you will see a yellow stripe in the center of the pavement, making a "fog line" to guide cars and bicycles when dense fog blankets the hills. A word of caution about the ridge on foggy days: a walk in the fog is a bracing experience, but stay on roads or well-defined trails. When visibility is close to zero, hikers can become disoriented and find themselves lost on these moors.

Where the service road reaches the ridgetop, you are in the GGNRA. Turn left for the Discovery Site, which is marked by a dark granite cylinder. Carved around it are the outlines of the landmarks in the sweeping views around you, such as Mt. Tamalpais, San Bruno Mountain, Mt. Diablo, and Montara Mountain.

From this point on the ridge Gaspar de Portolá's scouts saw "a great estuary . . . extending many leagues inland." They were in search of Monterey Bay, however, and felt misgivings that that bay and the ship they wished to rejoin might lie behind them. It was

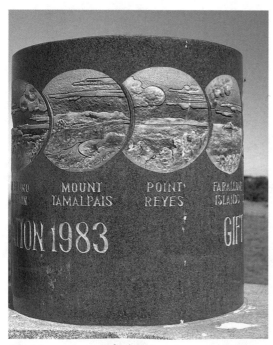

Marble monument depicts Bay Area mountains

only several years later, and after subsequent expeditions, that the Spaniards recognized the importance of San Francisco Bay and its magnificent harbor.

From the Discovery Site the Sweeney Ridge Trail heads south toward the boundary of the preserve. For more than a mile you go over grasslands, past rock outcroppings, and through patches of coastal scrub. In spring this is a flowery way, with carpets of goldfields, patches of blue lupine, and great clumps of blue coastal iris. On fine days you can see forever. The dark outline of Montara Mountain is before you, and on either side the views open up over the ocean and the Bay. As you go along, listen for the sharp cries of a kestrel, a small hawk with white undersides that searches the meadows for field mice and gophers.

Toward the south end of the preserve are a spring-fed marsh and a small reed-rimmed pond. The trail splits at the marsh; your route goes left of it. Follow this trail to the San Francisco Watershed's Portola Gate in the southeast corner of the preserve. You pass through a thicket of coastal scrub enlivened by apricot-colored monkey flowers, white heads of pearly everlastings, and here and there clumps of bright red and yellow Indian paintbrush. The trail going right at the marsh is an equestrian trail that takes off steeply downhill to stables at the end of Linda Mar Valley.

At the Watershed gate, your route turns north back to the Discovery Site where the Baquiano Trail, named for Portolá's scout, heads left (southwest). This trail goes down a ridge to end a mile below at a gate to private property beyond the preserve boundary. GGNRA rangers occasionally lead walks up into the preserve from Pacifica.

As of 2004 you can sign up for docent-led hikes, horse rides, and bike rides from Highway 92 to the Portola Gate and on to Sneath Lane or Skyline College. To sign up for one of these hikes, see the San Francisco Watershed's website: http://sfwater.org. The 9.5-mile trip through the Watershed to the Portola Gate and 3.5 miles to Sneath Lane parking requires a shuttle for hikers; bicyclists and equestrians probably can do a round trip.

SEE MAP ON PAGE 32

UP MORI RIDGE
TO THE DISCOVERY SITE

This trail heads straight up the steep grassy slope of Mori Ridge with superb views of the coast along the way.

Distance: 5 miles round trip

Time: 3 hours

Elevation Change: 1000' gain

From the Mori Ridge trailhead, access point (2), go to the preserve entrance gate where a service-road trail begins a steep, steady ascent up a grassy slope. Views open out over the Pacific Ocean and north to the Farallons, Point Reyes, and Mt. Tamalpais. In the foreground is an extension of this ridge, GGNRA's Mori Point, surrounded by the suburban community of Pacifica. To the south are the austere outlines of Pedro Point that give way to the high ridge headlands that take its name.

In spring the grasslands are bright with flowers. You will be glad to stop the stiff climb now and then to look at them more closely. A half-hour's hike brings you to scattered old plantings of Monterey pines. One by the trailside provides a welcome shady stop on a bright day. Often, however, this exposed ridge is swept by winds and fog.

Soon you are on a gentler slope where grasses give way to low bushes. On Sweeney Ridge is one of the best examples of the lively combination of low shrubs and flowers called coastal scrub. In spring and summer this scrub takes on a brilliance that belies the harsh, negative connotation of its name. It blooms then with white pearly everlastings; patches of blue coast iris; Indian paintbrush in red and yellow; daisies in yellow, lavender, and white; yellow yarrow; coffeeberry; greasewood; and blue wild lilac. The ever-present poison oak is bright red by the end of summer.

After 1.3 miles, you reach the Sweeney Ridge Trail, the Bay Area Ridge Trail route. Here the ridge flattens out and San Francisco comes into view, including the antenna on Sutro Heights and the towers of the Golden Gate Bridge. East are San Bruno Mountain and beyond, the East Bay Hills. At this intersection you bear right (southeast) on the Sweeney Ridge Trail (left goes north to Skyline College; open to hikers only). After 0.8 mile you skirt an old Nike site with blocky cement buildings and battered fences. This trail, surfaced and fairly level, is the upper end of Sneath Lane, and continues for 0.5 mile to the Discovery Site (described above).

SEE MAP
ON PAGE
32

SWEENEY RIDGE TRAIL FROM SKYLINE COLLEGE TO THE DISCOVERY SITE

A short ascent to a protected ridgetop with wide views leads to stairs into and out of a steep ravine and a final gentle climb past the Nike site to Portolá's Discovery Site.

Distance: 0.6 mile round trip to knoll; 4.6 miles round trip to Discovery Site

Time: 2½ hours

Elevation Change: 500' gain, plus gain of 300' out of the ravine

On a clear day the view is unlimited—all around the compass. However, this bald hilltop can get the full force of the wind from the ocean, so be prepared. On the other hand, if the day is clear and warm, take a lunch up to this hilltop, where you can look down at the coast from Mussel Rock to San Pedro Point. Pacifica is below you, and the green of Sharp Park Golf Course contrasts with the deep blue of the ocean. White breakers curl into the sandy curves of the beaches.

But, if the Discovery Site is your destination, continue into and out of the ravine ahead on a trail with stairs for hikers only and take the Sweeney Ridge Trail to the Discovery Site.

⬧ San Pedro Valley County Park ⬧

The park's 1140 acres include the narrow valley along San Pedro Creek's middle fork and the steep ridges draining the south fork. San Pedro Valley has a significant place in early Bay Area history as the site of Indian villages and the site of Gaspar de Portolá's camp from which his scouts climbed the ridge to get their first view of San Francisco Bay. An early outpost for Mission Dolores was in this valley, as was the adobe home of Francisco Sanchez, still standing and now a San Mateo County museum.

Park trails offer a number of easy, level strolls and some vigorous climbs to the ridges above the valley. The creeks run clear, and are still spawning grounds for the steelhead trout that migrate upstream to the park each winter. The creeks furnish a substantial part of Pacifica's water supply.

Ocean fogs often roll in to shroud surrounding ridgetops, but San Pedro Mountain tempers winds from the west, sheltering the sunny valley. The same

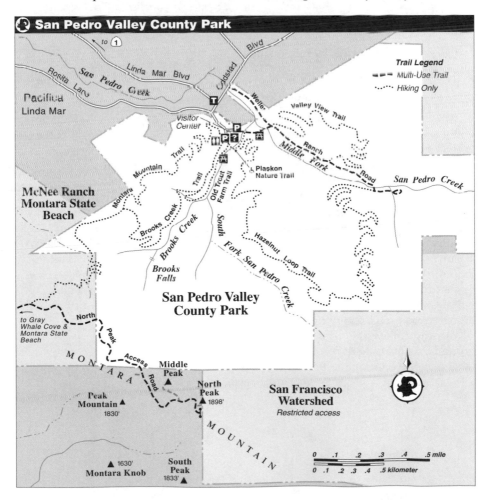

mild climate that led the Ohlone Indians to build their village by the creek makes San Pedro Valley Park a place to return to in all seasons.

Jurisdiction: San Mateo County: 650-363-4020

Facilities: Visitor center, picnic tables, and barbecues for families and groups; trails for hikers; self-guiding nature trail, wheelchair accessible; wheelchairs for day use offered free

Rules: Open 8 A.M. to dusk; bicycles permitted on Weiler Road only; no dogs; fee

Maps: San Mateo County *San Pedro Valley Park*; USGS topo *Montara Mountain*

How to Get There: From Hwy 1 in the south end of Pacifica turn east on Linda Mar Blvd. and drive to the park entrance.

A LOOP TRIP TO THE OLD TROUT FARM AND THE WESTERN HILLSIDE

SEE MAP ON PAGE 39

A short, shady walk along both sides of San Pedro Creek's South Fork passes the Old Trout Farm and returns on the western hillside.

Distance: 1.25-mile loop

Time: 30–45 minutes

Elevation Change: Relatively level

After exploring the visitor center, which has something for the whole family, you'll find this trip is just right for a bit of exercise before a picnic lunch at the Old Trout Farm Picnic Area. Children will enjoy display cases of the park's animals, and botany buffs will delight in the well-mounted specimens of a surprising variety of plants. Photographs trace San Pedro Valley's long history.

Shortly beyond the beginning of the Old Trout Farm Loop Trail, look to your right for the tanks that are the remnants of John Gay's trout farm, washed away in the floods of 1962. Under overhanging trees draped with German ivy and tangles of berry brambles that almost obscure the view of the creek, the trail continues for about ⅓ mile. Turn back when you will, or bear right at a park gate to continue the loop through a narrow canyon that once was a domestic garden. Stone steps lead to a sturdy bridge that crosses intermittent Brooks Creek where horsetails, ferns, willows, and currants flourish. After the bridge the trail continues uphill beside new redwood trees emerging through the dense eucalyptus forest.

You can follow this trail along the park's western hillside back to the picnic grounds, or bear sharp left at the first intersection to climb to the northwestern heights of the park on the Brooks Creek Trail.

NORTH RIDGE LOOP

SEE MAP ON PAGE 39

This trip climbs a west-facing slope on the Valley View Trail and then descends to join Weiler Ranch Road farther up the valley.

Distance: 2.2-mile loop

Time: 1 hour

Elevation Change: 600' gain

Cross the creek on a bridge from the main parking lot to the left of the visitor center. Continue past the group picnic area under venerable walnut trees. Turn right on Weiler Ranch Road, then almost immediately veer left on the Valley View Trail, which takes off uphill.

If you want a short level walk, continue on the road to one of the two picnic tables between the beginning and the end of the Valley View Trail. But for a brisk walk up the ridge before lunch, you can take the Valley View Trail and be back in less than an hour. In spring the meadow-side tables look out over a field of poppies, lupines, buttercups, and wild mustard.

The Valley View Trail climbs a sunny slope, then enters a eucalyptus grove and emerges in fragrant chaparral. From here you can look south to the heights of Montara Mountain. In April blue coast iris blooms in the grasslands. From the ridgetop easy switchbacks take you down to Weiler Ranch Road, on which you can return to the park office. For a longer walk you can follow this easy road to the upper end of the valley, where hills rise steeply to Sweeney Ridge a thousand feet above.

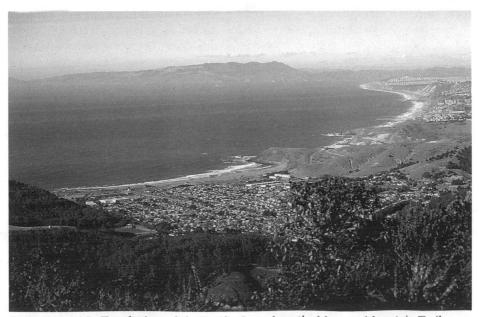

Point Reyes, Mt. Tamalpais, and the Pacific Coast from the Montara Mountain Trail

Or you can walk 0.4 mile east and climb the south ridge on the Hazelnut Ridge Trail for a longer loop; see the following trip.

An extension of the Valley View Trail is proposed to meet the Sweeney Ridge Trail in the GGNRA.

THE HAZELNUT RIDGE LOOP

After a climb up the high ridge on the Hazelnut Trail, return on a west-facing slope to the visitor center.

Distance: 4.3-mile loop

Time: 3 hours

Elevation Change: 800′ gain

On the Weiler Ranch Road, walk about 0.75 mile up the valley and cross the Middle Fork of San Pedro Creek on a bridge installed to facilitate steelhead navigation to spawning grounds on the upper reaches of this creek. Just after the bridge, the Hazelnut Trail turns off on your right. On this trail you make a wide swing west, then continue on switchbacks up the canyon wall. After a wide traverse east, you zigzag up a ridge, gaining 400 feet in elevation.

At the high point of the trail you come to a gentler grade in tall chaparral of coffeeberry, Montara manzanita, wild lilac, and scrub oak. You soon reach a high saddle between San Pedro Creek's middle and south forks. A huge eucalyptus grove dominates the northwest end of the flat just before you begin the steep pitch downhill.

As the trail turns down in earnest, it doubles back and forth through a thicket of hazelnut, the shrub that gives the trail its name. You are soon at the foot of the hillside and crossing a sloping, flower-filled little meadow behind the visitor center, the end of the trip.

MONTARA MOUNTAIN TRAIL

Climb the park's western ridge for dramatic ocean views.

Distance: 5 miles round trip

Time: 3 hours

Elevation Change: 1000′ gain

After the 1987 purchase of a strategic parcel of land between the adjoining McNee Ranch State Park and San Pedro Valley Park, San Mateo County built this trail. It crosses the steep southwestern slopes of the park and joins McNee Ranch State Park high on the saddle between San Pedro Mountain and Montara's peaks.

Leaving from just west of the visitor center, this trail for hikers only zigzags uphill, at first traversing a eucalyptus grove on east-facing slopes. It then goes through coastal scrub—huckleberry, manzanita, ceanothus, chinquapin, silk-tassel bush, and the ubiquitous poison oak. From notches in the hills one has glimpses of the ocean; higher up are splendid views of the coastline from Point Reyes to Half Moon Bay, and east to Sweeney Ridge and Mt. Diablo. In spring, irises bloom beside the trail and waterfalls drop into steep-sided canyons. At the junction with the trail from McNee Ranch, a left turn onto this wide service road, open to bicyclists also, leads to the North Peak of Montara Mountain, about 2.4 miles farther uphill. A right turn leads downhill through the state park to its gate at Highway 1.

BROOKS CREEK/MONTARA MOUNTAIN TRAILS LOOP

Find the falls on the way to the ridge between two deep canyons.

Distance: 4.2-mile loop

Time: 2½ hours

Elevation Change: 460' gain

Begin this trip on the hikers-only trail beside the restrooms at the picnic area west of the visitor center. Mount a few steps and turn left (west) on the other leg of the Old Trout Farm Trail, which makes a gentle climb along the base of the south-facing hillside. At each junction thereafter, bear right on the Brooks Creek Trail. You rise slowly up the hillside under tall pines, occasional redwoods, and many eucalyptus. When you leave the forest and get out into the chaparral, the views across the canyon open up and you see the Hazelnut Trail's route on the opposite hill.

With sounds of water tumbling down the canyon and the scent of flowering shrubs and wildflowers in the air, you find a bench at the much-heralded waterfall viewing area. If you want to see the waterfall, come right after a winter storm clears and you will see and hear the triple falls dropping down the sheer mountainside. The great force of the water creates its own mist, which sometimes shrouds the canyon wall. At other times, the stream is not full enough to put on a big display. However, the hike to the bench is pleasant with dramatic vegetation changes as you climb.

To complete the loop trail, keep climbing on the Brooks Creek Trail in and out of ravines on the southeast-facing ridge. Beautiful specimens of gray-green silk tassel trees and veritable forests of mahogany-trunked manzanita crowd the trailside and several benches offer places to rest. You head into a deep ravine and around some switchbacks, and pass little streams gurgling down the mountain. You soon reach the ridgetop and join the Montara Mountain Trail. From vistas of a misty, forested canyon you switch to splendid views of the ocean and the flanks of Montara Mountain. Turn right (east) on this trail and steadily descend around the bends and return to the floor of the park.

◆ McNee Ranch ◆

Rising steeply from rocky seacliffs, McNee Ranch's rugged slopes reach an elevation of 1500 feet near Montara Mountain's peaks. The 700-acre park includes the saddle between San Pedro Mountain and Montara Mountain. Over this saddle went the Indian trail followed by Gaspar de Portolá's party in 1769. Later it was the route of early wagon roads between coastal ranches. And in the 20th century the winding old San Pedro Road carried automobiles over the saddle until it was abandoned for the cliff-side Devils Slide route. Today the old road serves as a trail for hikers, bicyclists, and equestrians.

In McNee Ranch, a part of Montara State Beach, you can explore its steep hillsides and enjoy its wide coastal views from trails along the lower hillsides and on the trips described here following Old Pedro Mountain Road and a service road up the mountain. The southern leg of Old Pedro Mountain Road, partially paved and open to hikers, equestrians, and bicyclists, and the Farallone Cut-off path, for hikers only, link the park to the nearby community of Montara. (There is no parking at either Montara terminus, but the Farallone Cut-off path terminates at 2nd Street just across Highway 1 from the southern parking area at the restaurant on the south end of Montara State Beach.)

The State of California Department of Parks and Recreation purchased the McNee Ranch land in two parcels to accommodate a right-of-way for a possible Highway 1 bypass. In November 1996 citizens passed an initiative, Measure T, that substitutes a tunnel through San Pedro Mountain as the preferred route and gives it priority for federal and state highway funding. This route will preserve the park's trails and scenic values.

In 2001 the Peninsula Open Space Trust purchased the 4262-acre Rancho Corral de Tierra lands south and east of McNee Ranch. These lands share more than three miles of boundary with the San Francisco Watershed, which extends over the hills to I-280 and beyond. When Congress agrees to pay the remaining half of the purchase price, this remarkable piece of undeveloped land could be added to the Golden Gate National Recreation Area.

Jurisdiction: State of California, Department of Parks and Recreation: 650-726-8819

Facilities: Trails for hikers, equestrians, and bicyclists; emergency phone, restrooms, and picnic table near ranger residence; restroom and ample parking across from Gray Whale Cove

Rules: Open from 8 A.M. to sunset

Maps: McNee Ranch brochure, Pease Press *Trails of the Coastside and Northern Peninsula*, and USGS topo *Montara Mountain*

How to Get There: From the north, take Hwy 1 south from Pacifica past Devils Slide to large parking area on east side of Hwy 1 opposite Gray Whale Cove State Beach or continue 0.5 mile to ample parking area at beach on west side of highway. From the south, drive 8 miles north from Half Moon Bay to ample parking at Montara State Beach or across from 2nd St. at small parking area just south of the restaurant at the beach. Limited parking near park gate.

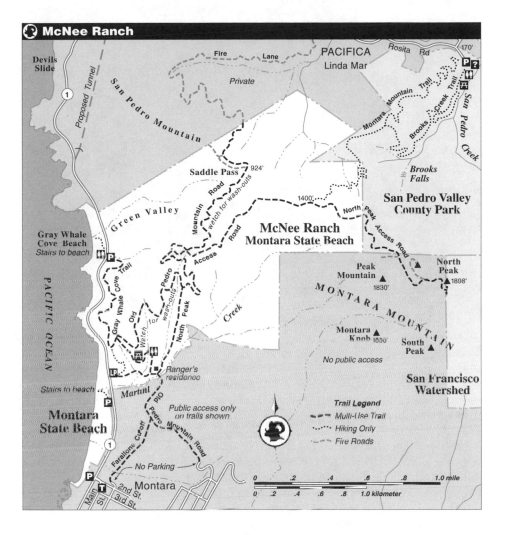

OLD PEDRO MOUNTAIN ROAD TO THE SADDLE

SEE MAP ON PAGE 45

For fine views of the ocean and coastal hills take this route on a clear day.

Distance: 6.4 miles round trip

Time: 3½ hours

Elevation Change: 925′ gain

From the entrance gate on Highway 1, walk ahead 0.2 mile on the cypress-lined road to the ranger's residence, then bear left on the Old Pedro Mountain Road. The first section of this old road can be gullied after heavy rains, though less steep than the service road, passable on foot, and therefore much better for foot and bicycle

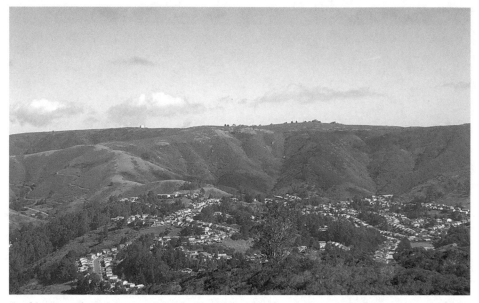

Looking east from Montara Mountain to Watershed and Sweeney Ridge

travel. The old road you take upward was for many years the principal north-south highway along the coast. Its pavement is now worn and eroded, but yellow and blue bush lupine and sagebrush cover its banks. There are serious washouts along this road, but non-motorized travel can maneuver around them with caution. After 1.1 miles you join the service road, the North Peak Access Road, and continue upward on it.

From this junction you see fields planted with rows of vegetables and flowers on the far side of Martini Creek. Above you tower Montara's peaks, chaparral-covered and formidable. Broad Montara State Beach stretches south, and on a rise out of sight is Montara Lighthouse. Now operated by Hostelling International, it is an appealing place for an overnight stay while exploring the park.

A half mile past the junction, the steep North Access Road turns right up the mountain to communications installations on its peaks, the route of another trip in the park. Keep left on Old San Pedro Mountain Road, colloquially known as Old Pedro Mountain Road. A short section of this road is washed out beyond this junction, but with caution it is possible to scramble down and back up to the old road level. From there the next 0.5 mile is on an easy grade.

It is worth the climb to reach the high flower garden that this old roadway becomes in late spring and summer. Its banks then bloom in brilliant variety, with red and yellow Indian paintbrush, purple pussy paws, orange wallflowers, blue-eyed grass, buttercups, and more. West over the steeply descending hillside is the blue of the Pacific Ocean.

As you continue around the hillside, you come to large outcrops of granitic rocks. This light-colored igneous rock is exposed on this mountain and in only a few other places in the Bay Area, such as the Farallon Islands and Inverness Ridge.

This is the same kind of rock you see at Yosemite Valley, formed beneath the surface many eons ago.

Old Pedro Mountain Road winds around the mountain, veers left at the Saddle Pass, the bypass section Caltrans once proposed for deep cuts, and continues to a gate marking the park's boundary. From the gate Old Pedro Mountain Road passes through private property and down to San Pedro Valley, but you retrace your steps from the gate. When the day is clear, you will have views northeast from the saddle toward Sweeney Ridge and up the coast toward San Francisco.

SEE MAP ON PAGE 45

To Montara Mountain's North Peak

A steady, 3.9-mile climb takes you to rewarding top-of-the-world views.

Distance: 7.8 miles round trip

Time: 5 hours

Elevation Change: 1798' gain

Start from the Highway 1 entrance as in the previous trip, but pass to the right of the ranger's residence, and continue to the North Peak Access Road as it veers north up Montara Mountain. On this steep service road you are soon in tall chaparral of wild lilac, coffeeberry, scrub oak, and here and there a few chinquapins— that sturdy tree with burrs and yellow-backed leaves that occurs on some dry slopes like these.

As you rise along the road and round the mountain, views are to the north and the east. Mileages differ for this trip: a sign at the junction with the Montara Mountain Trail coming up from San Pedro Valley County Park to the northeast says it is 2.4 miles to the summit and 2.1 miles to the beach. Local hikers say it is 3.9 miles from Highway 1 to North Peak. Nonetheless, from this junction on this wide, gravelly road you round many curves, sometimes it flattens out and then climbs again.

When you cross a flat where giant outcrops of granitic rock stand like medieval monuments, you may see the indigenous, rare Montara Mountain manzanita growing low between the rocks. Where there is less wind this native shrub can grow up to ten feet tall. Its white, bell-shaped flowers dangle in clusters at the end of its upright branches. From this high plateau you are 0.5 mile from Montara's peaks.

Continue up the mountain to North Peak, pass the private road leading to communications stations on the summit (1898 feet above sea level), and find a sunny, protected place to enjoy the view. On a clear day, views from the mountaintop are awesome. Southeast are the green heights of Scarpers Peak and the ridges of the Santa Cruz Mountains. Below lie the coastal terrace of Half Moon Bay and its beaches. West and north you see Mt. Tamalpais across the Golden Gate, the Bay, and the skyscrapers of San Francisco; east are the bridges, the East Bay hills, and Mt. Diablo in Contra Costa County. Below are the eastern ridges of adjoining San Pedro Valley County Park.

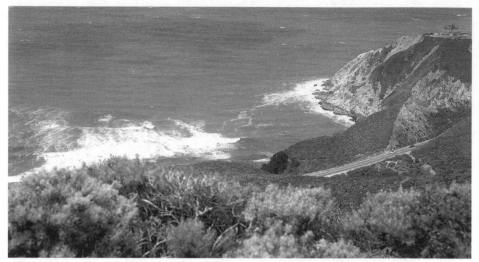

Gray Whale Cove seen from Montara Mountain on a crystal clear day

Your return to sea level is faster than the upward climb. In fact, the descent on the gravelly surface may be faster than you wish! Beware of speeding bicyclists around blind curves.

SEE MAP
ON PAGE
45

A SHORT TRIP TO GRAY WHALE COVE

A springtime treat on a trail festooned with flowers.

Distance: Hikers—less than 2 miles round trip; bicyclists and equestrians—2.5 miles round trip

Time: ¾ hour

Elevation Change: Relatively level

Just inside the entrance gate to McNee Ranch, hikers go left, uphill (north) onto a narrow foot trail that skirts the cypress trees and emerges on an open hillside blossoming with myriad shades of spring wildflowers. Bicyclists and equestrians follow the entrance road and bear left at the ranger station on Old Pedro Mountain Road as in as in the first trip, Old Pedro Mountain Road to the Saddle. All modes meet where Old Pedro Mountain Road veers sharply right in the ravine and a narrow trail climbs left to reach the bluff trail.

On a clear, bright day the views up and down the Coast and out to sea are superb. The Gray Whale Cove Trail meanders along above Highway 1 traffic with detours to several benches at strategic viewpoints. Toward the end of this short trail there is a dramatic view of the southernmost cove of Gray Whale Cove State Beach—deep azure blue, almost green at times, washed with the white curls of incoming waves.

As you reach the Gray Whale Cove parking area, descend around several switchbacks through lush coastal vegetation. Ferns, tall mustard, cow's parsnip, California bee plant, blue iris, and pink Clarkia add color and fragrance. Return the way you came for views south and east, especially the uncluttered, golden strand of Montara State Beach stretching a mile along the Pacific's edge.

✦ Junipero Serra County Park ✦

This 100-acre wooded park in the curve of Junipero Serra Freeway (I-280), just minutes from homes in San Bruno, provides a quick retreat from the urban scene into protected meadows and woods. The park, situated on a long ridge, once quarried for its Franciscan sandstone, offers several miles of trails, attractive picnic sites, and a visitor center.

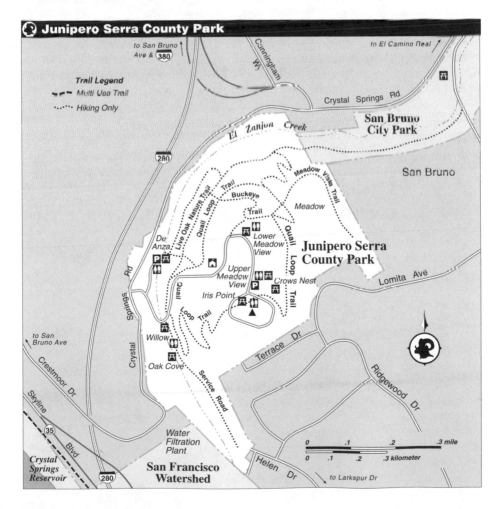

From the park entrance, meadows, picnic grounds, and parking areas extend left and right. On weekends families and groups gravitate to this sheltered canyon. The entrance road winds uphill past park headquarters and the picnic tables, continuing to the very top, where still more picnic tables nestle in a eucalyptus grove. This hilltop site offers spectacular views. From these wide views of mountains and Bay, the eye and the ear are drawn to the San Francisco Airport. Air-age, flight-minded children (and others too) delight in the bird's-eye view of planes taking off and landing.

At park headquarters, which serves as a visitor and information center, there are maps, exhibits, and information about long-ago inhabitants of this park—the Buri Buri tribe of Ohlones. A self-guiding nature trail through a wooded glade and a loop trail to the park's summit make good warm-up trips before a picnic spread at one of the many tables in this attractive setting.

Jurisdiction: San Mateo County: 650-363-4020

Facilities: Trails for hikers and a nature trail; picnic areas with barbecues; covered shelters and group picnic areas available by reservation only; visitor center at park headquarters; youth-group camp by reservation

Rules: Open 8 A.M. to sunset; fees; no bikes on trails

Maps: San Mateo County *Junipero Serra Park*, USGS topo *Montara Mountain*

How to Get There: From I-280: Southbound—Take Crystal Springs Rd. exit, go under freeway, turn right on Crystal Springs Rd. and go 0.7 mile to park entrance on left. Park at lower picnic areas or continue to more parking on hilltop. Northbound—Take San Bruno Ave. exit and turn left onto San Bruno Ave. West. Go under freeway and turn left back onto 280 south. Immediately exit at Crystal Springs Road and follow directions for southbound above.

HIKE TO THE HILLTOP
ON THE QUAIL LOOP TRAIL

Gaining altitude quickly on a zigzag climb, this trip leads to flowers in grasslands and woods and to protected slopes on the park's east side.

Distance: 1.4-mile loop

Time: Less than 1 hour

Elevation Change: 300' gain

To the right of the park entrance find the signed beginning of the Quail Loop Trail. You start climbing immediately, with oak trees overhead and patches of bright flowers at your feet. Early in spring, false Solomon's seal plants droop with clusters of small white flowers, which later form panicles of red-brown berries. Switchbacks take you up the mountain, first out into an open grassy slope where sun-loving orange poppies and yellow mule ears dot the hillside. At the next switchback you are under the cover of oaks and toyons with ferns and snowberry underneath.

Toward the top of the hill you encounter Monterey pines and a large grove of mature eucalyptuses. Here the trail crosses the picnic grounds to reach the wide meadow on an east-facing slope. On a clear day the brilliant Bay waters are set against the backdrop of East Bay cities and tree-topped hills. After taking in the sweep of Bay from north of San Francisco to its southern shores, continue on the Quail Loop Trail past the Crows Nest picnic shelter and bear left to descend across the meadow.

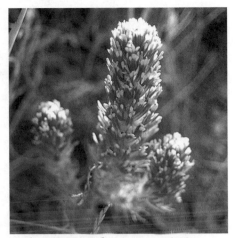

At the first trail junction you could turn left to reach the visitor center at park headquarters, but instead stay on

Pink owl's clover brightens trailsides

the Quail Loop Trail, which swings right. From the next trail junction the Quail Loop Trail goes left on a long traverse through woods of magnificent oaks back to the picnic areas near the park entrance.

If you would like to extend your trip, pass up the left Quail Loop Trail turnoff and continue down the hill for around two short zigzags to the next trail junction. Park signs offer the choice of going to San Bruno City Park or back to the park entrance on the Live Oak Nature Trail. If you take the San Bruno option, this trail, following El Zanjon Creek down to the park and back, adds 3 miles to this hike. When Native Americans, the Costanoans, lived in this area, they probably followed this trail along the creek to reach San Francisco Bay. Mollusks and fish were abundant and constituted a major part of their diet, along with herbs, bulbs, nuts, and berries. By means of snares and bow and arrows they hunted birds and small mammals to fill out a substantial diet.

If you ignore this side trip to San Bruno City Park, you will take the left turn to descend quickly on the Live Oak Nature Trail. In about 200 yards, take either leg of this trail to return to the meadows below.

Two Short Walks in the Canyon

The 0.5-mile Live Oak Nature Trail leaves the lower meadow parking area going left on the hillside just above El Zanjon Creek. The creek probably got its name from a Spanish word meaning "deep ditch" or "slough." Through an oak glade follow the trail in the shade of live oaks. In fall, poison oak bushes put on a brilliant red-orange display in the understory. Now crossing open grasslands, you see east to Mt. Diablo, the main reference point for surveying in northern California. The trail circles back on the shady upper hillside, then drops down to return to its starting point.

Another short walk goes by the Willow Shelter to the right of the park entrance on a service road above El Zanjon Creek, past picnic tables in the shade of oak groves. From the end of this road it is just a third mile back to the park entrance.

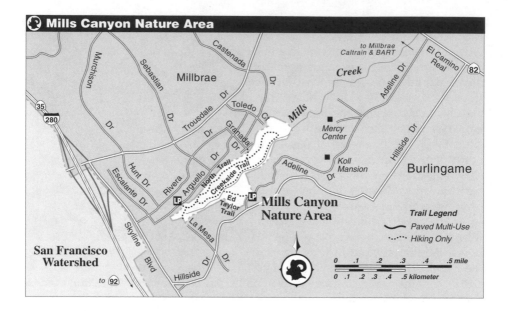

Mills Canyon Nature Area

◆ Mills Canyon Nature Area—Burlingame ◆

Under Mexican rule, Mills Canyon was part of Rancho Buri Buri, which included most of northeast San Mateo County, extending as far south as present-day San Mateo. In the early 1860s Darius Ogden Mills and his brother-in-law, Ansel Easton, each bought 1500 acres of Rancho Buri Buri. The division between their two holdings ran straight through this canyon. Most of Mills' estate was in contemporary Millbrae, but this land, including the upper part of this canyon which takes his name, was eventually annexed to Burlingame.

The city acquired the canyon as a park and wildlife area, and in 1978 volunteers built a delightful, hikers-only, 1.75-mile loop called the Ed Taylor Trail, in honor of the man who built the trail and inspired the volunteers. Dedicated in September 1983, the trail is maintained by local volunteers, the Friends of Mill Canyon, with the help of the city of Burlingame. This group offers a variety of hikes from the Adeline Street entrance on the second Saturday of every month, featuring topics on wildlife, native plants, geology, and insects, and a yearly nature treasure hunt for children. Eagle Scouts built the steps from Adeline Drive and other Scouts put up information boards at the trail entrance.

The Nature Area is open from 8 A.M. to dusk. To get to the Adeline Drive entrance, from El Camino or Skyline Blvd. in Burlingame take Hillside Drive and turn northeast on Adeline Drive to off-street parking. For the Arguello Drive entrance from I-280 or El Camino Real in Burlingame, take Trousdale Drive, and turn south on Sebastian Drive. In two blocks, turn right on Arguello Drive and go to the park entrance on the south side of the 3000 block.

This 1.75-mile loop trail through a tight little canyon in suburban Burlingame traverses open northwest slopes, then dips down into deep woods beside Mills Creek. On a summer day this canyon is a cool, sheltered place for a leisurely walk along a little watercourse, relatively unchanged since the early settlers came here. On fair winter days the southern sun shining on the northwest hillside will warm you while you enjoy the views down the canyon.

As you enter the preserve from Arguello Drive, a large sign tells you to start your trip on the Ed Taylor Trail which begins to your right about 25 feet from the entrance. This path descends gently through willows, live oaks, coyote bushes, and toyons for about 20 yards to a trail junction, marked by a sign post with arrows pointing to the Creekside Trail. This trail turns off sharply to the right, while the North Trail continues straight ahead on the upper hillside. By beginning on the North Trail, you have a shady uphill return on the Creekside Trail—best for warm summer days.

For Bay views, take the North Trail first, returning on the trail by the creek. On the North Trail you follow a shady path under huge, high-branched live oaks, then emerge into mixed grassland interspersed with young oaks. Then, descending along the upper edge of a tributary to Mills Creek, you follow the north bank of Mills Creek upstream winding in and out of little ravines. When you come upon a plank bridge with chain handrails that crosses to the south side of the creek at Adeline Drive, pass it to reach two tall and picturesque outcrops of graywacke, a rock formation associated with the San Andreas Fault. Then continue on the path upstream past mossy rocks and lacy wood ferns to a succession of miniature cascades and small pools. Before long the path to the main entrance turns uphill, and you leave this little creek, which below the park flows beside homes and schools, under streets and finally into the Bay at Burlingame's Shoreline Bird Sanctuary.

◆ Trails on Northern San Francisco Watershed Lands ◆

San Francisco Watershed— the Bay Area Ridge Trail Route

The 15-mile linear valley running through the Watershed was formed over the millennia by movements along the San Andreas Fault. For perhaps thousands of years before the coming of the Spanish this valley was the site of Native American villages. From then until the dams were built, it was a place of small, fertile farms and a few inns. The Crystal Springs Hotel, built in 1855, a popular spa of its day, gave the lakes their name.

In the northern Watershed between the San Francisco County line and Highway 92 there are two fine trails east of the San Andreas lakes and one long trail on the west side. Each of these trails is open to the public for hiking and horseback and bicycle riding. The Sawyer Camp Historic Trail and the San Andreas Trail on the east side of the lakes, longtime Peninsula favorites, are managed by San Mateo County and are the most used of any of the County parks.

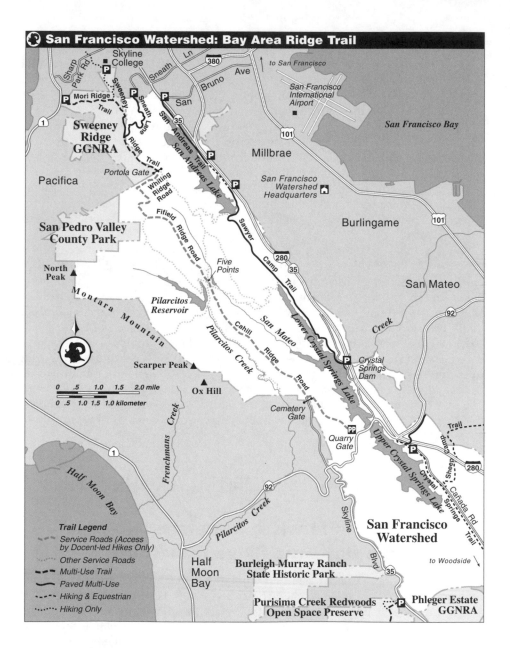

San Francisco Watershed: Bay Area Ridge Trail

Trail Legend
- – – – Service Roads (Access by Docent-led Hikes Only)
- · · · · · Other Service Roads
- ▬ ▬ ▬ Multi-Use Trail
- ▬▬▬ Paved Multi-Use
- – · – · Hiking & Equestrian
- · · · · · · Hiking Only

Negotiations over location of I-280 through the Watershed south of Highway 92 led to a 1969 agreement between the federal government, the State of California, the City and County of San Francisco, and San Mateo County to place the freeway farther east of the lakes than originally proposed. This agreement granted two easements affecting the Watershed lands and guaranteed certain scenic and recreation rights in perpetuity to the people of the United States.

Roughly 19,000 acres on the west side of the lakes are designated as a scenic easement. They must remain undeveloped—preserved for watershed capacity, scenic quality, and limited access. East of the lakes, 4000 acres of the Watershed will continue for their scenic value and watershed purposes, but may also be used for recreation, including trails someday.

The longest and newest trail is a 9.5-mile segment of the Bay Area Ridge Trail that starts beside the cemetery lands at the upper junction of Highways 92 and 35 (Skyline Boulevard) and follows Fifield/Cahill Ridge roads to the Portola Gate in Sweeney Ridge—Golden Gate National Recreation Area's open space lands south of Skyline College in San Bruno.

At this writing, the Ridge Trail hikes, bicycle rides, and horseback rides are open to docent-led trips only. Trips are available on Wednesdays, Saturdays, and Sundays. To sign up for one of these trips, to act as a docent, or to learn more about the Ridge Trail in the Watershed look at the website http://sfwater.org.

Presently, trips start from the old Watershed quarry, halfway up the mountain on the north side of Highway 92. From there it is a steep, approximately 1.5-mile climb to the Fifield/Cahill Ridge service road that meanders along the middle ridge of the Watershed lands. On this wide, fenced, gravel-surfaced road, you travel along Cahill Ridge through a tall, mature forest of Douglas firs interspersed with some redwoods. The understory is lush with bay trees, toyon bushes, and ferns draping old stumps and tree branches. There are too, occasional escapes from urban gardens, such as English holly.

From a few openings in the forest you can see San Francisco Bay, Mt. Diablo, and the East Bay hills. In the foreground are the San Andreas Lakes, though not as easily seen from this leg of the trip. A few patches of open grassland offer a view west across the canyon of Pilarcitos Creek to the upper ridges of Starker Peak. In less than 4 miles on the service road you reach the junction known as Five Points, which is the stopping point on the Ridge Trail route for the shorter trips.

However, the longer trip continues another 5 miles to the Portola Gate. This section beyond Five Points on Fifield Ridge becomes hilly and the trees fewer, but wildflowers in spring are glorious. At the top of the first hill beyond Five Points, you can look back to Pilarcitos Lake nestled in a wooded canyon on the west side of the ridge. The near view takes in the length of the San Andreas and Crystal Springs Lakes in the San Andreas Rift Valley. Beyond is the Bay shoreline curving south from San Bruno Point to Coyote Point. And farther off are the city of San Francisco, the Bay Bridge, and across the Bay, Mt. Diablo rising above the East Bay hills in the foreground.

For hikers there is a shuttle at the Portola Gate in Sweeney Ridge or at the Sneath Lane entrance 3.5 miles northeast. Check the website to sign up and see the Watershed on foot, on horseback, or by bicycle.

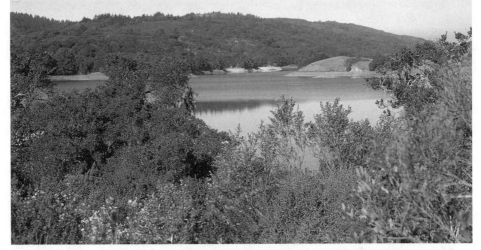

Looking northwest from old Watershed road, proposed extension of the Sawyer Camp Trail

San Andreas Trail

The wide, paved San Andreas Trail follows the eastern boundary of the San Francisco Watershed, giving views of the lakes and the wooded mountains. At Larkspur Drive it becomes a hiking and equestrian path, winding through the trees and underbrush in a fenced right-of-way until it reaches Hillcrest Boulevard.

Jurisdiction: San Mateo County: 650-363-4020

Facilities: Southern section of trail for hikers and equestrians; north section also open to bicyclists

Rules: Open dawn to dusk

Maps: See map on page 57. San Mateo County *Mid-County Trails*; USGS topo *Montara Mountain*

How to Get There: (1) North entrance: (a) Northbound—Take Skyline Blvd. to San Bruno Ave., turn east for streetside parking, use signalized crosswalk at corner of Skyline Blvd. and San Bruno Ave. to reach trail entrance on west side of road; (b) Southbound—from Skyline Blvd. follow directions above. (2) South entrance: (a) Northbound—from I-280 take Millbrae Ave. exit, go north on frontage road to Hillcrest Blvd., then west (left) under freeway to parking at trail entrance on right; (b) Southbound— from I-280 take Larkspur Dr. exit, go under freeway and turn south on frontage road to Hillcrest Blvd; turn right under freeway to trail entrance.

By Bus: One of the few trails with good bus access. The south entrance can be reached by Samtrans on weekdays and Saturdays.

Distance: 6 miles round trip

Time: 3 hours

Elevation Change: Relatively level

As you start down the 3-mile San Andreas Trail from the north entrance, you can see directly in the west the spot on the ridge from which Gaspar de Portolá first saw San Francisco Bay in 1769. A proposed extension of this trail would someday reach the trail to this "Discovery Site."

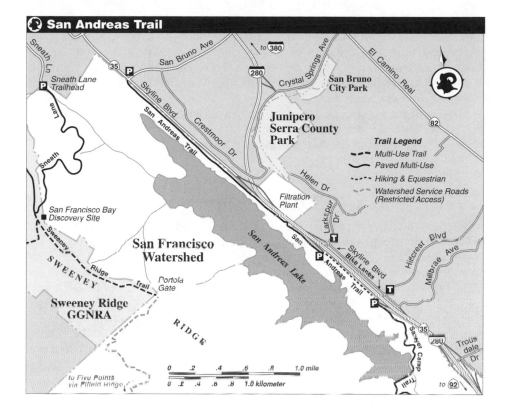

San Andreas Trail

Trail Legend
- **- -** *Multi-Use Trail*
- ⌒ *Paved Multi-Use*
- **-·-·** *Hiking & Equestrian*
- **- -** *Watershed Service Roads (Restricted Access)*

The San Andreas Reservoir now fills the valley, which for centuries before the coming of the Spaniards was the site of Native American villages. As Portolá's party was searching for a site for a mission and presidio in the northern part of the Peninsula, his diarist and historian, Father Francisco Palou, and his scout, Captain Fernando Rivera, went through this valley on November 30, 1774. Palou named it San Andrés, honoring that saint's feast day.

Later, the earthquake-fault valley north of the present dam site was included in the Rancho Feliz, where Spaniards grazed cattle and grew wheat. There were no Spanish settlements here, reportedly because of trouble with bears. It is now surmised that the bear population may have exploded when the cattle provided an increased food supply.

With the coming of the Anglos in the 19th century the valley became a place of small farms and a dairy. In the mid-1880s farmers and herdsmen were still hunting down marauding bears and mountain lions that were attacking their cattle. San Francisco's Spring Valley Water Company began buying up the farms in the valley in the late 1860s, and the lands have been kept as a watershed from that time. The bears are now gone, but the vast and still-wild watershed (also a State Fish and Game Refuge) harbors a great variety of animals, probably including mountain lions, a few eagles and some endangered species.

The first 2.4 miles of the San Andreas Trail are paved, from the San Bruno Avenue/Skyline Boulevard entrance to Larkspur Drive. From the end of this paved

path to the Sawyer Camp Trail entrance at Hillcrest Boulevard, hikers and equestrians take a cleared and maintained 0.6-mile path in a wooded corridor next to the
freeway. Runners use the trail frequently, perhaps because the forest floor is
springy underfoot and the air fragrant with the scent of pine needles. Bicyclists
must travel on Skyline Boulevard to Hillcrest Boulevard, where they turn right to
the paved Sawyer Camp Trail.

In spite of the noisy presence of the freeway, you can enjoy the outlook to the
west as the path winds through groves of Monterey pines and old plantings of
cypresses, with vistas of the lake below and the western hills beyond.

Sawyer Camp Trail

A historic road of singular beauty extends for 6 miles through the San Francisco
Watershed lands past the sparkling San Andreas and Crystal Springs lakes. The
road is paved, but open to hikers, equestrians, and bicyclists only. The camp that
gave the road its name was in a small flat in the San Andreas Valley where in the
1870s, Leander Sawyer trained performing horses for circuses. Later he ran an inn
here for travelers on their way to Half Moon Bay.

The sunny meadow by the creek where Sawyer had his camp had earlier been
home to the Shalshone Indians (a tribelet of the Ohlones), who hospitably offered
wild fruits and seed cakes to Gaspar de Portolá's expedition when it passed this
way in 1769. During Sawyer's day, wagons pulled by teams of eight horses hauled
wood over the road on their way to San Francisco and stage coaches used it as an
alternative route from San Francisco to Half Moon Bay.

When San Francisco took over the Watershed lands, narrow, winding Sawyer
Camp Road was kept open and later fenced on either side for protection of the
Watershed. San Mateo County closed the road to motorized vehicles in 1978, and
it is now officially the Sawyer Camp Historic Trail.

Jurisdiction: San Mateo County: 650-363-4020

Facilities: Trail for hikers, bicyclists, and equestrians; picnic tables, restrooms,
water at Jepson Laurel picnic area and north end of trail; telephones

Rules: Open dawn to sunset

Maps: See map on page 59, San Mateo County *Jogging, Exercise and Bicycle Trails*
and USGS topos *Montara Mountain* and *San Mateo*

How to Get There: By car from I-280: (1) North entrance at Hillcrest Blvd: (a)
Southbound—Take the Larkspur Dr. exit and go south on Skyline Blvd. to Hillcrest
Blvd., then west under freeway to trail entrance on right; (b) Northbound—Take
Millbrae Ave. exit and go north on Skyline Blvd., then west on Hillcrest Blvd. to
trail entrance. (2) South entrance at Crystal Springs Rd: (a) Southbound—Take
Hayne Rd. exit and go south on Skyline Blvd. to parking beside entrance gate on
west side of road; (b) Northbound—Take Bunker Hill Dr. exit, cross over freeway,
then go north on Skyline Blvd. past Crystal Springs Dam to entrance gate.

By Bicycle: Use the same approaches from Skyline Blvd. as for cars.

Distance: 6 miles one way

Time: 3 hours. A car shuttle is practical here. Shorter round trips on part of the
trail from either end make good hikes.

Elevation Change: 400' loss from north to south

Entering the trail at the north end, the first 1.75 miles descend from Skyline Boulevard to San Andreas Lake and its dam. The woods and lake are a pleasant introduction to the trail. Summer winds often ruffle the lake and drifts of fog sweep over the hills. On the far side of the dam look for a commemorative plaque that marks the hundredth anniversary of the dam's completion in 1869. From here the trail heads south along a shady walk between the creek and a hillside of bay trees. Fern-covered banks bloom with purple iris and scarlet columbine. You may see the very rare shrub leatherwood, with its small yellow blossoms. It is found in only a few places in San Mateo County (one of them is Edgewood Park). The Indians used its tough, flexible branches for lacings.

In a small clearing along the way, about 30 yards west of the trail, is the venerable Jepson Bay Laurel, thought to be the second-oldest and largest in the state. In

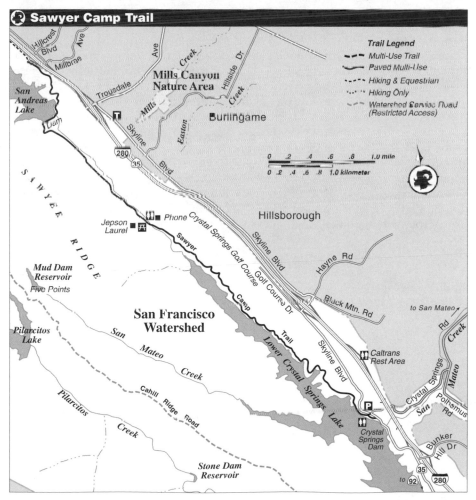

1923 it was named in honor of Willis Jepson, one of California's most noted botanists. The flowery little meadow around the tree was popular as a picnic spot in Mexican and early California times. Today the tree is fenced to protect it, and there is a picnic area nearby, and once again picnickers are enjoying this retreat beside the famous bay tree.

Here and there you will come to benches beside the trail for a place to rest, picnic, or enjoy the sound of a stream or a view of the lake. At about its halfway point, the trail crosses San Andreas Creek where it enters Lower Crystal Springs Lake. From here on, it borders the east side of the lake, giving a succession of views out over the bright waters to the wooded Watershed hills. The Peninsula's own "Lake District" has a special enchantment whether mists are shrouding the mountains or the lakes are reflecting a blue sky.

A few hawks sail overhead. Grebes, ducks, and other waterfowl bob on the water, and the oaks by the trail are alive with countless small birds—countless except to the Audubon Society, which enumerates the species meticulously in its annual Christmas bird count; a recent count totaled 190 species. Bring your binoculars and favorite bird guide.

Along the road cuts you will see the greenish-gray serpentine, a rock that occurs through the foothills in San Mateo County. It is frequently found in major earthquake fault zones, and is associated with some of our finest wildflower displays.

The south end of the trail is on Skyline Boulevard at the Crystal Springs Dam that crosses the gorge of San Mateo Creek. (A proposed extension to Highway 92 is planned in the near future.) This is a good starting point for a 3+ mile walk north by the lake, with vistas of the shimmering waters around each bend. Your return trip brings you new views as you retrace your steps. Walk here in late winter when clouds are moving across the sky and sunshine alternates with light showers. The hills are already green, drifts of magenta Indian warriors bloom under the trees, and the first buds of iris appear. This is one of the Peninsula's best walks for any time of the year and the most popular of San Mateo County parks.

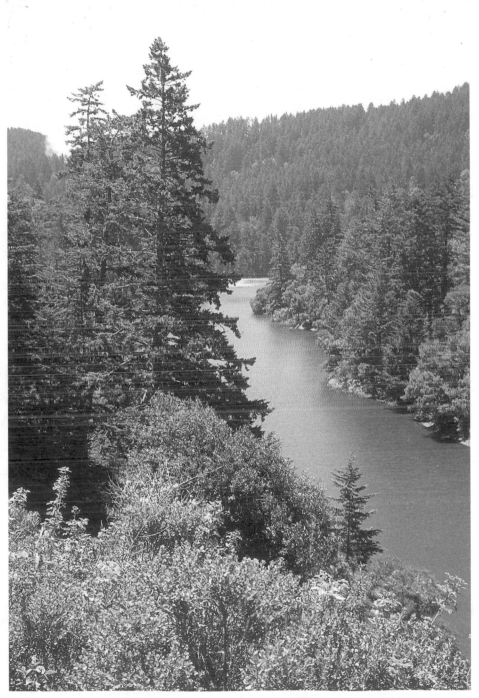

Pilarcitos Lake seen from Bay Area Ridge Trail route through the Watershed

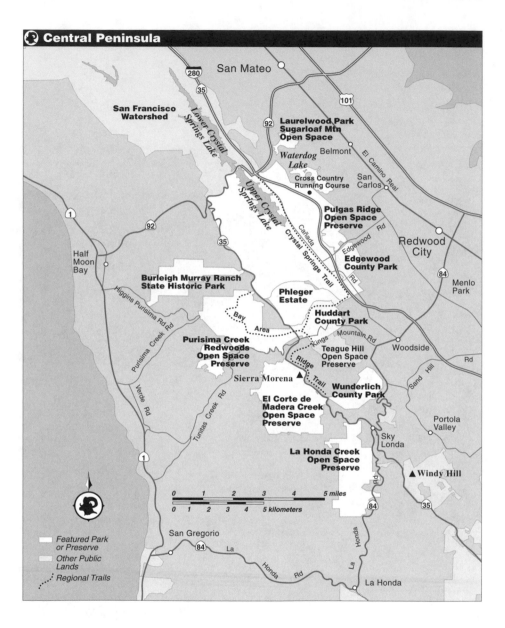

Central Peninsula

San Mateo

San Francisco
Watershed

Laurelwood Park
Sugarloaf Mtn
Open Space

Waterdog
Lake

Belmont

Cross Country
Running Course

San
Carlos

Redwood
City

Pulgas Ridge
Open Space
Preserve

Edgewood

Edgewood
County Park

Menlo
Park

Half
Moon
Bay

Burleigh Murray Ranch
State Historic Park

Phleger
Estate

Huddart
County Park

Woodside

Purisima Creek
Redwoods
Open Space
Preserve

Teague Hill
Open Space
Preserve

Sierra Morena

Wunderlich
County Park

El Corte de
Madera Creek
Open Space
Preserve

Portola
Valley

La Honda Creek
Open Space
Preserve

Sky
Londa

Windy Hill

San Gregorio

La Honda

0   1   2   3   4   5 miles
0 1 2 3 4 5 kilometers

Featured Park
or Preserve
Other Public
Lands
Regional Trails

◆ Central Peninsula ◆
From Highway 92 to Highway 84

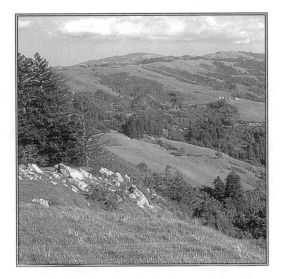

◆ Trails on Southern San Francisco Watershed Lands ◆

Crystal Springs Trail

Bordering Upper Crystal Springs Lake, this trail traverses the linear valley on the San Andreas Rift Zone known by the Spaniards as Cañada de Raimundo, then continues through a corner of the Watershed and up through Huddart Park to the Skyline. Views of lakes, mountains and hills make this a beautiful trail for short trips along its segments. Connections with trails east and west make it a useful route for longer expeditions. The trail is part of San Mateo County's north-south trail corridor, and it provides access to the regional Bay Area Ridge Trail

The Crystal Springs Trail follows the easement of the old California Riding and Hiking Trail between the boundary fence of the Watershed and Cañada Road, from Highway 92 to Huddart Park and up to the Skyline. Although the trail easement extends north to the Sawyer Camp Trail, a 1.3-mile segment from Highway 92 to the Crystal Springs Dam is proposed.

The nearly 10-mile Crystal Springs Trail appears in this book in three sections: (1) from Cañada Road at Highway 92 to Edgewood and Cañada roads, (2) from Edgewood Road to Huddart Park, and (3) through the park to the Skyline. The first trip in Huddart Park, An All-Day Hike Circling the Park, features this trail.

At the Pulgas Water Temple grounds there is a small parking area, open on weekdays from 9 A.M. TO 4 P.M. No roadside parking is allowed within a mile on either side. However, the lovely water temple and its reflecting pool and grounds, open to pedestrians and bicyclists, make a fine destination from either end of the trail.

Jurisdiction: San Mateo County: 650-363-4020

Facilities: Trail for hikers and equestrians

Rules: Open from 8 A.M. to sunset; no bicycles

Maps: San Mateo County *Mid-County Trails*; USGS topos *San Mateo* and *Woodside*

How to Get There: From I-280: (1) North entrance: (a) Southbound—Take Half Moon Bay exit to Skyline Blvd. (Hwy 35), go south to Hwy 92, and then turn east. Turn south on Cañada Rd. and go 0.2 mile to trail entrance on west side of road just opposite the Ralston Trail/I-280 Overcrossing Trail junction; (b) Northbound— Take Hwy 92 exit west to Cañada Rd. Turn south for 0.2 mile to trail entrance. (2) South entrance: Take Edgewood Rd. exit, go west to Edgewood/Cañada Rd. inter- section, where there is parking. No parking at Raymundo Drive cul-de-sac entrance to Huddart Park. Note: No parking is allowed on Cañada Rd. Canada Rd. is closed to motor-vehicle traffic from the intersection of Hwy 92 to Edgewood Rd. for "Bicycle Sunday," a popular event held every Sunday year-round.

prevous page:
West side of the Santa Cruz Mountains seen from La Honda Creek Open Space Preserve

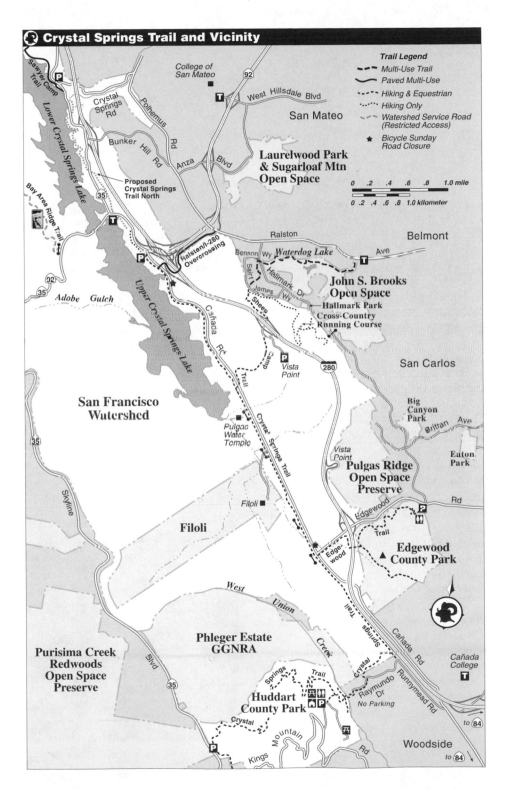

Crystal Springs Trail and Vicinity

College of
San Mateo

92

West Hillsdale Blvd

San Mateo

Sawyer Camp Trail

P

Crystal
Springs
Rd

Polhemus Rd

Bunker Hill Rd

Anza Blvd

Lower Crystal Springs Lake

35

Proposed
Crystal Springs
Trail North

**Laurelwood Park
& Sugarloaf Mtn
Open Space**

Trail Legend

- - - Multi-Use Trail

Paved Multi-Use

- - - - Hiking & Equestrian

· · · · Hiking Only

- · - Watershed Service Road
(Restricted Access)

★ Bicycle Sunday
Road Closure

| 0 | .2 | .4 | .6 | .8 | 1.0 mile |

| 0 | .2 | .4 | .6 | .8 | 1.0 kilometer |

Bay Area Ridge Trail

T

Ralston

Belmont

Benson Wy

Waterdog Lake

Ave

T

92

35

Adobe Gulch

Upper Crystal Springs Lake

Cañada Rd

Hallmark Dr

Sair

James Wy

Shee

**John S. Brooks
Open Space**

Hallmark Park
Cross-Country
Running Course

Camp Trail

P
Vista
Point

280

San Carlos

**San Francisco
Watershed**

35

Pulgas
Water
Temple

Crystal Springs Trail

Big
Canyon
Park

Brittan Ave

Vista
Point

Eaton
Park

**Pulgas Ridge
Open Space
Preserve**

Rd

Skyline

Filoli

Filoli

Edgewood

Trail

P

ᵢ⫟

Edge-
wood

▲ **Edgewood
County Park**

West

Union Creek

Crystal Springs Trail

Cañada Rd

Runnymead Rd

Cañada
College

T

**Purisima Creek
Redwoods
Open Space
Preserve**

Blvd

35

**Phleger Estate
GGNRA**

Springs

Trail

Raymundo
Dr
No Parking

to 84

**Huddart
County Park**

Crystal

Mountain

Rd

Kings Blvd

P

Woodside

to 84

SEE MAP
ON PAGE
65

HIGHWAY 92 TO EDGEWOOD AND CAÑADA ROADS

Lakeside views give way to broad, parklike meadows set against a back-drop of wooded slopes of the Santa Cruz Mountains.

Distance: 4 miles one way

Time: 2 hours

Elevation Change: Relatively level

The trip south begins on a path departing from a point on Cañada Road, 0.2 mile south of Highway 92 and just across the road from the western entrance to the Ralston Trail/I-280 Overcrossing. You can also walk north along this unimproved lakeside trail as far as the intersection of Highway 92 and Skyline Boulevard. At times the trail swings away from the road, coming close to the lake, or leads down below road level through oak groves.

The lake is a resting place for water birds on the Pacific Flyway, so take your binoculars. Even without them you will easily identify the big, brownish Canada geese that winter here. Flocks of them often gather along the shores. In the early morning and evening you may see herds of deer grazing in the fields or drinking at the water's edge.

Soon after the trail leaves the lakeside, it passes the point where the Sheep Camp Trail joins the east side of Cañada Road. From here to the Pulgas Water Temple the trail is on a bank above the road. The Water Temple grounds, re-opened on October 25, 2004, the temple's 70th birthday, are open to the public from 9 A.M. to 4 P.M. daily, and include lawns for picnicking and sunning, and the Water Temple itself. At the end of a long reflecting pool is the classic little Pulgas Water Temple, where waters from high in the Sierra thunder into the sluiceway to the Crystal Springs lakes. Inscribed around the pediment are words from the Book of Isaiah, "I give waters in the wilderness and rivers in the desert to give drink to my people."

Continuing south you see on the valley floor to the west open fields and groves of stately oaks, a part of the Filoli estate, which once belonged to W.B. Bourn, president of the Spring Valley Water Company. The name for the estate was coined by Bourn from "Fight," "Love," and "Live," taken from "Fight for a just cause, love your fellow man, and live a good life." A later owner, Mrs. William

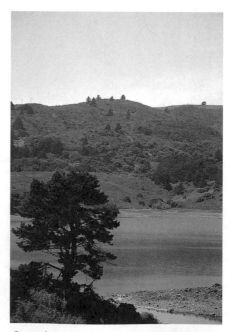

Crystal Springs Trail from Cañada Road

Roth, changed the "fight" to "fidelity." Designed by Willis Polk and completed in 1917, Filoli was the last of the great mansions built in San Mateo County.

Filoli was purchased by the Roth family in 1934, and Mrs. Roth gave the estate to the National Trust for Historic Preservation in 1975. The Filoli Center, a non-profit organization, operates the center. The mansion is hardly visible from the trail, but its beautiful formal gardens and the mansion itself, as well as its nature trails, are open for tours by arrangement with the Filoli Center.

From the Filoli gates your trail passes more oak-bordered meadows to reach the stone gates at the foot of Edgewood Road, the end of this trip. From there the Crystal Springs Trail continues on to Huddart Park.

SEE MAP ON PAGE 65

EDGEWOOD AND CAÑADA ROADS TO HUDDART PARK

A short trip over a hill through the Watershed and down to West Union Creek in Huddart Park.

Distance: 2.4 miles one way

Time: 1¼ hours

Elevation Change: 200′ gain

As you pass the stone gates at the foot of Edgewood Road, fields extend on either side of Cañada Road. Come this way in April and May to see some of the Peninsula's most dazzling displays of wildflowers. They thrive on the thin, magnesium-rich soil over serpentine rock outcroppings. Swatches of intense blue larkspur bloom against great drifts of cream cups, goldfields, poppies, lupines, and owl's clover. Admire these flowers from the roadside paths, photograph or paint them, but do not cross the fence and walk among them. The fields have been set aside as a preserve in the Watershed, and these flowers, if left undisturbed, will continue to bloom year after year to amaze and delight your great-grandchildren.

Where Cañada Road turns east to cross under the freeway, the trail continues south beside the freeway for nearly a mile between wire fences, the freeway on one side and the Watershed lands on the other. It's not so attractive a stretch for walkers, but the cinderpath surface is popular with equestrians and joggers.

The Crystal Springs Trail emerges from the cinderpath at Runnymede Road at the Woodside town boundary. From here another fenced trail goes about a mile across a corner of the Watershed and south on an easement to Raymundo Drive. From this point walk west on Raymundo Drive 0.2 mile to its cul-de-sac.

The trail leaves the south side of the cul-de-sac, descending into oak woods on switchbacks for 0.3 mile to the redwood groves beside West Union Creek. Here a footbridge takes you across to forested Huddart Park. The Crystal Springs Trail continues upstream by the creek, then turns up through the park on the 3.5-mile trip to the Skyline described in An All-Day Hike Circling the Park, the first trip in the section on Huddart Park. Access to the Phleger Estate also is possible from this trail.

For groups with a backpack excursion in mind, there is a trail camp (by reservation) about 1.25 miles up the trail on the park's secluded north side. From there you can explore the miles of trail in the park, or climb up the mountainside to the Skyline Trail (and Bay Area Ridge Trail route) across to Purisima Creek Redwoods Open Space Preserve.

The Ralston Bike Trail/I-280 Overcrossing

A wide, mile-long pedestrian, equestrian, and bicycle path and freeway overpass crosses high above 10-lane Junipero Serra Freeway, I-280, at its interchange with Highway 92. It connects the bike path on Ralston Avenue in Belmont to Cañada Road north of the Sheep Camp Trail junction.

Jurisdiction: San Mateo County: 650-363-4020
Facilities: Pedestrian, equestrian, and bicycle path
Rules: Open sunrise to sunset
Map: See map on page 65; USGS topo *San Mateo*
How to Get There: From I-280: (1) East entrance—Take Hwy 92 exit east, then take Ralston Ave. exit. At first traffic signal, 1.13 miles east of Ralston/Polhemus/Hwy 92 interchange, park on south side of Ralston Ave. (2) West entrance: (a) Northbound—Take Hwy 92 west to Cañada Rd. Go south on it 0.2 mile to gate on east side. Parking is on either side of road. (b) Southbound—Take Half Moon Bay exit to Skyline Blvd. (Hwy 35) and continue south to Hwy 92, then turn east to Cañada Rd. Go south on it 0.2 mile to gate on east side.
Distance: 2 miles round trip
Time: 1 hour
Elevation Change: 125' loss

This is no quiet country trail, but a paved, fenced path and concrete structure vaulting over the freeway. At this writing, the surface is a bit rough and cracked, but it is the only way to cross the freeway on foot, horse, or bicycle at this point. From Ralston Avenue the path goes through a gate to the Watershed lands and descends along chaparral-covered slopes. It curves south and then rises steeply to the arched structure over the freeway. A swift drop on the other side and a sharp right turn take you down to Cañada Road. On the west side you can pick up the roadside Crystal Springs Trail.

An interesting 6.2-mile circle hike starting at the Ralston Avenue entrance combines the Overcrossing Trail, part of the Crystal Springs Trail, the Sheep Camp Trail, and the upper part of the Waterdog Lake Trail. When the Waterdog Lake Trail reaches Hallmark Drive, walk north on it to Ralston Avenue, then west on the Ralston bike path to where you started. These trails are described more fully in their separate chapters.

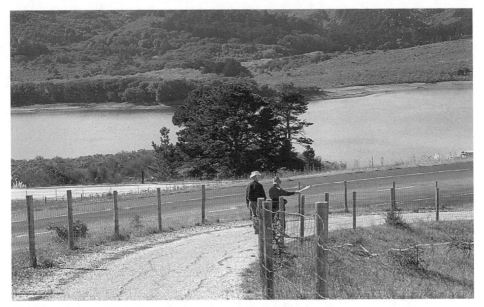

Ralston Bike Trail/I-280 Overcrossing nearing Cañada Road

Sheep Camp Trail

A scenic downhill trip from the eastern crest of the Watershed winds downhill to cross under I-280. On the far side the trail meanders through sheltered oak groves and small meadows to join the Crystal Springs Trail at Cañada Road.

Jurisdiction: San Mateo County; 650-363-4020

Facilities: Trail for hikers and equestrians

Rules: Open 8 A.M. to sunset; no dogs or bicycles

Maps: See map on page 65; USGS topos *San Mateo* and *Woodside*

How to Get There: From I-280 take Hwy 92 east to Ralston Ave., turn south on Hallmark Dr., west on Benson Way and south on St. James Rd. Gate to Watershed is on right.

Distance: 2 miles round trip

Time: 1 hour

Elevation Change: 400′ loss

Enter through the green gates to the Watershed. Walk straight ahead on the graveled road over the grassy slope to the sign SHEEP CAMP TRAIL,. CAÑADA ROAD 1.6 KM. No sheep are in sight, but around the bend is a view of eight or ten concrete lanes of the Junipero Serra Freeway, which would surprise its namesake, the Franciscan Father who trod a more modest path between his missions.

Keep going downhill on the road and cross under the freeway. As the road starts up the hill to the vista point, go instead through a gate on the right. From here a dirt and gravel road takes you away from the freeway roar into the Watershed's quiet oak woods and small meadows. About 0.5 mile from the gate you reach Cañada Road. On the far side is the Crystal Springs Trail, which goes south to

Huddart Park and north to Highway 92. Just 0.4 mile south is the Pulgas Water Temple, a pleasant picnic destination.

For an interesting 6.2-mile loop trip on the Sheep Camp Trail and other trails in this area, see the description of the Ralston Trail/I-280 Overcrossing, page 68. Someday it may be possible to make a 9-mile loop hike using the Sheep Camp, Crystal Springs, Edgewood, Pulgas Ridge, and Watershed boundary trails. Only a short connection from Pulgas Ridge Open Space Preserve to the eastern Watershed boundary trail is missing at this writing.

Cross Country Running Course

Considered one of the best running courses in the Bay Area, this course has a location on the eastern crest of the Watershed that makes it a good walking trail as well. Here is a chance to check your pace on carefully measured and marked loop paths.

Jurisdiction: San Francisco Water Department; maintained by College of San Mateo, 650-574-6448.

Facilities: Trails for runners, joggers, and hikers; drinking fountains at trail entrance

Rules: Open to runners, joggers, and hikers except during competition events; no dogs; no bicycles; no smoking

Maps: See map on page 65, city of Belmont *Jogging Trails*, available at the Parks Department, USGS topo *San Mateo*

How to Get There: From I-280 take Hwy 92 east. Take Ralston Ave. exit, turn right on Hallmark Dr. and continue to Hallmark Park on west side of street just before Wakefield Dr. Park along street. Take path through trees by tennis courts to running course.

Distance: 0.5 to 7.5 miles

Time: 15 minutes to 4 hours, or as long as you like

Elevation Change: Relatively level

This championship course, started some 40 years ago by two College of San Mateo coaches, had to be rerouted because of the construction of I-280. Its popularity continues to increase. Local, regional and state high-school and community-college competitions held during the months of September, October, and November, draw large crowds, both runners and spectators.

Care of the course is under the direction of the College of San Mateo track and cross-country coaches. Volunteers do cleanup, mowing, and course conditioning. Walkers, hikers, and joggers can use the course, but should respect competitions by staying off the course during races.

From the start of the course at Hallmark Park the paths extend in loops west and south. The openness of the rolling hillsides and the views over Crystal Springs lakes to the Santa Cruz Mountains make this an exhilarating walk at any time of the year. In spring, poppies, lupines, daisies, blue-eyed grass, and brodiaeas bloom at your feet. In summer, coastal breezes cool what could be a hot, sunny path. And with these breezes come drifts of fog curling over the mountains to the west.

For other walks along the Watershed ridge from Hallmark Park you can take the graveled service roads of the San Francisco Water Department that follow the Watershed boundary. Good for walks in wet weather, these surfaced roads extend more than a mile west and southeast. Going west from Hallmark Park, you will come to the upper entrance to the Sheep Camp Trail at the St. James Road watershed gate.

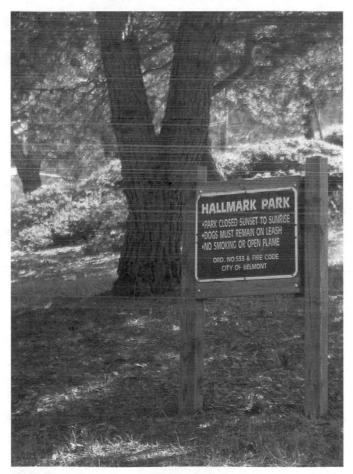

Entrance to Cross Country Running Course

✦ Foothills Parks Adjoining ✦ Southern San Francisco Watershed

Pulgas Ridge Open Space Preserve

In the foothills west of San Carlos and just north of Edgewood Park is the 293-acre Midpeninsula Regional Open Space District preserve, featuring a broad central meadow flanked by two wooded canyons. Cordilleras Creek originates in the preserve's canyons and then flows east to the Bay near the end of Whipple Road, picking up volume from the streams in Edgewood Park.

Formerly the site of a tuberculosis hospital owned by the city of San Francisco, the area was purchased by MROSD in 1983. Residents of San Carlos approved a local tax on their assessed valuation to help fund the purchase.

Restoration efforts on this preserve have succeeded in reducing the number of non-native, invasive plant species, particularly eucalyptus, acacia, and broom. Volunteers and the California Conservation Corps worked with District personnel to re-seed several areas with native species to restore them to a more natural state. This project, begun in 1996, is an ongoing, probably 20-year effort.

Jurisdiction: Midpeninsula Regional Open Space District: 650-691-1200

Facilities: Trails for hikers and an off-leash area for dogs; Cordilleras Trail accessible to wheelchairs and hikers (no dogs)

Rules: Open dawn to dusk; dogs allowed on all trails and must be on maximum 6-foot leash, except in designated off-leash areas, where they must be under voice control; owners must clean up after their dogs

Maps: MROSD *Pulgas Ridge OSP*, USGS topo *Woodside*

How to Get There: From I-280 take Edgewood Rd. exit east and go 0.75 mile. Turn left on Crestview Dr. and immediately left again on Edmonds Rd. Around first curve, park at roadside turnout.

SEE MAP ON PAGE 73

HIGH MEADOWLANDS LOOP

Hikers and their dogs will sample the best trails in this preserve.

Distance: 3-mile loop

Time: 1½ hours

Elevation Change: 400′ gain

From parking on Edmonds Road, walk through the entrance gate onto the 0.6-mile, fenced Cordilleras Trail on an easement beside the San Francisco Water Department road. This surfaced trail, accessible to wheelchairs, meets the paved service road that rises to the top of the preserve.

However, at this junction an unpaved trail goes right through a little glade on the east side of Cordilleras Creek. Here is a bench, installed by local Boy Scouts, in a willow-shaded clearing. From the bench, hikers can continue on the east side of the creek to the George Seagar Memorial Grove, where a plaque commemorates the first MROSD Ward 7 Director. He was instrumental in preserving this land for open space. Native live oaks, maples, and willows shade the peaceful scene, a pleasant destination for a short trip on a hot day

Returning toward the junction of the Cordilleras Trail, bear right on a small bridge across the creek and head uphill on the Polly Geraci Trail. This trail follows the creek near its west bank and then ascends on switchbacks through an oak forest. Ferns cover the hillside, and shade-loving flowers blossom here in spring. The authors try to visit this trail every spring to see the profusion of small, white, star-shaped blossoms of fetid adders tongue growing beside the trail.

Leaving the creek far below, the trail rounds a ridge where madrones and large, shiny-barked manzanitas appear in a tall chaparral cover. Here is a wooden bench shaded by evergreen oaks facing due north toward the chaparral-covered ridge across the canyon, now part of this preserve. A trail northeast along this ridge will someday join the San Francisco Watershed lands.

Farther along the trail you can look across the headwaters canyon of Cordilleras Creek and in rainy winters see a small waterfall tumbling over its headwall. The

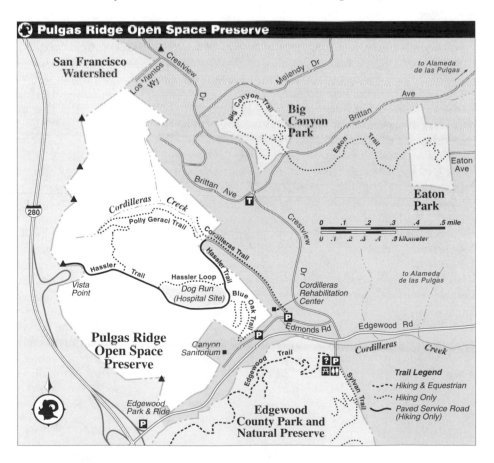

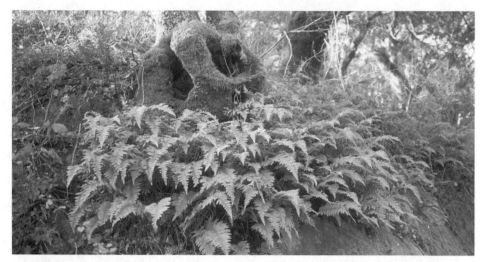

Graceful ferns on a rotting tree stump in Pulgas Ridge Open Space Preserve

trail zigzags west and uphill until it finally breaks out in full chaparral scrub and joins the Hassler Trail at the top of the preserve's high meadow. Some tall eucalyptus, remnants of the dense forest planted here years ago, still border this trail. If you turn right at this junction, you can walk 0.2 mile uphill to a clearing beside the Caltrans triple-fenced, circular Vista Point rest area.

Returning to the paved Hassler Trail you will see immense oaks filling the deep canyons on the west side of the ridge. The trails planned for this canyon will someday bring a more intimate look at these lush forests.

On the left side of the trail is the site of the former health home, now a sloping meadow, capped by tall eucalyptus—a place to picnic and enjoy the views of San Francisco Bay through a notch in the foothills. South are Edgewood Park's grasslands and wooded hilltop; west are the forested Santa Cruz Mountains.

Below the meadow is an off-leash dog run fenced with split-rails and circled by a surfaced road. Signs caution both dogs and dog owners to be on their best behavior.

Opposite the dog run and just off the edge of the trail are two large plots of cactus, probably remnants of a garden adjoining the site of the chief doctor's former home.

As the surfaced Hassler Trail curves left downhill, watch for the Blue Oak Trail on your right. Take this trail down switchbacks through a lovely, mixed oak forest. Look for deep-red Indian Warriors and blue hound's tongue as early as January—early augurs of spring. This delightful, 0.4-mile trail switchbacks down the canyon passing rivulets edged with moss-covered boulders and trailsides draped with maidenhair fern. A thoughtful Eagle Scout, Daemen Merrill, constructed a bench at a wide spot where you can rest, listen to many bird calls, and observe the differences in oak species. The dominant species is the live oak, *Quercus agrifolia*. The blue oak, *Quercus douglasii*, is deciduous, usually a much smaller tree, and has blue-green leaves that are not as prickly as the live oak. It is usually found on dry hillsides.

When the Blue Oak Trail emerges at Edmonds Road, on which you entered the preserve, turn left (northeast) to the parking area.

For a 1.1-mile loop, start from Edmonds Road on the Blue Oak Trail, bear right downhill on the Hassler Trail, and return to your car on the Cordilleras Trail. The shady ascent is just right for a hot day.

Edgewood County Park and Natural Preserve

This San Mateo County park of hilltops, gentle meadows, oak groves, and canyons faces the green expanse of the Skyline ridge to the west and looks out over the Bay to the east. It adjoins Pulgas Ridge Open Space Preserve just across Edgewood Road and the southern San Francisco Watershed lands across I 280. You can picnic here on a knoll listening to meadowlarks in the grass, climb a hill, or walk in cool, secluded glades.

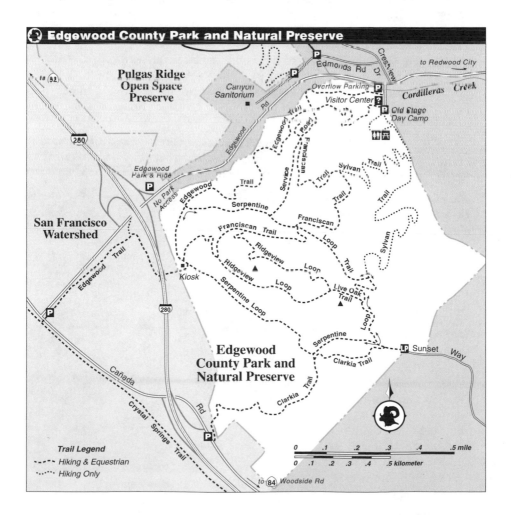

Edgewood Park's 467 acres, crowned by a wooded hill rising steeply from the surrounding meadows, had been set aside for a state college. After years of negotiation, the land was finally acquired for a park by San Mateo County and the Midpeninsula Regional Open Space District in 1980. The county originally planned a golf course on the park's grasslands with trails on the periphery, but in 1994 changed plans and declared Edgewood a park and natural preserve.

Implementation of the park's 1996 master plan is under way: the Friends of Edgewood Natural Preserve lead hikes from March through mid-June; volunteers continue the work of eliminating exotic plants; all trails are in good shape and a new map shows all trails and contour lines; plans for an interpretive center are complete and the site chosen.

From the park's main entrance on Edgewood Road, more than 7 miles of trail lead through wooded, fern-filled canyons to the rolling grasslands that surround the central wooded ridge. Beyond the entrance near the trailhead are a day camp and an amphitheatre beside Cordilleras Creek. Close by are attractive picnic sites nestled on terraces under the shade of huge oaks and redwoods, open to the public except during summer day-camp. Other entrances also open onto trails that reach flower fields, the wooded hilltop, and the northern canyons of the park.

This is a park for all seasons. Its closeness to the hundreds of thousands who live in neighboring communities makes it a good choice for short outings. In winter, rain-washed air and north winds bring clear views and cold days for brisk hiking. In spring, the meadows underlain with serpentine are thick with goldfields, poppies, cream cups, lupines, and owl's clover. From March to June, volunteer members of the California Native Plant Society lead free weekend wildflower walks. On summer and fall days, shady oak groves provide good picnicking and inviting walks on the wooded northeast slopes.

Jurisdiction: San Mateo County: 650-363-4020

Facilities: Trails for hikers and equestrians; picnic areas with barbecues, restrooms, day camp, and amphitheatre

Rules: Open from 8 A.M. to sunset; no dogs or bicycles; horses on all trails but Sylvan Loop

Maps: San Mateo County *Edgewood Park* and USGS topo *Woodside*

How to Get There: From I-280: (1) Main entrance on Edgewood Rd. at Old Stage Day Camp—Take the Edgewood Rd. exit and go east 1 mile; turn right at Edgewood Park and Day Camp sign, cross bridge to

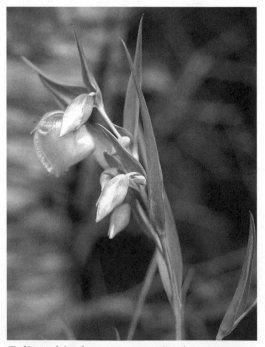

Delicate fairy lanterns are springtime treats

park. Overflow parking uses unpaved area beside Edgewood Rd. (2) West of I-280 on Edgewood Rd—Take Edgewood Rd. exit, go west under freeway. Park on south side of Edgewood Rd. near freeway or at Cañada and Edgewood roads. (3) Cañada Rd—Take Edgewood Rd. exit, go west under freeway, turn south on Cañada Rd., go through freeway underpass and park beside Cañada Rd. opposite PG&E switch-yard. The Clarkia Trail entrance is immediately north of this installation. (4) Sunset Way—Follow directions for (3) above, but continue on Cañada Rd. 1.2 more miles and turn left on Jefferson Ave. Turn left on California Way (not West California Way) and then right on Sunset Way to park entrance at Hillcrest Way. Limited parking beside road.

LOOP TRIP TO THE WOODED HILLTOP THAT CROWNS THIS PARK

Take this trip across the park's wooded ridge for views over the Santa Cruz Mountains and out to the Bay.

Distance: 5-mile loop

Time: 2½ hours

Elevation Change: 600' gain

Starting from the Old Stage Day Camp entrance, you enter the park across a narrow old bridge over Cordilleras Creek framed by spreading valley oaks. Just beyond the bridge, a rustic brown sign points to Old Stage Road, a section of a mid-1800s route to lumber mills and camps in Woodside. Ahead are the parking area and the trailheads for the Edgewood and Sylvan trails. Near this entrance too, will be the new interpretive center.

Start uphill on the Edgewood Trail to the right of the parking area on switchbacks that take you up the north side of a steep canyon. Shading your way are woods of buckeye, madrone, and oak, with an understory of toyon, snowberry, and poison oak.

Skirting a sloping meadow accented by immense spreading oaks, you continue uphill, crossing a service road to stay on the shady, tree-lined Edgewood Trail. At the next junction take the Franciscan Trail to your left. Now you traverse the steep canyon's rim and look across it to the southern San Francisco Bay and the East Bay hills. From a rocky outcrop beside the trail you can see into the canyon where once stood a Victorian house, part of the 1915 San Francisco Panama Pacific Exposition. It was disassembled and barged down to Redwood City, then reassembled on this site. Only the foundations of the house and vestiges of the garden walls remain today, artfully used to support terraced areas of the day-camp and picnic areas.

Continue around the hillside on the Franciscan Trail to its intersection with the Sylvan Trail. If you turn left here, you will return to the park entrance and make this a 1+ mile loop trip. But if you stay on the Franciscan Trail, you first cross a high grassy plateau, and then take the Serpentine Loop Trail left, pass another Sylvan Trail turnoff on the left. Hidden in the tall grasses are the homes of gophers, field

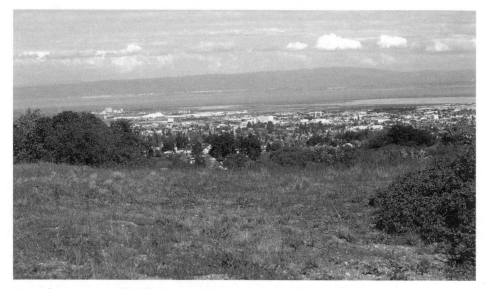

From the Serpentine Trail looking over Redwood City to the Bay

mice, and other rodents that make up the diet of the hawks you may see soaring overhead.

After the second Sylvan Trail junction, you round two bends, leave the Serpentine Trail, and turn right onto the Live Oak Trail. Under a canopy of live oaks and buckeyes you soon come to a fork in the trail. Take the right-hand fork and walk over the wooded crown of this hill and out into the chaparral. From a wide clearing, views stretch up and down along fifty miles of the San Andreas Rift Zone. Looking northwest you see a vista relatively unchanged from early times (disregarding the multi-laned concrete ribbon by which you reached this idyllic spot). In San Francisco Watershed lands you see thousands of acres of unbroken forests, from the Skyline ridge to the lakes along the fault line.

To continue on your trip, follow the Ridgeview Loop Trail around the hill, bearing left at two trail intersections. Then, contouring around the south side of the hill, you look down on the serpentine grasslands, aglow with dazzling wildflower displays in spring.

At a saddle on the ridge you complete the Ridgeview Loop. Walk left on the Live Oak Trail for another 500 feet and turn left onto the Serpentine Trail at the junction where you left it. Along this short stretch of trail look for clumps of the low-growing blue-eyed grass and drifts of clarkia that bloom from early spring into summer.

Almost 3 miles from the beginning of your trip, you come to the Sylvan Trail on your right. Take it for a different way back. Around wide switchbacks you descend deep into a canyon. A spring high up the headwall feeds a perennial stream, which you cross and then follow along its fern-covered banks.

Emerging from the canyon, you pass the other leg of the Sylvan Trail on your left. Go straight ahead and downhill for 0.2 mile. Then pass to the right of the Old Stage Day Camp or take the left-hand trail, which curves around the camp's picnic tables and barbecues on the landscaped borders of Cordilleras Creek. The park entrance is just beyond the day camp.

For a shorter route to the park's central ridge, take the Edgewood Trail from the parking area at Edgewood and Cañada roads on the west side of I-280. This trail runs through a corridor paralleling the south side of Edgewood Road. It goes around a fenced-off, large meadow, and leads to a passageway under the freeway. After going through the passage, continue to a kiosk that displays maps, photos and current news about the preserve and volunteer work opportunities. Turn left on the Serpentine Loop and in 200 feet turn right on the Franciscan Trail, which you follow to the Ridgeview Loop. Turn either left or right to circle the hilltop. This makes a 2.75-mile loop trip with an elevation gain of 430'.

SEE MAP
ON PAGE
75

A SUMMER SUPPER HIKE

Some warm summer evening, take the Edgewood Trail out to the grassy knolls northwest of the park's wooded hilltop.

Distance: 2 miles round trip

Time: 1 hour

Elevation Change: 400' gain

Starting from the Old Stage Day Camp entrance, you enter the park across a narrow wooden bridge over Cordilleras Creek framed by spreading valley oaks. Just beyond the bridge, a rustic brown sign points to Old Stage Road, a section of a mid-1800s route to lumber mills and camps in Woodside. Ahead are the parking area and the trailheads for the Edgewood and Sylvan trails. Near this entrance too, will be the new interpretive center.

Starting from the trailhead at the main park entrance, follow the Edgewood Trail and continue past the Franciscan Trail junction. Then, for the next 0.5 mile, there is little change of elevation as the trail contours around several steep-sided ravines.

When you get out into the grasslands, choose a trailside picnic spot with a view of the western hills. If your picnic supper is accompanied by a flutelike bird call, it may be the meadowlark's song filling the evening air. These once-common, pale-yellow birds with a black cravat are becoming rare as development continues to diminish their grasslands habitat.

Rare, too, except in some protected grasslands, are the lemon-yellow blossoms of mariposa lilies, which dot these meadows in early summer. Their centers blotched with magenta, these delicate, bowl-shaped flowers bloom in surprising profusion for flowers of such elegance.

The rosy glow of the summer sun setting over the Skyline ridge will remind you to allow time for the 1-mile hike back to your car in the lowering light.

SEE MAP ON PAGE 75

A SHADY CANYON HIKE

Measured and marked as an exercise loop, the Sylvan Trail Loop circles the canyon south of the day camp. In shade for most of the way, it is a favorite warm-day trip for hikers and runners.

Distance: 2-mile loop

Time: 1+ hours

Elevation Change: 500' gain

Starting from the Old Stage Day Camp entrance, you enter the park across a narrow old bridge over Cordilleras Creek framed by spreading valley oaks. Just beyond the bridge, a rustic brown sign points to Old Stage Road, a section of a mid-1800s route to lumber mills and camps in Woodside. Ahead are the parking area and the trailheads for the Edgewood and Sylvan trails. Near this entrance too, will be the new interpretive center.

This loop, closed to equestrians, starts by going straight ahead uphill from the parking area staying to the left of the greensward. In less than 0.2 mile you turn right on the Sylvan Trail and zigzag up the north side of the steep canyon. These switchbacks, at least eight of them, take you through shady woodland to the edge of a high meadow, where you meet the Serpentine Trail. Turn left on it, and weave in and out of the woods for 0.5 mile.

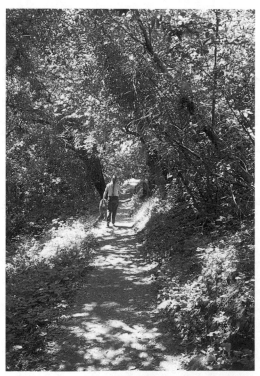

Now pick up the Sylvan Trail on your left and follow its wide switchbacks downhill. This trail at first descends an exposed, south-facing slope, but soon drops into deep woods. In spring, watch for some of the season's first flowers, the deep-red Indian warriors, blooming under patches of oaks. Watch too for the part of the Sylvan Trail that arcs far back into the canyon to a perennial stream crossing. If you linger for a moment here in the depths of this canyon on the urban fringe, the only sounds to break the stillness are those of flowing water and woodland birds.

Then, continuing on for a few minutes, you pass the other leg of the Sylvan Trail and go straight ahead to the park entrance.

Edgewood's shady Sylvan Trail

TRAILS TO THE SERPENTINE MEADOWS

For a spring wildflower pilgrimage take these short trails and glory in masses of colorful blossoms.

Distance: 0.5 mile to 3.5 miles round trip

Time: 1-2 hours, or linger as long as you can

Elevation Change: From 100' to 400' gain

After you have been on one of the Native Plant Society's guided walks, return on your own to test your memory of names and species. No matter if you've forgotten the names; the glorious displays in the grasslands will more than suffice for a little memory loss.

Both the Edgewood and the Clarkia trails lead to the park service road, one leg of the Serpentine Loop that crosses the main flower display. The quickest way to reach the flower fields is from the trail below the south side of Edgewood Road west of I-280. This trail leaves from the corner of Edgewood and Cañada roads and goes east, crosses under the freeway and joins the Serpentine Loop.

Take the fenced trail south to the passage under the freeway and thence to the service road, the Serpentine Loop, in a grassy swale. Walk east for the best wildflower displays. Around the outcroppings of serpentine you will see goldfields, tidy tips, cream cups, owl's clover, lupines, and many more annuals. Where there is more moisture, look for blue larkspur. Bring your flower guide.

These serpentine meadows produce lovely carpets of flowers each spring. They were home to the very rare checkerspot butterfly, although their numbers have decreased in recent years. The are found only here and on the extensions of this meadow west of the freeway, on San Bruno Mountain, on Jasper Ridge Biological Preserve, and on a private site in Santa Clara County. The presence of this butterfly, now on the federal list of threatened species, is marked on the accompanying map as protected area, the main habitat of the checkerspot.

If you have the time, walk along the length of the Serpentine Loop road and up on the Ridgeview Loop Trail, from where you can look down on the sea of color. In the shaded woodlands of this loop you will find different species, such as red Indian warriors, white milkmaids, and blue hound's-tongue.

If you enter from Cañada Road, the Clarkia Trail contours around a south-facing hillside past some large serpentine outcrops and through a scattering of oak trees to reach the east end of the service road, the Serpentine Loop. As its name implies, you will find a show of magenta clarkias here in early summer. This 0.75-mile trail, closed to horses in winter, circles the grasslands, and makes a good starting point for a trans-park trip.

Another entrance to the park's flower fields is from Sunset Way, but there is little parking there. For those with limited walking ability, this entrance offers a short route to an overlook of the colorful display.

◆ City Parks and Trails in the Foothills ◆

Many beautiful parks, large and small, dot the Peninsula landscape east of I-280. Nestled among residential neighborhoods, they provide a welcome green space, attractive children's play equipment and welcome meeting places within walking distance of many suburban dwellers. In previous editions of *Peninsula Trails* we described walks in several cities' parks. In this fourth edition of *Peninsula Trails* we again call attention to these pretty havens of open space ranging from 40 to 250 acres and remind our readers of their local interest.

A special feature of this fourth edition is a complete write-up of those city parks in the foothills that connect to county, regional, state, or federal parks. Belmont's Waterdog Lake Park and John S. Brooks Memorial Open Space is the only park that answers that criterion entirely. However, Laurelwood Park in San Mateo is planning new trails that link its Laurelwood Park to its spacious Sugarloaf Mountain and to the trails in Belmont. Big Canyon and Eaton parks in San Carlos connect by sidewalks through residential neighborhoods to Pulgas Ridge Open Space Preserve and thence to Edgewood Park. As San Mateo County and its cities plan for the future, it is quite possible that links will be created, thus forming a vast complex of public open space accessible to Bayside residents on foot, horse, or bicycle trails.

In the area covered in this guidebook, trails in four towns on the southern Peninsula—Portola Valley, Palo Alto, Los Altos Hills, and Cupertino—reach parks and preserves in the foothills or on the Skyline. Some are paved off-road trails paralleling roads and others are unpaved paths that wander through residential areas, but all pass pockets of woodland, grassy meadows, or small neighborhood open spaces.

Laurelwood Park and Sugarloaf Mountain

Pleasant paths through the 227-acre park surrounding Sugarloaf Mountain invite young and old to wander along the shaded canyon of Laurel Creek and climb its sunny hillsides.

Jurisdiction: City of San Mateo: 650-522-7400

Facilites: trails for hikers; picnic tables; children's play equipment; paved bicycle path

Rules: Open from sunrise to sunset, but occasionally closed for resource and fire protection

How to Get There: From I-280 take Hwy 92 east, exit east on De Anza Blvd. and go to Glendora Dr. Parking is on east side of Glendora Dr., where two paths enter the park.

The paved path from Glendora Drive enters the upper canyon in a sunny natural amphitheater shaded by several wide-spreading oaks. This main path continues to Laurelwood Drive under the giant bay trees that gave the creek its name. Another path, a foot trail, descends on steps from Glendora Drive and then

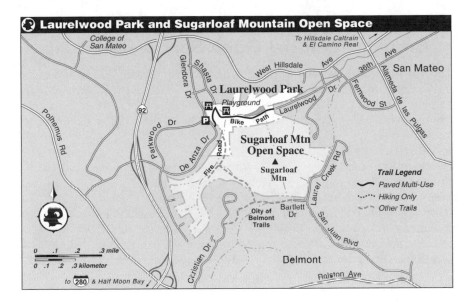

meanders through a handsome old grove of buckeye trees to reach the park's large turfed area on the south side of Laurel Creek.

The city of San Mateo acquired Sugarloaf Mountain in 1988 and retained it for passive open space. In June 2004, the city submitted a Master Plan for Sugarloaf Mountain, which proposes a trail that leaves the park's southwest corner and zigzags up the west side of the mountain to its summit. This trail will be accessible to the physically limited as well as to hikers and joggers. Another trail will traverse the mountain's east side after reaching the summit and then circle back to the trail entrance along the east and north sides of the mountain. These well-designed trails will supplant the various informal trails that entail scurrying through the poison oak and overhanging brush on poor gradients over unstable ground. An extension of one of these new trails will reach an existing trail in the city of Belmont on the mountain's east side. From this trail one could follow several of Belmont's trails leading to the Waterdog Lake Trail and the Sheep Camp Trail, and the Cross Country Running Course in the San Francisco Watershed.

Presently, a wide, unsurfaced, informal trail leaves the southwest corner of the park to follow Laurel Creek west and uphill for approximately 0.75 mile. It is open to hikers and bicyclists.

Waterdog Lake Park and Trail/John S. Brooks Memorial Open Space—Belmont

The trail through Belmont's wooded Diablo Canyon passes Waterdog Lake and comes out on the crest of the hill at the eastern boundary of the Watershed, where panoramic views of Crystal Springs Lakes and the Santa Cruz Mountains spread out before you. Here it joins a trail that leads to San Mateo County's long north-south trail.

Jurisdiction: City of Belmont
Facilities: Trail for hikers, joggers; lake for fishing and picnicking
Rules: Open dawn to dusk; no swimming; no boating
Maps: City of Belmont *Jogging Trails* and USGS topo *San Mateo*
How to Get There: From I-280 take Hwy 92 east and turn on Ralston Ave. to (1) East entrance: turn south on Lyall Way. Look for gate and sign just beyond Lake Rd. intersection. (2) West entrance: turn south on Hallmark Dr., go west on Benson Way, and then south on St. James Rd. Find trail entrance across street from gate to Watershed, just past Rinconada Circle.

Distance: 3 miles round trip
Time: 1½ hours
Elevation Change: 300′ gain

Enter the Waterdog Lake Trail through a narrow opening in a chain-link fence on the south side of Lyall Way at Lake Road. This trail was the old road over the

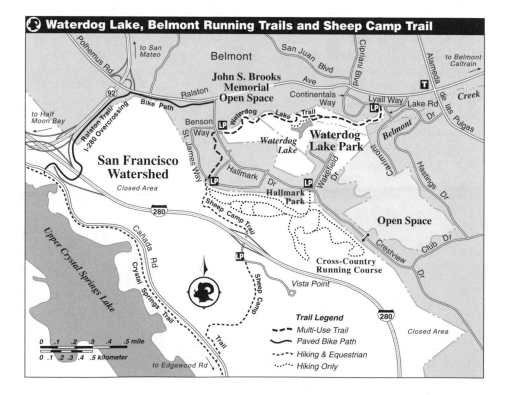

hill to Laguna de Raimundo, now beneath the waters of Crystal Springs Lakes. In 1969 San Mateo County, using federal funds, rebuilt the road as an urban trail. Now, under the jurisdiction of the City of Belmont, the trail traverses the north side of Belmont's Waterdog Lake Park and John S. Brooks Memorial Open Space.

At first the trail winds up a hill past apartments; then, under a canopy of oaks you are in Cañada del Diablo, which the Spanish unaccountably called this woodsy place. A walk of about 0.5 mile brings you to Waterdog Lake, a little reservoir that in earlier days was the water supply for Belmont, now a good stopping place for a rest or a picnic.

From the dam at the end of the lake, the road climbs gently for another 0.5 mile along the north side of the John S. Brooks Memorial Open Space, with views across the wooded canyon, now rimmed with houses and extending into the canyon. In spring, a roadside garden of blue lupine, yellow California poppies, scarlet Indian paintbrush, and purple brodiaea graces your way.

When you emerge from the canyon at Hallmark Drive, cross the street to a gated easement, a steeper 0.5-mile stretch through oaks and behind backyards, to the highest point of the trail at St. James Road. Just across the street is a gate to the grassy slopes of the San Francisco Watershed.

Here you have several choices of other walks. You can follow the graveled service road to the left along the upper boundary of the Watershed. Or the Cross Country Running Course to the southeast may tempt you to stretch your legs. A third choice takes you south for a 1-mile walk on the broad Sheep Camp Trail to join the Crystal Springs Trail beside Cañada Road.

Big Canyon and Eaton Parks—San Carlos

Trails in two city parks—Big Canyon and Eaton parks—climb to high vantage points and descend to meet at Brittan Avenue

How to Get There: From I-280 take Edgewood Road east, turn left (north) on Crestview Drive and then go right (east) on Brittan Ave. After 0.2 mile find the trail entrances on either side of the street. Or, From El Camino Real in San Carlos go west on Brittan Ave. for 2 miles. There is on-street parking.

Big Canyon Park is marked by a prominent, wooden sign. Across the street the City of San Carlos sign on a tall post marks the entrance to Eaton Park.

BIG CANYON PARK

This little gem of open space is actually a small canyon of 28 acres with steep, narrow sides. One side is so shaded and cool that it supports a surprising variety of ferns, while the other side is a bright, sunny sagebrush slope. You enter the park from the north side of Brittan Avenue and climb a winding trail along its shady side to its upper reaches. Several creeks tumble down the hillside, nourishing dense collections of native plants—buckeye, live oaks, ocean spray, brodiaea, and many other spring wildflowers. At the highest point of the trip there is a bench placed to view San Carlos, Redwood City, and, farther south, the dark slopes of Black Mountain and Loma Prieta.

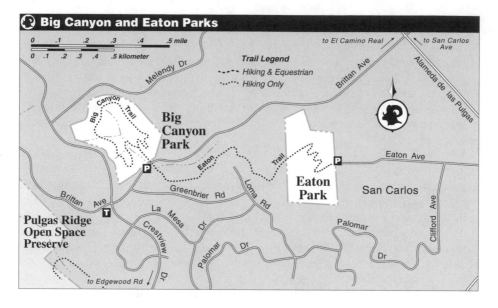

EATON PARK

Across from Big Canyon Park on the south side of Brittan Avenue are sturdy railroad-tie steps that lead up to a narrow, mile-long trail built by Sierra Club volunteers. This delightful, well–laid-out trail meanders along a north-facing hillside under live oak and bay trees, crosses several creek canyons, and traverses occasional grasslands en route to Eaton Park. When numerous spring wildflowers are in bloom and ferns grace the shady hillsides, this is a delightful, 2-mile round trip from Brittan Avenue. Even on warm summer days, the shady trail is pleasant to travel.

✦ Mountainside Parks and Preserves ✦ on the Central Peninsula

Forests cover most of the steep slopes on both sides of the Santa Cruz Mountains' crest. Those on the east slopes in the watersheds and in Huddart, Phleger, and Wunderlich parks are familiar to Baysiders as a backdrop of their communities.

Today, Peninsula residents visit and appreciate the many parks and preserves on the west slopes of the Santa Cruz Mountains encompassing the 9100 acres open to the public—Burleigh Murray Ranch State Park, Purisima Creek Redwoods, El Corte de Madera, and La Honda Creek open space preserves. They enjoy the spectacular views of the Coastside and the ocean from high ridges in these preserves.

Two centuries ago, majestic redwood forests extended from the Peninsula's valley floor over the ridge of the Santa Cruz Mountains and down the west slopes. In the forests on the east slopes, known to the Spanish as Pulgas Redwoods, Spanish soldiers, with the help of Indians, felled trees and dragged them by oxen to build missions in San Francisco and Santa Clara.

In 1840 the Mexican Governor of California, Luis Alvarado, granted to his friend John Coppinger the 12,545-acre Rancho Cañada de Raimundo, which included most of the Pulgas Redwoods, extending from the Woodside valley floor to the Skyline. During the decade in which Gold Rush San Francisco was built, the great trees were cut, and the lumber hauled down to the Embarcadero in Redwood City and sailed by schooner up the Bay to San Francisco.

By 1870 hardly a redwood tree remained uncut in the Pulgas Redwoods. Logging began then in the primeval forests along the Skyline and down the steep west slopes, and continued into this century until the old forests were almost completely cut over. In the years since, second-growth trees have been cut sporadically.

However, in the 1980s the Midpeninsula Regional Open Space District acquired much of these upper slopes west of the Skyline as preserves. The State of California purchased historic farmlands—the Burleigh Murray Ranch and lands extending to the Skyline ridge. Logging ceased in Purisima Creek Redwoods, El Corte de Madera, and La Honda Creek open space preserves. In 1995 the Peninsula Open Space Trust secured 1232 acres of the former Phleger Estate and this beautiful forest is now in the Golden Gate National Recreation Area.

In these preserves and parklands, extensive trail systems are in place on old logging and farm roads. Trails in canyons, along creeks, and over the ridges are now open to hikers, equestrians, and bicyclists.

Important trail links join these western parklands to the parks and trail systems on the east slopes that reach down to cities on the Bayside. A long-distance ridge trail extending north and south along the Skyline is part of the Bay Area Ridge Trail initiated in 1987. In the central section of San Mateo County, 12 miles of this trail system are already in place, many more are complete in the north and south sections of the county and a trail corridor has been designated to complete the gaps in the Ridge Trail through the county.

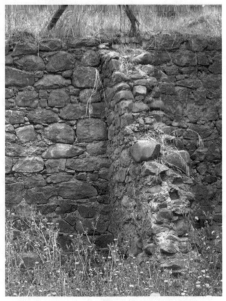

Future trail connections from Purisima Creek Redwoods and La Honda Creek open space preserves to Burleigh Murray Ranch State Park and thence to the coast may make it possible some day to walk from the Bay over the Santa Cruz Mountains to the ocean.

A historic stone wall in Burleigh Murray

Burleigh Murray Ranch State Park

A historic ranch tucked away in a valley south of Half Moon Bay now belongs to the California State Park system. In the 1860s this was a working ranch, growing hay and grazing cattle. Mills Creek, named for Robert P. Mills, the first owner of the ranch, flows through the narrow valley. An arched stone bridge crosses this creek to an old barn and a bunkhouse remaining from the ranching days. The State of California received the donated property in 1983 and later added a parcel known as Rancho Raymundo extending east to Skyline Boulevard. The ranch is named for one of the last of many owners of the property, Burleigh Hall Murray.

The state is preserving the 1121-acre park for its historical interest, with an emphasis on interpreting early San Mateo County ranch life. The historic buildings, unparalleled on the north San Mateo County coast, will be restored; they made roof repairs and preserved the stone walls and arched stone bridge. The farm lands are returning to their natural state and protecting the sensitive riparian habitat is a priority.

The state collected all historic artifacts, and catalogued and stored them. Besides historic preservation, the major use of the park is for hiking, bicycling, and horseback riding. An old farm road runs from the entrance on Higgins Purisima Road about 2 miles northeast, roughly following Mills Creek. This perennial steelhead stream rises near the Skyline ridge and flows through the heart of the park. The state is re-evaluating the trail system as it relates to the ranch's history.

Jurisdiction: State of California, Department of Parks and Recreation: 650-726-8819

Facilities: Trails for hikers, equestrians, and bicyclists; a picnic table is situated under the eucalyptus trees approximately 0.75 mile from the park entrance; portable restrooms are at the parking area and above the creek crossing

Rules: Open 8 A.M. to sunset; no dogs

Maps: USGS topos *Half Moon Bay* and *Woodside*

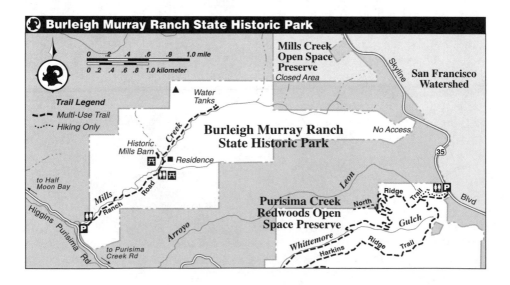

How to Get There: From Hwy 1/92 intersection go south on Hwy 1 for 1.2 miles to Higgins Purisima Rd. Turn left (east) and go 1.7 miles to park entrance on left. Park in graveled area just inside gate.

EXPLORE THE HISTORIC RANCH

Follow an old ranch road into a secluded coastal valley where a historic barn and bridge remain from early San Mateo County ranching days.

Distance: 2 miles round trip to barn; 4 miles round trip to water tanks

Time: 1 hour round trip to barn; 2 hours round trip to water tanks

Elevation Change: 680' gain

Leave the park entrance at the mouth of the valley on the farm road now used as a trail. As you near alder-bordered Mills Creek in the stillness of this secluded valley, you can hear the sounds of the stream accompanied by the songs of birds. This perennial steelhead stream rises near the Skyline ridge and flows through the heart of the park. Former orchards and farm fields border the trail and rounded hills rise on both sides of the canyon.

Upstream, where the valley narrows, you cross two bridges at a bend in the creek. Beyond, in a semicircular meadow between the creek and the trail, you find wildflowers blooming profusely in spring. On shady, north-facing road banks, wild currant bushes blossom in winter.

One mile from the park entrance a small tributary enters the creek from the east and the trail veers left, following the creek into a broad flat near the old ranch headquarters. Past a 1930s bungalow that serves as a park residence, you cross a bridge from which you can note the original rock work lining the curve in the creek banks. Downstream is an arched stone bridge built with Italian masonry techniques dating back to the Romans. This bridge is often overgrown, but in late spring the area is usually cleared and the bridge is quite visible. On the far side of the creek is a great wooden barn dating from the 1890s, built to house 100 cows. Its roof no longer sags and its locked doors work. The state plans call for more restoration as funds become available. Another fine stone wall holds the bank beyond the barn.

Continuing on the road beyond the barn and its corrals, you pass a small wooden bunkhouse by the creek. In a tangle of blackberry bushes stand pumps, outbuildings, cattle chutes, and gates, all no longer used.

The trail continues up the narrowing valley between steep, chaparral-covered hills to the east and high, old farm fields to the west. Then, about a mile above the barn, the old road used as a trail ends at the water tanks. In the future, however, trail volunteers hope to clear this trail up the steep ridge to the next creek crossing. Someday a trail may join other parks and preserves in this beautiful area.

Heading back down the valley, you see the creek, rounded hills, and valleys from a different perspective.

At the picnic tables under the trees you can stop for lunch in the shade, then perhaps visit one of the state beaches nearby.

Visitors to this park should be aware that there is a shooting range near the park residence, reserved for police and sheriffs' practice.

Purisima Creek Redwoods Open Space Preserve

This MROSD preserve is a 3117-acre treasure of redwood forests, clear-flowing streams, steep-sided canyons and long ridges. Its size and its rugged terrain make it a place to find both quiet seclusion and long trails for strenuous hiking trips. This northernmost redwood forest in San Mateo County is just minutes from the urban San Francisco Peninsula.

The preserve extends westward for 3 miles from the 2000-foot-high crest of the Santa Cruz Mountains. East across Skyline Boulevard are the San Francisco Watershed lands, Huddart Park, and the Phleger Estate. From the Skyline crest, three ridges divide the preserve into two main canyons trending west. Between Harkins and Tunitas ridges flows Purisima Creek, the centerpiece of the preserve.

Purisima Creek, a beautiful, year-round stream fed by many tributaries, rises along the Skyline ridge and flows west for 3 miles through the preserve. In the lower end of the preserve, large second-growth redwoods line its banks and side slopes. Leaving the preserve, Purisima Creek runs through rolling grasslands and the 2200-acre Cowell Ranch to reach the ocean in a waterfall over sandstone cliffs. The ranch, purchased in 1987 by the Peninsula Open Space Trust, included some bluffs and a beach which are now the Cowell Ranch State Beach.

Between Harkins Ridge and the next ridge north is Whittemore Gulch, where an intermittent creek flows through a lovely wooded canyon to join Purisima Creek at the preserve's west entrance.

In the 1860s, when redwoods were first cut here, the logs proved too large to drag up the steep canyons. Although the west end of the canyon was open, there was little need for lumber on the Coastside and no port from which to ship it to San Francisco. Therefore, the trees were cut for shingles, which pack animals could haul out of the gulches over steep, winding trails. As many as eight shingle mills operated here during the late 1800s.

Logging was back-breaking, dangerous work, but some ingenious techniques were developed to hoist the heavy logs out of the canyon. One such device used a cable to operate a tramway rising one thousand feet from the creek to the ridgetop.

Lumbering ventures came and went in the narrow, steep canyon of the Purisima. Last logged in the 1970s, now stands of second-growth redwoods fill most of the canyon.

Since 1982 when MROSD bought 849 acres in Whittemore Gulch, land purchases aided by the Save-the-Redwoods League and gifts of land, the preserve has grown to 3117 acres. These acres include the headwaters of Purisima Creek, substantial acreage south and west of Bald Knob, and a few primeval redwoods. One redwood is said to be 1200 years old. Purisima also harbors one of a few remaining critical habitats of the marbled murrelet, a seagoing bird now on the list of threatened species, which nests in old-growth trees.

Some of the most challenging hikes on the Peninsula are trips down Purisima's canyons and up its ridges. The old county road, now the Purisima Creek Trail, descends from Skyline Boulevard to follow the creek to the lower end of the canyon. New trails and old logging roads form a 21-mile trail network.

Several narrow trails are exclusively for hikers, others on logging roads are also open to equestrians and bicyclists. The 0.25-mile Redwood Trail for the physically limited, funded by POST, meanders through tall redwoods along the Skyline ridge. From several turnouts for picnic tables one can look out toward the coast.

A short walk on an easy grade from the preserve's west entrance on Higgins Purisima Road reaches groves of the largest redwoods beside Purisima Creek. Starting long loop hikes from this entrance gives you the advantage of gaining altitude while you and the day are both still fresh.

Trails in Purisima Creek Redwoods link with adjoining Huddart Park and Phleger Estate trails, making it possible to walk from Bayside cities over the Santa Cruz Mountains to the west end of the preserve, only a few miles from the ocean— a "city-to-sea" trail. With advance reservations, backpacking groups can camp in Huddart Park.

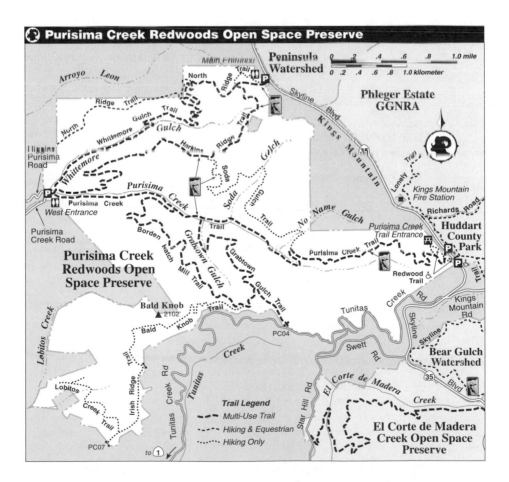

Be weather-wise when visiting Purisima Creek Redwoods Preserve. Because it is several miles back from the ocean, the preserve often has sun when fog hangs on the coast. However, on the days when fog sweeps in from the sea to reach the redwoods along the Skyline, condensed moisture falls from the tree branches like rain.

Jurisdiction: Midpeninsula Regional Open Space District: 650-691-1200

Facilities: Trails for hikers, equestrians, and bicyclists; one trail for the physically limited; picnic tables, restroom and special parking; equestrian parking

Rules: Open dawn to dusk; no bicycles on Soda Gulch or North Ridge foot trail; no dogs

Map: MROSD brochure *Purisima Creek Redwoods O.S.P,* USGS topo *Woodside*

How to Get There: There are four entrances: (1) Main entrance is on Skyline Blvd. 4.5 miles south of Hwy 92; (2) Purisima Creek Trail entrance is 2.0 miles farther south; (3) Redwood Trail entrance and wheelchair parking are 0.2 mile south of Purisima Creek Trail entrance; (4) West entrance is off Higgins Purisima Rd., reached from Hwy 1 just 1.2 mile south of its intersection with Hwy 92 in Half Moon Bay.

PURISIMA CREEK TRAIL

Follow the old 19th century Purisima Creek Road down a deep canyon beside Purisima Creek to the preserve's west entrance. Today's travelers can enjoy tall trees, beautiful flowers and the sight and sound of a year-round stream.

Distance: 8.2 miles round trip

Time: 4½ hours

Elevation Change: 1600' loss

Downhill all the way makes for a relatively easy trip if you arrange a shuttle at the west entrance. Hardy hikers can combine the first leg with the Soda Gulch and Harkins Ridge trails to make a 10-mile loop trip.

Starting from the southern Skyline Boulevard entrance (2) opposite Huddart Park, go over the hiker's stile and down the wide trail through a redwood and fir forest. Note to the left of the stile the wheelchair gate to the specially surfaced Redwood Trail. Before long, you come to switchbacks, where logging operations cleared the trees to make level platforms or landings. Wild lilacs, spring-flowering in shades of blue and purple, and young tan oak trees are thriving in this clearing. The climax trees, Douglas fir and redwood, will eventually shade out these hardy early plants.

After about a mile down the trail you begin to hear Purisima Creek, and before long you see it through the trees. Soon you are walking close to it. At a sharp turn in the trail, the Soda Gulch Trail, for hikers only, takes off to the right up a heavily wooded canyon to join the Harkins Ridge Trail. Continuing on the Purisima Trail you cross the ever-widening creek at the next turn, where fern fronds and horsetails edge clear pools.

Around the next bend on the south side is the site of a mile-long cable tramway that in the 1870s lifted logs from Purdy Pharis' shingle mill out of the canyon to a location near present-day Kings Mountain School. This ingenious device, a forerunner of modern cable-logging, had a short existence, but its location appeared on maps for many years.

From here to the west entrance the old road is close to the creek, which stair–steps down the canyon over rocks and under bridges of fallen logs. Some logs, still rooted, are sprouting new shoots. A heavy-timbered bridge used to cross the creek to a trail leading to Grabtown, an old logging settlement on top of Tunitas Ridge. (The bridge is slated for replacement in 2004.) Where the canyon widens, two shingle mills operated by Borden and Hartley in the early 1900s were some of

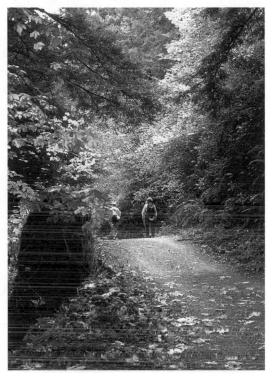

Bigleaf maples glow in Purisima Creek Redwoods

the last in the canyon. This is an open, sunny place to stop for lunch and to speculate on the rugged life of those loggers, who had to deal with floods, fires, and accidents.

The remaining 1.3 miles of your trip are less steep and more heavily wooded. Small streams trickle down the canyon sides, and flowers bloom at every season, from the deep red trillium of early spring to the lavender asters of fall. Soon your way is completely enclosed by forest. Some immense redwoods remain near the creek at the lower end of the preserve. On the north side is a grove of memorial trees, dedicated by a contributor to the Save-the-Redwoods League, which helped purchase this beautiful preserve.

Now you are near the preserve's west entrance. Before starting your return trip to Skyline Boulevard, find a log to sit on beside the creek to enjoy its clear waters and the light filtering through the redwood trees. If you have a car shuttle waiting, continue to gate PC02. The west entrance is a popular and convenient way to the Santa Cruz Mountains for Coastside residents, and with its ample parking, can be the starting point for the first three trips in this section in reverse. If you are doing the loop trip, cross the creek and start up the Harkins Ridge Trail.

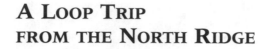

A LOOP TRIP
FROM THE NORTH RIDGE

This vigorous trip from the north ridgetop to the west entrance descends to Purisima Creek on the North Ridge and Harkins Ridge trails and returns on the Whittemore Gulch Trail.

Distance: 6.9-mile loop

Time: 4+ hours

Elevation Change: 1630' loss and subsequent gain

Alternate routes of the North Ridge Trail leave the north Skyline Boulevard parking area: (1) hikers watch for the foot-trail turnoff about 100 feet from the entrance on the right, which bypasses the steep grade of the service road; (2) bicyclists and equestrians use the North Ridge service road for this 0.3-mile stretch to reach the Harkins Ridge Trail junction. The foot-trail zigzags 0.5 mile down the mountainside just below the ridgetop under Douglas firs, wide-spreading tan oaks, madrones, and a scattering of live oaks. If the day is clear, the views west present a sweep of the San Mateo coast from Half Moon Bay north and south.

When the hikers-only trail intersects the service road, all users go south on the Harkins Ridge Trail. On a bench created by long-ago landslides, this path traverses the hillside above a steep canyon filled with clumps of sizable redwood trees and a thick stand of Douglas firs. Abundant flowers brighten the trailside—iris in spring, lavender asters, a purple mint, and apricot-colored sticky monkey flower in late summer.

After a 0.6-mile contour around the canyon headwall, the route turns right on an old fire road down the spine of Harkins Ridge and descends more than 1300 feet in 2.1 miles. The ridge is predominantly chaparral-covered, although some tan oaks and bay laurels grow on the steep mountainside. Small stands of firs and redwoods on the north side of Harkins Ridge give late afternoon shade. From here you look north down into Whittemore Gulch, the route of your climb back to the Skyline ridge.

In 0.3 mile down Harkins Ridge, the Soda Gulch Trail (for hikers only) takes off south to meet the Purisima Creek Trail in the canyon below. However, you continue your descent on the Harkins Ridge Trail, passing knolls densely covered with ceanothus, which forms a showy blue cloud in spring.

After the trail arcs left off the open ridge, it makes four switchbacks into the cool shade of the Purisima Creek redwoods, and then follows the creek downstream for about 0.5 mile. Just a few steps before the bridge to the south side of the creek, you find the Whittemore Gulch Trail junction on the right. About 300 feet beyond the bridge is the preserve gate at Higgins Purisima Road. You could leave a car here and avoid the hike back up the mountain, or you could start the hike here and do the steep climb first. In any case, first step down to the creek to see its pools and cascades at close range.

The Whittemore Gulch Trail offers a 3.5-mile (3.8 on hikers-only route) return to the Skyline ridge. This trail's soils are heavily eroded, and it is closed in wet weather to bicyclists and equestrians, who should return on the Harkins Ridge Trail. In the lower gulch, redwoods deemed too small or irregular to cut in the logging days are now grown to handsome large trees. Alders and big-leaf maples fill openings among the redwoods and firs, and the canyon walls are lush with ferns. After crossing the creek, the trail passes close to the shell of a redwood tree, which was at least 15 feet in diameter. There are venerable Douglas firs too. One old giant has sent out a branch that rises vertically after its first horizontal 8 feet, becoming an immense tree itself.

After about 2 miles, this well-designed trail leaves the canyon depths and zigzags more than a mile up the mountainside, crossing a thickly covered chaparral slope. Poison oak dominates the hillside, its fall colors brilliant reds and oranges. The southern exposure here is welcome on a winter's day, but can be hot in summer.

When you reach the old jeep road, the North Ridge Trail, turn right and follow it for 0.5 mile. Then watch for the trail junction where hikers turn left into the forest on the 0.5-mile foot trail on which they started their trip. Bicyclists and equestrians continue 0.3 mile uphill on the North Ridge service road.

GRABTOWN GULCH LOOP

Explore the southern ridgetops of the preserve where a colony of timber cutters once lived.

Distance: 7.4-mile loop

Time: 3 hours

Elevation Change: 1200' gain

Grabtown Gulch takes its name from the settlement that sprang up on a small flat off of Tunitas Creek Road. It was the first level spot that logging wagons reached on their three- or four-day trip to the embarcadero at Redwood City. According to legend, a boy named it Grabtown because settlers grabbed whatever lodging or garden space became available.

Begin this trip on the Purisima Creek Trail at the parking area on Higgins Purisima Road. Go uphill on the Purisima Creek Trail for 1 mile to the Borden Hatch Mill Trail (or, to take the loop trip in the opposite direction, continue down the canyon 0.3 mile to a trail on the right that climbs south on the ridge west of Grabtown Gulch). The Borden Hatch Mill Trail gains 1200+ feet of elevation as it snakes 2.5 miles up the north-facing side of the mountain below Bald Knob. You cross a tributary of Grabtown Gulch, sometimes quite damp in winter, rising ever upward. In spring, trillium and occasional globe lilies bloom, and in fall, tall creek maple leaves turn golden, enlivening this deep green forest trail. Pass the abrupt, sharp right turn onto the Bald Knob Trail and continue northeast for 0.2 mile to the Grabtown Gulch Trail and follow it west along the southern border of the preserve.

You come to a junction in a large opening in the forest which had been a landing for logging operations. At this clearing, trails take off left and right. To the right is a little rise along the flank of the ridge (possibly the Grabtown site). You take the left-hand trail, the 1.4-mile Grabtown Gulch Trail, which descends through Douglas firs and young redwoods that are surely overtaking the tan oaks and madrones that sprang up after previous logging. At this stage of re-growth, there is still some space and light between trees for ceanothus, wild roses, toyon, and honeysuckle. From openings in the trees it may be possible to look out to the ocean—though it can be shrouded with fog.

Your trail continues downhill, cuts east across the ridge and then reverses direction to descend a very steep slope into Grabtown Gulch. You follow a path lined with ferns and ocean spray, where the creek is well below the trail. Continuing on the creek's shady east side, you can find 3-foot-tall orange tiger lilies in midsummer.

Shortly, Grabtown Gulch Creek enters Purisima Creek, which you cross on a recently reconstructed old logging bridge. You have reached the widest part of Purisima Canyon. Of the shingle mills that flourished here, no vestiges remain to be seen, but you can sit on the bridge to watch the water and listen to the birds at the confluence of these creeks.

To complete this loop, turn left on the Purisima Creek Trail, go 0.3 mile downhill, pass the Borden Hatch Mill Trail you climbed to the southern ridgetop and head for the gate at Higgins Purisima Road, one mile farther downhill.

SEE MAP
ON PAGE
91

BALD KNOB
AND IRISH RIDGE EXPLORATION

Discover the heights and depths of the preserve's southwestern corner on a long day's hike.

Distance: 14.4 miles

Time: 8 or 9 hours

Elevation Change: 1600' gain to Bald Knob, 800' loss to Lobitos Creek Trail

Take plenty of water and some extra food and snacks and get an early start. Then start this trip from the lower Purisima Creek trailhead, gate PC03 and follow the directions in the Grabtown Gulch Loop trip to the Borden Hatch Mill Trail, continue uphill and turn sharp right onto the hikers-only Bald Knob Trail. On this sometimes-narrow trail that hugs the steep hillside, you wind through tan oaks and young, second-growth redwoods. Soon the summit of Bald Knob is visible through the trees. As the trail switchbacks around the south side of Bald Knob, redwoods give way to firs, some of giant proportions amid several huge stumps.

After about a mile, you walk through a dense grove of chinquapins searching for light in a tall fir forest and emerge onto grassy slopes dotted with young trees. Here is one of the most glorious vistas on the Coast. You are at the steep upper end of Irish Ridge, which divides Tunitas Creek from Lobitos Creek. The view to the south and west encompasses the west side of the Santa Cruz Mountains sloping down to miles of surf breaking on the shore, with the Pacific Ocean spreading out to Hawaii and beyond. You have just traversed the south side of Bald Knob, which is private, but not bald. A dense grove of young firs is flourishing on its summit.

After 1.3 miles on the Bald Knob Trail you turn sharply south and follow the rough, gravel track down Irish Ridge. Continue on this old patrol road with splendid views to the south. Shortly before you reach the preserve boundary, look for the somewhat overgrown Lobitos Creek Trail, which winds along the lower edges of the preserve. It crosses a tributary of Lobitos Creek but winds in and out of the woods and eventually stops at the western preserve boundary. As yet there is neither connection west nor trail that loops up the west side of this southwest addition to Purisima Creek Redwoods, so you need to retrace your steps up the mountain.

As you climb along Irish Ridge toward Bald Knob, look downslope (south) to an open, brushy area to see the rooftops of private homes in the Kings Grove community. At the junction with the Borden Hatch Mill Trail, you retrace your steps downhill, grateful for the relief from the arduous climb to the east flank of Bald Knob.

SEE MAP
ON PAGE
91

THE BAY AREA RIDGE TRAIL

Sample all the preserve's habitats on four different trails.

Distance: 5.6 miles—hikers; 7.7 miles—bicyclists and equestrians

Time: 3½ hours

Elevation Change: 1000' loss—hikers; 1400' loss—bicyclists and equestrians

This route is one segment of the already 267 completed miles of the Bay Area Ridge Trail. Starting from the preserve's southeast entrance on the Purisima Creek Trail, as described in the first trip in this section, head downhill through a mixed forest of fir, redwood and tan oak trees. Descending steadily for 1.6 miles to the junction of the Soda Gulch Trail, hikers turn off on this narrow trail and bicyclists and equestrians continue on the Purisima Creek Trail to the Harkins Ridge Trail junction and ascend on it to the ridgetop (see the Purisima Creek Trail).

Although this hillside was logged sporadically into the 20th century, the redwood forest has regrown beautifully. A few trees of majestic size, scarred by fires of long ago, remain along the route, reminding one that this species has incredible vitality.

On the Soda Gulch Trail you wind back into No Name Gulch and other little canyons where bridges cross small creeks that can become rushing torrents in winter. Springtime brings wildflowers with delightful splashes of color to brighten the trail—especially the clusters of rosy-red blossoms of Clintonia and the tall, delicate flowers of crimson columbine.

You then traverse a south-facing slope, drier and warmer, before returning to the cool shade of a deep redwood forest in Soda Gulch. Here are some of the largest redwoods on your trip, lovely circles or fairy rings of second-growth trees

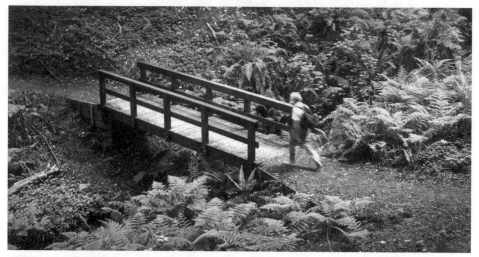

No Name Gulch Bridge, one of many on the Soda Gulch Trail

surrounding a space where an ancient tree once stood. After hiking deep into the upper reaches of Soda Gulch Creek, you cross a fine, sturdy bridge, and head west to emerge in chaparral. Climbing a bit, you bend north and reach the Harkins Ridge Trail, on which you join the equestrians and bicyclists going right uphill (northeast).

From here you are following the route described in A Loop Trip from the North Ridge in reverse. After a steady 0.9-mile ascent on the Harkins Ridge Trail, hikers cross the service road to take the 0.5-mile foot trail segment of the North Ridge Trail, while equestrians and bicyclists bear right (east) to follow the unpaved North Ridge service road 0.3 mile uphill to the north preserve entrance.

You could have a shuttle car waiting here or return over the same route to make a long day's trip. From here to Milagra Ridge there is only one gap in the Bay Area Ridge Trail—a 4-mile stretch to the Highway 92 junction with Skyline Boulevard. Beyond Highway 92, the 9.5-mile route through the San Francisco Watershed is open three days a week for docent-led trips for bicyclists, equestrians, and hikers. Check the Watershed's website and the trail description earlier in this guidebook.

Phleger Estate

These 1232 acres of redwood and oak/madrone forest lie on the east side of the Skyline ridge immediately north of San Mateo County's Huddart Park. Situated at the southern end of the San Francisco Watershed, over which the Golden Gate National Recreation Area has a scenic easement, this newest addition to the GGNRA becomes a vital link in a 56-mile-long, 40-mile wide tapestry of permanent open space from San Francisco south to San Jose. Trails for hikers and equestrians ascend through the forest from Huddart Park to the Skyline ridge, gaining 1400 feet in elevation en route.

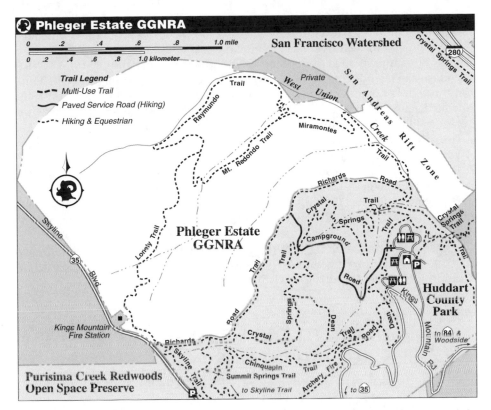

Once the domain of Herman and Mary Elena Phleger, who bought most of the land from George Eastman in 1935 and the balance in 1946, this property has changed little since that time. Redwood forests cut during the building and rebuilding of San Francisco after the Gold Rush are now achieving considerable girth and height. West Union Creek and its tributaries flow clear and clean and woodland spring wildflowers adorn the forest floor.

The Ohlones camped near here, hunting game and fishing the waters of West Union Creek, leaving little impact upon the land. Loggers established camps and built the town of Union Creek nearby. They cut the giant trees, skidded them down U-shaped ditches known as skid roads to mills downstream, and then hauled the lumber by oxen to Redwood City to be barged to San Francisco.

In 1927 when George Eastman built his home, designed by San Francisco architect Gardner Dailey, this area of the Peninsula was sparsely inhabited. But as the Peninsula population grew, the Phleger lands became prize development property. With 1990 zoning there could have been 550 homes, each built on a 2.5-acre parcel. From the earliest days of its founding, the private, nonprofit Peninsula Open Space Trust had hoped to keep this key piece of land in open space.

After the death of Mrs. Phleger in 1990, POST met with her trustees to work out terms of a purchase. POST agreed to raise $14.5 million by August 1991, and to meet the total purchase price of $25 million by December 1994. A member of the POST Advisory Council, Gordon Moore, purchased the Phleger home and 24.5

surrounding acres, subject to a conservation easement restricting building, subdivision and commercial development. The Save-the-Redwoods League contributed $2.5 million and the Midpeninsula Regional Open Space District gave $6 million. Private donations made up another $3 million. After expanding the GGNRA boundaries to include this parcel, Congress appropriated the remaining $10.5 million through Land and Water Conservation Funds and by December of 1994, the Phleger Estate addition to the National Park Service was completed. It was the largest public-private acquisition in national-park history.

Jurisdiction: Golden Gate National Recreation Area: 415-561-4700; 415-239-2366

Facilities: Trails for hikers and equestrians

Rules: Open 8 A.M. to sunset; fee for parking at Huddart Park; no dogs, pets, fires, camping, vehicles, or bicycles

How to Get There: (1) Huddart Park entrance—From I-280 take Woodside Rd. (Hwy 84) west 1.5 miles to Kings Mountain Rd., turn right, and go 1.5 miles to Huddart Park entrance on right side of road. (2) From Skyline Boulevard—take Kings Mountain road as in (1), turn right on Skyline Boulevard and go to Purisima Creek Redwoods parking on east side of road. Cross to northwest corner of Huddart Park, enter through gate H15, turn left (north).

CLIMB TO THE CREST OF THE SANTA CRUZ MOUNTAINS

SEE MAP ON PAGE 99

Make a circuit of the forested estate on four different trails.

Distance: 10.4 miles returning on Raymundo trail; 9.6 miles returning on Mt. Redondo Trail

Time: 5 hours

Elevation Change: 1400' gain

Two circle trips start on the Crystal Springs Trail in Huddart Park, one taking that trail uphill through the park and returning downhill through the Phleger Estate, the other going both up and down through the Phleger Estate. Described here is the latter route, starting from the trailhead south of the restrooms at the Zwierlein Picnic Area in Huddart Park. A signpost marking the Crystal Springs Trail points left (north), and says 0.7 MILES to the Phleger Estate and each turn thereafter is clearly marked.

This beautiful trail winds downward through redwoods and Douglas firs along banks lush with fern fronds and woodland shade-loving plants. After 0.2 mile you bear right, switchbacking downhill around a fairy ring of redwoods grown in a circle around the cavity where once an ancient redwood stood. In the depths of McGarvey Gulch you parallel the creek, but do not cross the first bridge over the creek. Follow the creek downstream (right) for 0.1 mile, and then turn sharply left to cross over it as it flows through a culvert. Now you head uphill left on wide Richards Road, watching for the right turn on the Miramontes Trail, marked by a prominent sign, THE PHLEGER ESTATE.

In spring the trailside banks are brightened by white violets and in summer by sticky monkey flower's apricot blossoms. Keeping West Union Creek on your right, you bear left at a fork, and soon come to a wooden sign hanging from a post topped by a metal cutout of a tired Indian warrior on his horse announcing that you are indeed on the Miramontes Trail. Follow the lovely, clear creek on its course over gravel bars, around meanders, and past pools beneath redwood roots or behind fallen trees.

After going through a metal gate in a fence, the trail starts uphill, switchbacking through an area of madrone trees and chaparral. Here on a flat are clusters of cream-colored Fremont lilies on tall stalks blooming in spring and healthy, ubiquitous poison oak bushes close to the trail.

At the next junction, 1.4 miles from the entrance to the Phleger Estate, you come to a crossroads, again marked by the Indian warrior atop his horse. The Woodside Trail Club, which formerly built and managed these trails, originally installed distinctive trail markers which have been replicated by POST. Take the Mt. Redondo Trail uphill 0.8 mile along the south side of the steep canyon carved by a tributary of West Union Creek. Here you see very few old redwoods, but you travel under tall second-growth trees interspersed with Douglas firs and clumps of madrone and tan oak trees. Underfoot you may meet a five- or six-inch-long, slimy yellow banana slug, especially in rainy weather. Do avoid crushing this slow-moving, important decomposer of forest litter.

After a series of switchbacks in a predominantly madrone-tree forest, you come to yet another metal sign marking the junction of the Lonely and Raymundo trails with the Mt. Redondo Trail. To continue upward to the Skyline ridge, take the Lonely Trail left (southwest), and climb 0.6 mile up and around the heads of several small ravines before reaching a wooden bench in a small clearing. The bench, installed by POST, is inscribed with the words, "Rest and Be Filled with the Grace of the Forest"; take that advice and stop for a snack while enjoying the quiet broken only by sounds of woodpeckers and blue jays in the forest.

Climbing ever upward on the narrow, 0.9-mile trail, you traverse the steep canyonside of a West Union Creek tributary until you cross it in an opening in the forest. Look uphill on the right for another wooden bench—no inscription but quite a pleasant, cool place on a hot summer day. From here meander around and up more zigzags, pass an obscure gated trail on the right and then take another trail ambling left below the Skyline ridge on a much more gentle grade. After more than 0.4 mile on this trail, you come to the upper Crystal Springs Trail entrance to Huddart Park.

Now that you have achieved the summit of the Phleger Estate at 2000 feet, you can continue into Huddart Park and follow the beautiful Crystal Springs Trail downhill through vigorous second-growth redwoods to the Zwierlein Picnic Area where you started this trip. See Huddart Park's An All-Day Hike Circling the Park, in reverse, page 104.

However, if you retrace your steps on the Lonely Trail to its junction with the Mt. Redondo and Raymundo trails, you can peel off left (north) on the 1.6-mile Raymundo Trail, and walk beside the banks of West Union Creek as it burbles along under alders, redwoods and occasional firs. Then after rejoining the Miramontes Trail, you head back to the Crystal Springs Trail to complete a trip on all the estate's trails. You will have crossed or walked beside each of the three branches of West Union Creek on a 10.6-mile trip up, down, and around this splendid addition to the Golden Gate National Recreation Area.

SEE MAP
ON PAGE
99

A CREEKSIDE WALK

You could spend a day exploring the riches of this riparian landscape.

Distance: 4.2 miles round trip to Miramontes/Raymundo-Mt. Redondo junction

Time: 2 hours

Elevation Change: 200′ loss to creek, 200′ gain to Phleger, 140′ loss to creek in Phleger

Follow directions in previous trip and descend to the banks of lovely West Union Creek. Saunter along its verdant edges, look for tadpoles, little green tree frogs, and myriad insects. Ferns thrive under the redwood, Douglas fir canopy and the creek is lined with fallen logs. When the creek is low in the fall, look for animal tracks on sandy flats by the creek.

Shade-loving plants and wildflowers surround you in this cool, moist environment. Look for fetid adder's tongue, a lily that sends out half-inch white flowers on the end of 4–5-inch fragile stems. As its name implies, its fragrance is not pleasant. Its dark green splotched leaves distinguish it even when it has no blossoms.

After crossing a little tributary that tumbles over a steep hillside edged with large, moss-covered rocks, the trail veers left and begins the climb to the Mt. Redondo/Raymundo junction. However, the main creek canyon is the destination of this trip so linger as long as you like.

Huddart County Park

In Huddart County Park not only do stumps of the big redwood trees and vestiges of skid trails remind us of the early logging days, but many place names recall that era. Up on the mountain near the little logging town of Summit Springs, Frank King's Saloon flourished until the beginning of the 20th century, giving his name to the road that goes through the park. From Richards sawmill on the Skyline ridge, wagons carried lumber down a steep road that is now Richards Road Trail. Owen McGarvey had wood-cutting rights on the gulch that traverses the park and now bears his name.

But a far more significant heritage for us is the handsome second-growth redwood and fir forest and the woodland of oaks, madrones, and California bay trees in this 972-acre park.

In addition to its picnic areas and playfields there are 18 miles of trails through its redwoods, along its creeks, and up its mountainsides. A disabilities-access and a

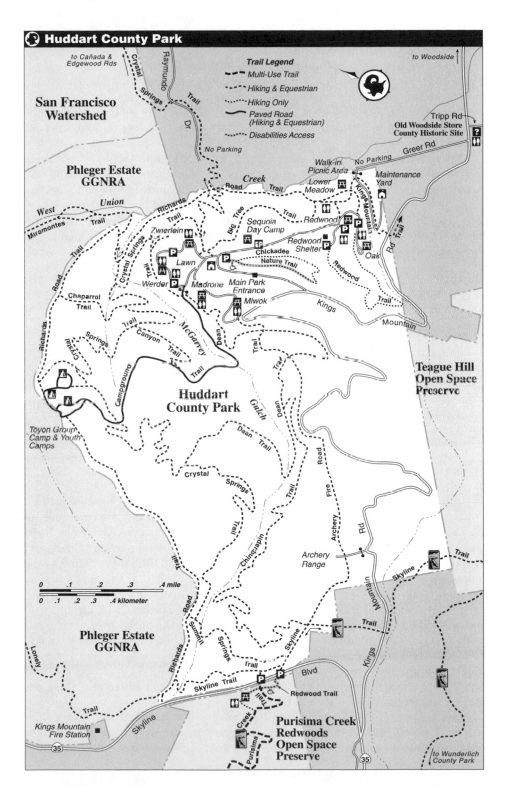

Huddart County Park

Trail Legend
- Multi-Use Trail
- Hiking & Equestrian
- Hiking Only
- Paved Road (Hiking & Equestrian)
- Disabilities Access

to Cañada & Edgewood Rds

to Woodside

San Francisco Watershed

Phleger Estate GGNRA

Tripp Rd
Old Woodside Store County Historic Site

No Parking

West Miramontes Trail

Union Trail

Richards Trail

Crystal Springs Dr

Raymundo Trail

Creek Road

Creek Trail

No Parking

Greer Rd

Walk-in Picnic Area

Lower Meadow

Maintenance Yard

Big Tree Trail

Sequoia Day Camp

Redwood

Kings Mountain

Zwierlein

Chickadee

Redwood Shelter

Crystal Springs Trail

Lawn

Nature Trail

Oak

Redwood

Werder

Madrone

Main Park Entrance

Miwok

Kings Mountain

Chaparral Trail

Crystal Springs Trail

Canyon Trail

McGarvey Trail

Dean Trail

Rd Trail

Richards Road

Campground Trail

Huddart County Park

Dean Gulch

Teague Hill Open Space Preserve

Toyon Group Camp & Youth Camps

Crystal Springs Trail

Dean Trail

Archery Fire Road

Skyline Trail

Phleger Estate GGNRA

Crystal Springs Trail

Chinquapin Trail

Archery Range

Kings Mountain Rd

Skyline Trail

0 .1 .2 .3 .4 mile
0 .1 .2 .3 .4 kilometer

Richards Road

Summit Springs Trail

Skyline Trail

Redwood Trail

Blvd

Lonely Trail

Skyline Trail

Kings Mountain Fire Station

Purisima Creek Trail

Purisima Creek Redwoods Open Space Preserve

35

35

to Wunderlich County Park

nature trail with special parking offer short, easy walks. A group camp on the park's remote northern boundary is available by reservation.

Jurisdiction: San Mateo County: 650-363-4020

Facilities: Trails for hikers, equestrians, and the physically limited; equestrian parking; picnic grounds; group camping facilities; children's play area

Rules: Open 8 A.M. to sunset; group picnics and camping by reservation only; some trails open to hikers only, some closed to equestrians in wet weather; no pets; no bicycles on trails; fees

Maps: San Mateo County *Huddart County Park*, USGS topo *Woodside*

How to Get There: There are two entrances: (1) Main Entrance—from I-280 take Woodside Rd. (Hwy 84) west 1.5 miles to Kings Mountain Rd., turn right, and go 1.5 miles to main park entrance on right side of road. (2) Skyline Blvd. entrance— turn right from Kings Mountain Rd. onto Skyline Blvd. and go 0.3 mile. Use parking area on west side of Skyline Blvd. at Purisima Creek Redwoods Open Space Preserve and cross to Huddart County Park entrance.

SEE MAP
ON PAGE
103

AN ALL-DAY HIKE
CIRCLING THE PARK

Take a history tour along a woodcutter's claim to the site of a logger's ridgetop saloon.

Distance: 8.2-mile loop, 7.2 miles without the Toyon Camp Loop

Time: 5 to 6 hours

Elevation Change: 1500' gain

This loop takes you from the Miwok Picnic Area down to West Union Creek and up the magnificent Crystal Springs Trail to the Skyline heights, ending with a downhill return on the Chinquapin Trail on the south side of McGarvey Gulch.

Starting at the Miwok Picnic Area, walk west from the parking area and pick up the Dean Trail heading downhill. (Don't take the wide unpaved Archery Fire Road taking off to the left.) The Dean Trail crosses Toyon Road (Campground Road) and descends through redwoods, tan oaks and madrones for a little more than 0.5 mile to join the Crystal Springs Trail headed to McGarvey Gulch. At the next junction, bear left, walk across the McGarvey Gulch bridge upstream from West Union Creek and continue on a zigzag course up the Crystal Springs Trail. On this trail you will explore some of the most beautiful features of the park's north side.

At first in an oak-madrone woodland, you are soon in redwoods on the far side of McGarvey Gulch. Cross a small bridge over a tributary creek and continue uphill around wide switchbacks through a sizable second-growth redwood forest. Ferns, native iris, and spring wildflowers line the trail and here and there are immense stumps from the ancient forest.

After 1.4 miles the trail leaves the gulch, passing the Chaparral Trail on the right and the Canyon Trail on the left. Then zigzagging up the steep mountainside you reach the junction where the Crystal Springs Trail splits; one fork goes straight to the Toyon Group Camp and Richards Road, the other goes left (if no camp is in session, you could find a table on which to spread out your lunch, then circle the camp and return on Toyon Road to rejoin the Crystal Springs Trail farther west—adding another mile to your trip). Bear left on the Crystal Springs Trail at this junction and continue on the trail, which soon crosses the service road (Toyon Road) to begin a 2-mile climb to the Skyline. Gates bar horses from this segment of the Crystal Springs Trail when storms make the ground muddy.

Redwoods, firs, and madrones cover the mountainside and birds fill the air with their songs. The trail winds in and out of small canyons and crosses grassy meadows, beguiling the hiker with new vistas around each bend. Springs dampen fern-covered ravines, and in spring wildflowers bloom where small clearings let in the sun.

At 3.13 miles the trail climbs steeply to meet the Dean Trail. Here you could shorten the hike by returning to your starting point via the Dean Trail. But this trip continues up the ridge on comfortably graded switchbacks through a glade of madrones. Their summer leaf fall makes a rustling carpet underfoot in a delicately colored pattern of lemon-yellow, pink, and cream.

The trail levels off in a huckleberry flat under redwoods where the Crystal Springs and the Richards Road trails converge at the Summit Springs Trail. A plank bench makes a good seat for your picnic lunch.

From this intersection take the wide, steep Summit Springs Trail (fire road) to the left and follow it toward Skyline Boulevard. The redwoods here have not been cut for over a century. Heavy winter rains (as much as 40 inches a season) and summer fog drip give these trees the moisture on which they thrive. Widely spaced trees, many of them 4 feet in diameter, have a handsome understory of shiny-leaved huckleberry and a ground cover of wood fern and oxalis. In spring you will find yellow violets, mauve mission bells, and irises in many shades of blue and purple. For a short expedition to this part of the park, you can drive to the Skyline Boulevard entrance and get to this fine forest without the climb from below.

At 2000-feet elevation (a sign informs you), the Summit Springs Trail meets the Skyline Trail. Here you can bear right and cross Skyline Boulevard to Purisima Creek Redwoods O.S.P. But to continue this trip, take the Skyline Trail left (southeast) an eighth mile farther. From this point the Skyline Trail bears right to Kings Mountain Road and continues south to Wunderlich Park, the service road (now becomes the Archery Fire Road) descends to park headquarters, and your route turns left (northwest) onto the Chinquapin Trail.

Your return trip on the nearly 2-mile Chinquapin Trail descends a ridge below the Summit Springs Trail through a handsome second-growth forest. A scattering of great stumps gives you a measure of the stately forest that grew on this mountainside until it was logged in the 1860s. The trail winds down a steep hillside into McGarvey Gulch, but before it reaches the creek it turns south, then doubles back north, and abruptly switchbacks again to make a long traverse southeast along the side of McGarvey Gulch. From several bridges and culverts you hear water falling over huge boulders in spring; in summer you see little pools nestled at the base of huge, moss-covered rocks. This well-engineered trail ends at the Dean Trail, which then crosses the Archery Fire Road twice. After 0.75 mile on the Dean Trail you see the gated Toyon Road and the Miwok picnic areas on your right.

A LOOP THROUGH
THE CENTER OF THE PARK

A half-day hike takes you up McGarvey Gulch and down the other side.

Distance: 4.3-mile loop

Time: 2½ hours

Elevation Change: 400′ gain

Find the Dean Trail west of the Miwok Picnic Area and head uphill. Less than a half hour's walk along the side of McGarvey Gulch brings you to a bridge over the creek, a cool spot to linger on a hot day. In winter and early spring you can enjoy the creek waters cascading over huge boulders and mossy rocks. The logging road near the trail and the great redwood stumps recall the history of logging, but now second-growth trees reach high overhead. Where there is underground water near the creek, giant chain ferns are taking hold again and bigleaf maples are growing on the bank.

Leaving the creek, the Dean Trail contours around a ridge on an easy grade. In a half hour a hiker should reach an intersection with the Crystal Springs Trail. Turn right on it, and after rounding another bend the trail turns downward through a handsome redwood forest.

From here the trip down repeats in reverse the journey up the Crystal Springs Trail described in An All-Day Hike Circling the Park. In 1.1 miles from the Dean Trail you come to the Toyon Group Camp. After passing it, there are another 1.3 forested miles to the lower end of the park. Turn up there on the other end of the Dean Trail to complete your trip to the Miwok Picnic Area.

A LOOP TRIP
IN LOWER MCGARVEY GULCH

Explore the forest and the chaparral-covered slope in the park's lower, northeastern corner to find tall forests, wide vistas, and a walk down the old road from Richard's lumber mill.

Distance: 3.5-mile loop

Time: 2 hours

Elevation Change: 360′ loss

This easy trip takes one steep stretch going downhill. From the Werder Flat Area proceed past the Childrens Playground to the gated service road, Toyon Road (used only for service vehicles). On this road you will cross the Dean Trail. On a slight rise in grade you go into and out of McGarvey Gulch. A little less than 0.25 mile past the creek, turn right down the Canyon Trail. You switchback down the side of McGarvey Gulch in a transitional forest where redwoods are growing high enough to shade out the madrones and tanbark oaks that took over after these slopes were logged.

From the Canyon Trail jog right onto the Crystal Springs Trail and go downhill a few hundred feet to pick up the Chaparral Trail. At this point you leave the forest to traverse a ridge where scattered oaks, madrones, and a few toyons cast light shade. Native bunchgrass covers open areas along with spring-blooming iris and snowberry. In 0.5 mile the trail approaches the park's northern boundary, beside which Richards Road Trail makes its steep way down to West Union Creek. In the 1850s this road carried logs down to Whipple's sawmill on the creek.

You start down Richards Road Trail on an open ridge among shrubby manzanita and blue-blossomed wild lilac. The view is toward Emerald Lake Hills, topped by a cross, and to the Bay plain beyond. To the right of the trail and paralleling it, the old skid road where oxen dragged logs to the mill is still visible.

Below the chaparral area, great canyon oaks meet above the trail. Then as you approach the creek through groves of redwoods, you pass the left turn-off to the Phleger Estate. Shortly the trail veers right to cross McGarvey Gulch Creek running in a culvert. After crossing over this culvert, immediately bear left (west) uphill on the Crystal Springs Trail. In 0.1 mile take the Dean Trail to the right, and make an easy climb through redwoods back to Werder Flat.

SEE MAP ON PAGE 103

A SHADY WALK BY WEST UNION CREEK

A warm summer day is a good time to explore these cool trails by the creek.

Distance: 2-mile loop

Time: 1½ hours

Elevation Change: 500' gain

The park's creekside trails, shaded by spreading big-leaf maples and tall redwoods, are a peaceful retreat. But over a century ago, in the 1850s, three sawmills operated along West Union Creek, handling logs cut from forests extending to the Skyline above.

For an easy, leisurely walk by the creek and a short loop up into the forest, start from the Redwood Picnic Area in the southeast corner of the park. Go east past tables filled on weekends with groups of picnickers down into the west meadow walk-in area through a pedestrian stile at the gate. Walk a few yards north and pick up the Richards Road Trail to the right of the Bay Tree Trail on which you will return. Richards Road, a broad service road, forms the north boundary of the park. It continues its nearly level way beside the creek where thimbleberries, bull rushes, and bigleaf maple trees thrive in the shade. Sounds from the picnic area begin to fade as you round the first bend and enter the quiet of the tall forest.

West Union Creek runs year-round, though dry years leave the water level low. Ferns and lush shrubs line its banks. Here and there are inviting spots for a creekside picnic. About one-half mile upstream from the Meadow on the Richards Road

Trail you come to a crossroads to which the Crystal Springs Trail (which you take on the returning leg of the trip) descends from the picnic area above and goes 3 miles east to Cañada Road and Edgewood Park. Along this part of Richards Road Trail by the creek are some of the park's largest trees.

Pass the first intersection with the Crystal Springs Trail on your left and then after another 0.75 mile on the Richards Road Trail you arrive at McGarvey Gulch Creek. Fed by springs along the Skyline, it flows down a deep-sided canyon through the center of the park. Here you go straight for a few steps on the Crystal Springs Trail following the creek's south side for 0.1 mile. Continue on the Crystal Springs Trail uphill past the Dean Trail for a lovely walk through the redwoods to the vicinity of the Zwierlein Group Picnic Area on Werder Flat.

To complete this loop, find the Bay Tree Trail near the Crystal Springs trailhead below the Zwierlein area. Take this trail, for hikers only, bearing left downhill. Native bunchgrasses grace the hillside under the oak and madrone trees. You cross several small streams on plank bridges and then swing wide to the left. Ferns carpet the hillside and more small streams flow down to join the creek below. This 0.7-mile trail is quiet, well-graded and soon arrives at the top of the meadow next to the Richards Road Trail on which you started this hike.

SEE MAP
ON PAGE
103

CHICKADEE TRAIL
INTO THE FOREST

This pleasant, nearly level trail, suitable for the physically limited, goes through tall chaparral and oaks and past fern-lined banks to reach a redwood grove.

Distance: 1-mile loop

Time: ½ hour or more

Elevation Change: Nearly level

This self-guiding nature trail, designed for wheelchair use, has a well-compacted surface and a grade of less than 5%. For the sight-impaired there is a guide wire. A brochure is available at the trail entrance. Though suitably graded and surfaced for wheelchairs, this trail also provides a pleasant short walk for anyone who would enjoy an easy trip into the forest.

From a level parking space in the southwest corner of the main parking lot by the park entrance, the trail takes off around a hillside covered with wild lilac, coyote bush, and toyon. A short bridge spans an old log chute left from early timber-cutting days. The path soon comes into the deep shade of redwoods. Here a bench, dedicated to former park planner Harry Dean, is strategically placed for viewing the Bay Area while resting before you retrace your steps. Or you can turn downhill and return to the parking lot on an unpaved, lower trail through oak woods to the parking lot.

The Skyline Trail

THE BAY AREA RIDGE TRAIL ROUTE BETWEEN TWO PARKS

A beautiful and varied trail through the Bear Gulch Watershed links Huddart and Wunderlich county parks. This long trail follows the Skyline ridge, where frequent fogs make it a cool trip in hot weather.

Jurisdiction: San Mateo County: 650-363-4020
Facilities: Trail for hikers and equestrians
Rules: Open 8 A.M. to sunset; no dogs or bicycles

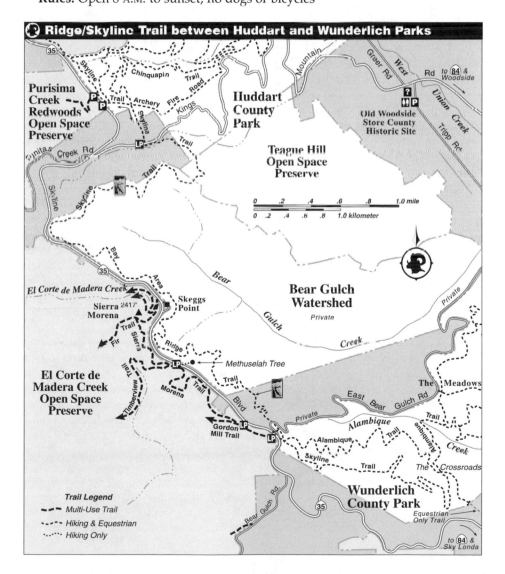

Maps: San Mateo County *Huddart Park* and *Wunderlich Park*, USGS topo *Woodside*

How to Get There: (1) Huddart Park entrance—Take Skyline Blvd. (Hwy 35) 6.5 miles south from Half Moon Bay Rd. (Hwy 92) or 6.5 miles north from La Honda Rd. (Hwy 84) to parking at Purisima Creek trailhead on west side of Skyline Blvd. Cross road to trail entrance; alternate northern entrance at the Phleger entrance (gate 15) (2) Kings Mtn. Rd. entrance—From Skyline Blvd. take Kings Mtn. Rd. 0.3 mile east to limited roadside parking; (3) Wunderlich Park entrance—Take Skyline Blvd. 3 miles north of La Honda/Skyline Blvd. intersection to entrance at Bear Gulch Road East (private, gated road); limited parking on west side of Skyline across from private road.

Distance: 5.8 miles one way

Time: 3+ hours

Elevation Change: 580′ loss

In 1989 the Bay Area Ridge Trail Council dedicated this trail as an official segment (and the first in San Mateo County) of the proposed long-distance Ridge Trail. This segment runs from the west boundary of Huddart Park to Wunderlich Park's west gate. Today there are 267 completed miles of this regional trail that will encircle the nine-county Bay Area along its 400-mile ridgetop route.

Following the crest of the Santa Cruz Mountains, the Skyline Trail passes under tall second-growth redwoods and Douglas firs, through two county parks, an open space preserve and a watershed. A part of the old California Riding and Hiking Trail, it is also a segment of San Mateo County's north-south trail system.

With a car shuttle you can start at the north end and make this a one-way trip. Starting from Huddart Park's Skyline Boulevard entrance [(1) in directions], hikers and equestrians follow the graveled service road southeast through open woodland to a park crossroads with connections to Purisima Creek Redwoods west and the Crystal Springs and Chinquapin trails east through Huddart. To continue on the Skyline Trail you turn right (south) here. On the east side of this trail is lush redwood forest, and on the west is a large private inholding of several new homes on rolling grassland and evergreen forest. After 0.3 mile from your start, you reach Kings Mountain Road, which you cross to find the narrow path running beside the road, well-marked with Bay Area Ridge Trail signs.

Climbing under redwoods through low-growing huckleberries, you then swing south and cross a corner of Teague Hill Open Space Preserve in oak-madrone woodland. As the trail heads west it emerges on chaparral slopes at a sunny crossroads from which a watershed service road goes downhill. However, the Skyline Trail continues straight ahead beside a property-line fence. Although the trail now runs through a fenced easement in the California Water Company's Bear Gulch Watershed paralleling Skyline Boulevard, for the most part the fencing is barely apparent and does not give a closed-in feeling.

Circling around a meadow you come to a view south to Monte Bello Ridge, recently almost obliterated by new growth. In spring and summer some tall, yellow-flowered bush poppies brighten this spot. Soon the trail heads south, enters a forest of redwoods, then one of Douglas firs. As the trail contours around the ridges, you find redwoods growing especially tall in the deep, moist canyons below. Some of the Douglas firs are huge trees of the old-growth forest, but an occasional thicket of younger trees has sprung up, perhaps after some past fire.

From here to Wunderlich Park the trail often goes out on ridges some distance from Skyline Boulevard. At times it brings you close enough to hear the sounds of traffic, but most of the way all you hear is the wind in the treetops, the call of birds, and, in summer, the fog drip hitting leaves on the forest floor.

At about the halfway point you come to a part of the forest where very large redwoods once grew. Note the size of some old stumps—6 to 8 feet in diameter. Look for slots cut into the trees about 6 feet off the ground, signs of the early logging method. Loggers wedged boards in these slots to support the planks they stood on while sawing the trees. Uphill from the trail you may catch a glimpse of the "Methuselah" tree, one of the few surviving giants of the old forest on the east slope of the Santa Cruz Mountains. According to a sign at its base, it is 14 feet in diameter and 1800 years old. Its crown was lost in some long-ago storm, but its lower branches are still flourishing. Can you imagine the timber-cutters' awe at the sight of the old forest with many majestic trees like Methuselah?

The trail continues in and out of canyons, here and there giving you a view out over the Bay. Wildflowers seen include many of the less common ones of the deep conifer forest. You can't miss the Clintonia in late spring, with its deep rosy-red blooms borne in clusters on 20-inch stalks above large basal leaves. Its unusual bright-blue berries glisten in the summer sun. However, you will have to watch very closely for the rare coral-root orchid, a plant bearing brownish flowers on foot-high stalks without any green leaves. The cool, shaded forest environment prolongs the plentiful spring flower blooms into early summer.

In fall you will find the snowberry's inedible white balls on shrubs beside the trail, and the yellow leaves of the big-leaf maple that reflect the light in golden hues. This trail is seldom dusty because the tall redwoods capture the fog, which then drips down to the forest floor.

Nearing Wunderlich Park the trail descends in switchbacks that take it below a subdivision of very large homes. After this detour, you climb back out of the canyon to reach the park's west gate at Bear Gulch Road, the end of the Ridge Trail route. This road is currently

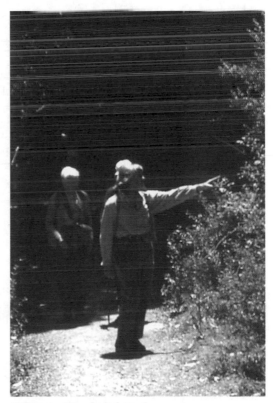

Hikers in Wunderlich Park

private, but the county has retained an easement on it for future trail use. From the west gate the old California Riding and Hiking Trail, the Skyline Trail, goes 2.7 miles east, downhill, to the southern boundary of Wunderlich Park (described in "Figure-Eight Loop Trip to Skyline Ridge from Park Office" of that park, see page 114). From the park boundary, a 0.6-mile trail on an easement for equestrians only continues to SkyLonda.

Across Skyline Boulevard is an entrance to El Corte de Madera Open Space Preserve, a possible trailhead for the continuation of the Bay Area Ridge Trail south. At this writing, the route between the Skyline Trail and La Honda Creek Open Space Preserve is under consideration, though not yet determined.

Wunderlich County Park

Before the coming of white settlers, the Pulgas Redwoods covered most of the mountainside of present-day Wunderlich Park. During the 1850s and 60s these forests, part of the Rancho Cañada de Raimundo, were heavily logged for building and re-building San Francisco. After the timber was cut, some of the lower hills were cleared for farming, but on the steeper mountainsides redwoods began to grow again.

The upper reaches of Wunderlich Park extend along the Skyline ridge at an elevation of about 2200 feet. East of the ridge the hillside falls away steeply, and the slope then flattens somewhat at a large meadow halfway down the mountainside. From this meadow smaller ridges and ravines descend to the lower park boundary along Woodside Road, making a total elevation change of nearly 1800 feet. Alambique Creek runs diagonally across the park, fed by streams in the precipitous wooded ravines to the north.

Alambique, which is the Spanish word for "still," reportedly was the site of a distillery in logging days. For a year the creek supplied water power for the Peninsula's first sawmill, built by Charles Brown in 1847, until a steam boiler was installed. A plaque marks the site at the intersection of La Honda and Portola roads. Early residents drew their water from Alambique Creek, eventually piping it to the reservoir at Salamander Flat.

In 1872 Simon Jones bought 1500 acres of the Rancho Cañada de Raimundo and turned some of the cutover land into a working ranch he named Hazelwood Farm. (You will see the graceful shrub, hazelnut, as an understory in the forests along the trails.) Vestiges of the orchards, vineyards, and olive groves Jones planted remain on the lower slopes of the park.

For the next owner, James A. Folger II, who bought the farm in 1902, it became the site of excursions, carriage trips, and weekend campouts in the woods. He built the handsome stable near the park entrance and a mansion that still stands, though not within the park. This historic stable, though in need of major repairs, still retains the flavor of its former elegance and continues as a boarding stable for horses. The graceful design by architect Arthur Brown Jr., the redwood paneling and the marble fireplace in the tack room recall the days when well-cared-for horses and carriages provided the transportation to trains and to mountain retreats. The

National Register of Historic Places granted historic status to the stable on April 16, 2004. A special committee of the Friends of Wunderlich and Huddart Parks, the Folger Estate Stable Committee, has pledged to secure the funding for its restoration as a place of national significance.

These lands changed hands again in 1956 when Martin Wunderlich acquired much of the Folger estate. In 1974 he generously gave 942 acres to San Mateo County for open space and park use.

In 1978 San Mateo County completed the present extensive trail system, using the old ranch and logging roads and constructing a few new trails for loop trips, making this an outstanding park for hikers and equestrians. These 15+ miles of trail, well laid out and clearly marked, lead through a mountainside wilderness of forest and meadow that can challenge hikers and horsemen with all-day trips to the Skyline or delight casual walkers with an hour or so of strolling under the trees.

It is possible to hike all day virtually without retracing any steps. A circle trip into the park from the main entrance on Woodside Road to "The Meadows" or from the Skyline Boulevard entrance down to "The Crossroads" and back is a good half-day's hike. Shady Alambique, Salamander, and Redwood flats, 2 miles or less from the park office, are fine summer destinations. A segment of the regional Bay

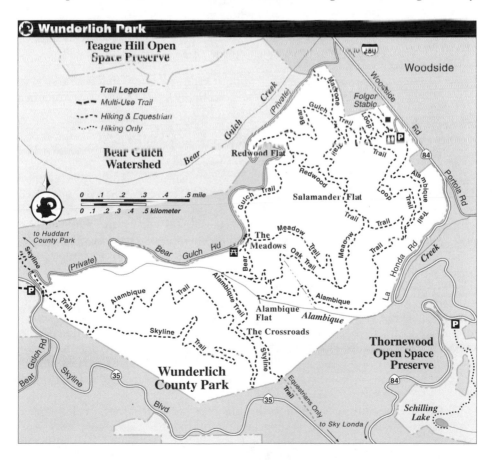

Area Ridge Trail begins on the Skyline Trail in the northwest corner of the park and continues to Huddart Park.

Once you have sampled some of these trails, you will want to return often to explore other routes. Following are more detailed descriptions of four suggested trips.

Jurisdiction: San Mateo County: 650-363-4020

Facilities: Trails for hikers and equestrians; at the parking area there is drinking water (none elsewhere, so carry your own) and a chemical toilet

Rules: Open 8 A.M. to sunset; no pets or bicycles allowed

Maps: San Mateo County *Wunderlich Park* and USGS topo *Woodside*

How to Get There: (1) Main entrance on Woodside Rd: From I-280 take Woodside Rd. (Hwy 84) southwest for 2 miles. Look for park sign on right. (2) Upper entrance on Skyline Blvd: Follow directions above, but continue on Woodside Rd. to right turn uphill onto La Honda Rd. Turn right off La Honda Rd. at Skyline Blvd. and go 3 miles to park entrance on east side of Skyline Blvd. near entrance to Bear Gulch Road East (private). Limited parking on both sides of Skyline Blvd.

SEE MAP ON PAGE 113

FIGURE-EIGHT LOOP TRIP TO SKYLINE RIDGE FROM PARK OFFICE

An ambitious all-day hike through the varied terrain and different ecosystems of the park includes sheltered, sunny meadows and cool streamsides.

Distance: 10.3-mile loop

Time: 6 to 7 hours

Elevation Change: 1080' gain

This hike follows the Alambique Trail to the Skyline ridge, then returns by the Skyline, Alambique, and Bear Gulch trails. Start on the Alambique Trail from the south side of the main parking lot on Woodside Road. For the most part, it is an easy grade along a former ranch road. For a short stretch you go up a hill through a redwood grove, but before long you note the invading "exotics"—eucalyptus, acacia, scotch broom, and other survivors of the ranch plantings, now gone wild. A project is under way to eradicate the eucalyptus and replant with redwoods, but you can see that that battle is far from won.

Rounding the ridges and climbing, the Alambique Trail goes through open mixed woodland. Some deciduous black oaks and the familiar combination of toyons, canyon oaks, and madrones are a friendly habitat for birds. Veteran birders will recognize many species, but even the novice will enjoy their songs and identify at least the insistent call of the scrub jay and the flash of its blue wings through the oaks.

The old road continues through the mixed woodland, where in late spring Douglas iris show their blue, purple, or creamy blooms along the banks. After passing the Loop and Meadow trails on the right, the Alambique Trail enters the redwoods above Alambique Creek, which forms the boundary of the park here. The redwoods near the creek have grown again to a good size since the logging of a century ago, making Alambique Flat a cool, shady place to pause on a hot day. A side trip down to the creek over the soft duff shows you a sample of the redwood plant community. Note the size of the stumps of the old trees of the virgin forest cut in the 1850s. Huge trees (the largest some 8 feet or more in diameter where the water is most plentiful) were widely spaced but their high crowns nearly touched.

After leaving Alambique Flat you soon come to a junction with the Oak and then the Bear Gulch Trail on the right, but you continue up the creek on the Alambique Trail. Soon you cross the creek and turn left to start a 0.6-mile climb out of the canyon along the forested hillside to "The Crossroads," where the Alambique and Skyline trails intersect, 2.8 miles from the start of your trip. In this circular clearing is a bench under the madrone and oak trees—a fine place to catch your breath for more uphill climbing.

You could take the Skyline Trail from here to the summit, but instead stay on the Alambique Trail, on which it's 2 miles and a good hour's walk to the top. This part of the trail winds in and out of steep ravines, which support sword fern and wood-wardia, the 4-foot-tall, feathery, giant chain fern. In the grove of big redwoods near the summit is an old loading platform from which logs were put on wagons for the mills below. As the trail goes through the cuts for powerlines, you have a glimpse northward to San Bruno Mountain, the San Francisco skyline, and Mt. Tamalpais in Marin County. Just beyond here is the gate to Skyline Boulevard at Bear Gulch Road. Note the trail connection going north to Huddart Park—the Skyline Trail, described in the previous section. It is a 5.8-mile segment of the Bay Area Ridge Trail.

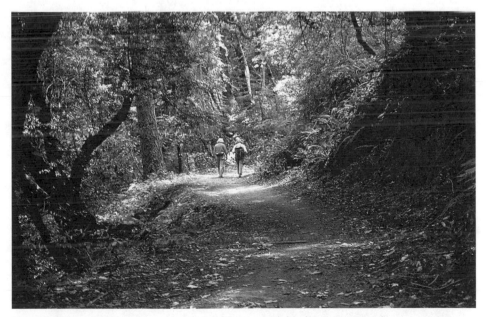

The Alambique Trail was once used to haul logs out of this forest

Turn left (southeast) at the trail convergence and follow the Skyline Trail through an avenue of magnificent Douglas firs and great oaks, which escaped the logger's saw of the last century. Soon the trail borders a long meadow where bunchgrass mixes with sedges and imported oat grasses. In spring the meadow is thick with flowers—baby blue eyes, rosy wild checkerbloom, and blue and purple lupines. The sloping terrain faces southeast, a welcome warm exposure for winter morning hikes. As you look down the meadow, the Bay and East Bay hills are before you. There are fine spots here for eating the lunch you carried uphill. Note: in recent years this meadow has been overgrown with yellow star thistle, an invasive, prickly weed. But, if you are here early in spring, the spines have not yet developed and the seating is pleasant.

Leaving the meadow, the trail leads again into fir forest, which is interspersed with huge specimens of madrone. Out from under the trees the trail emerges on a sunny ridge through a grove of chinquapin, a relative of the oak not commonly seen in San Mateo County but found in several of our hillside parks.

A hairpin turn brings you back into shady forest with an understory of buckeye, hazelnut, and gooseberry. Just ahead is "The Crossroads." From here retrace your steps along the Alambique Trail to the Bear Gulch Trail, on which you turn left, uphill, to "The Meadows." Once an expanse of rolling grasslands, these meadows now are overgrown with invasive broom and native coyote brush. San Mateo County Parks Department hopes to stop the advance of broom and yellow star thistle with the help of volunteers. You can still find the springtime yellow Mariposa lily growing beside the trail, see hawks soaring overhead on their hunt for prey, and get long views of the southern Santa Cruz Mountains where more trails abound.

Leaving "The Meadows" by the Bear Gulch Trail, go along a narrow track under Douglas firs. Some of the fallen trees give an idea of their great size at maturity, nearly 200 feet in height and 6 or more feet in diameter. In early spring this trail segment is adorned with bold, blue-flowered hound's tongue and a sprinkling of the little white blossoms of milkmaids. Hazelnut branches with pale green buds just showing make a lacelike tracery against the dark forest.

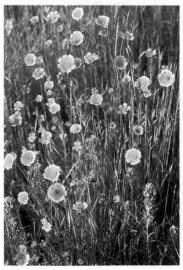

The trail soon crosses some old skid roads, those chutes where oxen dragged redwood logs down to the sawmills below. For a while the trail goes down the canyon close to Bear Gulch Road East on the northern boundary of the park, and then it veers away through Redwood Flat, a grove of tall second- and third-growth redwoods. Now the stump sprouts growing in circles around cut trees are as tall as 150 feet, making a lofty redwood grove again.

From Redwood Flat the trail winds down ravines through a fir forest, crosses the Madrone Trail, zigzags downhill for one mile, passes the Loop Trail, and then goes another 0.25 mile along brushy hillsides back to the stables and the parking lot.

Tidy tips

SEE MAP ON PAGE 113

LOOP TRIP TO "THE MEADOWS"

Climb gently to "The Meadows," the park's center, and return by way of Salamander Flat, the site of a little reservoir in the redwoods.

Distance: 5.7-mile loop

Time: 3½ hours

Elevation Change: 950′ gain

After leaving the park office on the Bear Gulch Trail, you walk (or ride) 0.3 mile along the lower slopes of the park through brush and oak woodlands. Then turn left onto the Loop Trail and make a gentle, 0.77-mile traverse to the Alambique Trail, which you follow for a very short distance (0.08 mile) before turning off to the right on the Meadow Trail. This is an old ranch road through the eucalyptus grove and orchards planted in Simon Jones's farming days. Beyond the Redwood Trail junction you are in a handsome stand of toyon and madrone, where flowers bloom beside the Meadow Trail. In spring look for purple shooting stars, yellow wood violets, and magenta Indian warriors. Under a canopy of tall black oaks you go uphill for 0.44 mile. In summer the monkey flower's apricot blossoms brighten the banks and golden stars edge the trail.

At the next trail junction turn left on the broad Oak Trail, which is shaded by oak woodland for another 0.52 mile. Next you turn right on a very short stretch of the Alambique Trail (0.24 mile). Follow the narrow track through a madrone, oak and fir woodland which filters the light falling on the ground cover of low-growing poison oak (fortunately kept away from the trail).

At the next junction, turn right on the Bear Gulch Trail, descending 0.3 mile through a small clearing and an oak glade before coming out in "The Meadows," where invasive plants have crowded the grasslands. At the top of the meadow, where perhaps there has been less plowing, you may find mounds where the grass grows in tufts, a sign that some of the ancient bunchgrass has survived here. This is one of the native perennial grasses that once covered the hills of California before being displaced by the annual European oat grass that now gives our state the famous golden look in summer.

Old clumps of bunchgrass are deep-rooted and may persist for hundreds of years (some say even thousands), spreading outward in circles. Indians burned it off in the fall to improve hunting. Although the Spaniards found the native grass to be good forage, the oat grass they inadvertently brought with them thrived in the dry California summers and soon took over.

After exploring "The Meadows," leave on the Meadow Trail going east and stroll 0.7 mile through rolling grasslands bordered by large madrones and spreading oaks. Sweeping views to the southeast show the broad flanks of Black Mountain, with the bare slopes of Monte Bello Ridge on its northwest. The trail makes a switchback bringing you back into oak woodlands, though eucalyptuses now have a good foothold here. You descend rapidly to the Meadow/Oak Trail junction and take the Meadow Trail left downhill for 0.4 mile of the trail you took on your way up. This brings you to the intersection of the Redwood Trail, on which you turn left.

From the sunlight of the intersection of the Meadow and Redwood trails you enter the deep shade of redwood forest. The soft forest duff muffles your footsteps on the narrow trail and the air is cool on even the warmest day. For 0.7 mile the Redwood Trail crosses the park, contouring along the hillside at about the 1100-foot elevation line. It goes in and out of small ravines where moss-covered rocks line streams that cascade down the mountain after winter rains. After 0.2-mile on this trail you reach Salamander Flat, in a thick grove of big trees. An oval reservoir fed by springs up the hill was once a water supply for the farm below; later it was reportedly used as a swimming pool, but now it is fenced. The deep shade of Salamander Flat is an inviting place to lunch on the stump of a giant redwood or pause for a while on a hot day.

To return to the park entrance from Salamander Flat, pick up the Madrone Trail going right, downhill. Keep the reservoir on your right. In wet weather the reservoir overflows its dam, creating rivulets along an old wagon road. The hiker takes the wagon road, too, passing fences and hand-fashioned gate posts left from the farming days of the park's past.

About 0.6 mile from Salamander Flat, the Madrone Trail intersects the Bear Gulch Trail and you turn right onto it, then descend the last 0.8 mile to the park office and the parking lot.

SEE MAP
ON PAGE
113

CIRCLE TRIP TO "THE CROSSROADS" FROM THE SKYLINE ENTRANCE

Swing down the Alambique Trail to "The Crossroads" and return by the Skyline Trail on a loop through the heart of the upper park.

Distance: 4.4-mile loop

Time: 2½ hours

Elevation Change: 700' loss (and subsequent gain)

Starting from Skyline Boulevard on the Alambique Trail, you can go downhill at a good clip around bend after bend on the old ranch road. On this, the most remote trail in the park, you may hear deer crashing through the brush, but no sounds of civilization reach you. For more details of these trails see Figure-Eight Loop Trip to Skyline Ridge from Park Office, above. When you get to "The Crossroads," you are in one of the coolest canyons of the park, a delightful woodsy destination for a hot day. A handsome bench invites you to rest and enjoy this clearing marked by a grand old madrone in its center. Here you pick up the Skyline Trail and start uphill. (The other segment of the Skyline Trail descends about 0.25 mile to the park's gated south boundary.) On the varied terrain of your uphill trip you will walk along a ridge covered with oaks and madrones, traverse the edge of a long, sloping meadow, and then reach the upper park entrance under giant Douglas fir trees.

A Short Loop Trip in the Lower Park to Salamander and Redwood Flats

This walk takes you to a small reservoir and shady redwood groves before circling back on the Bear Gulch Trail switchbacks.

Distance: 3.2-mile loop

Time: 1½ hours

Elevation Change: 600′ gain

This trip is in shade all the way, a delightful hot-weather walk. All the trail segments are described in earlier trips. Starting from the park office, follow the 0.7-mile Alambique Trail to the Meadow Trail junction and turn right on the Meadow Trail for 0.35 mile. Then turn right again on the Redwood Trail. On a gentle traverse at the 1100-foot level for 0.7 mile, you pass through both Salamander and Redwood flats, good stopping places for a leisurely lunch.

Turn right at the Bear Gulch Trail junction, from which the remainder of the trip is downhill, a quick 1.4 miles on easy switchbacks. At trail's end you might notice the handsome stone walls along the old roads and beside the stable, which attest to an early craftsman's art.

El Corte De Madera Open Space Preserve

The 2821 forested acres of El Corte de Madera Open Space Preserve, which include most of the drainage basin of El Corte de Madera Creek, lie west of Skyline Boulevard between Star Hill, Swett, and Bear Gulch roads. The creek rises from springs near the Skyline and flows between high ridges on the west side of the preserve, to be joined by its main tributary, Lawrence Creek, which flows through the southeast side. The preserve, from its 2400-foot high point, Sierra Morena, to the canyon where the creek leaves the lower boundary at an elevation of 700 feet, is a place of high ridges and precipitously steep, deep canyons. From some of these high ridges, views between the trees of Coastside and ocean are breathtaking.

The primeval forests of El Corte de Madera's canyons and ridges were logged in the most accessible areas as early as the 1860s, starting first near the creek close to the Skyline. Logging of the old forest continued into the 20th century, and second-growth forests have been cut sporadically since then. After the Midpeninsula Regional Open Space District acquired these lands in 1985, even limited timber cutting ceased by 1988. Although signs of logging are evident along certain roads, a handsome second-growth forest now covers the canyons and ridges.

Old logging roads, sometimes steep, form the basis for an extensive trail network for hikers, equestrians, and bicyclists. A former owner allowed a motorcycle club, the Pits, to use the land, and remnants of these trails can be seen striking off from the district-designed trails. In spring 1996 the District, after a study by a citizens'

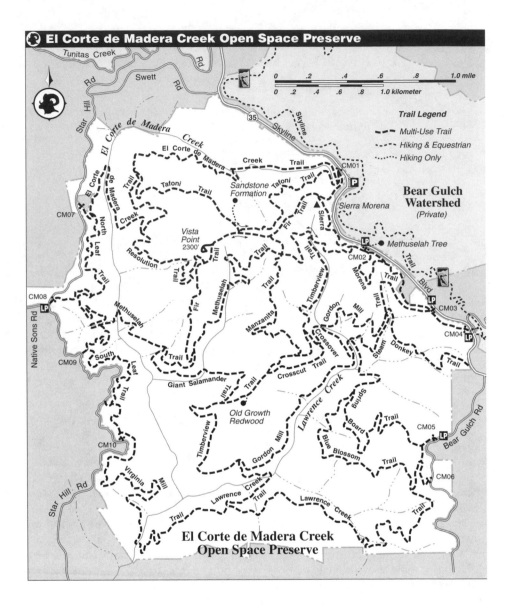

El Corte de Madera Creek Open Space Preserve

Tunitas Creek

Swett Rd

Rd

Star Hill Rd

0   .2   .4   .6   .8   1.0 mile
0   .2   .4   .6   .8   1.0 kilometer

35

Skyline

Skyline

Trail Legend

— ▪ — ▪ — ▪ Multi-Use Trail
– · – · – · Hiking & Equestrian
· · · · · · · Hiking Only

El Corte de Madera Creek

El Corte de Madera Creek Trail

Creek

Trail

CM01

P

Bear Gulch Watershed
(Private)

Tafoni Trail

Sandstone Formation

Tafoni Trail

Trail

Sierra Morena

El Corte de Madera Creek Trail

CM07

North Leaf Trail

Fir Trail

Sierra

Methuselah Tree

LP

CM02

Vista Point 2300'

Resolution Trail

Trail

Trail

Morena Trail

Trail

Trail

CM08

LP

Native Sons Rd

Methuselah Trail

Fir Trail

Manzanita Trail

Timberview Trail

Gordon

Mill

Steam

Trail

Donkey Trail

LP

CM03

CM04

LP

CM09

South Leaf Trail

Trail

Crossover Trail

CM05

LP

Giant Salamander Trail

Crosscut Trail

Lawrence Creek

Spring

Board

Trail

Bear Gulch Rd

Old Growth Redwood

Timberview Trail

Gordon Mill Trail

Blue Blossom Trail

Trail

CM10

CM06

Virginia Mill Trail

Lawrence Creek Trail

Lawrence Creek Trail

Trail

Star Hill Rd

El Corte de Madera Creek Open Space Preserve

task force, adopted a revised trails plan which offers 18 miles of challenging trails descending into the heart and around the periphery of this beautiful preserve. Mountain bicyclists favor this preserve, especially on weekends. However, on weekday hikes, the authors found themselves quite alone on these wonderful trails.

All trails in El Corte de Madera Open Space Preserve are subject to environmental review to determine possible sedimentation in El Corte de Madera Creek. Consult the maps at trail entrances or contact MROSD for updated information.

Jurisdiction: Midpeninsula Regional Open Space District: 650-691-1200

Facilities: Trails for hikers, equestrians, and bicyclists

Rules: Open dawn to dusk; no dogs; all trails except foot trail to Sandstone Formation open to bicyclists and equestrians

Maps: USGS topo *Woodside*, MROSD map *El Corte de Madera Open Space Preserve*

How to Get There: On Skyline Blvd. there are four entrances: (1) at gate CM03 (Gordon Mill trailhead) 3.0 miles north of Skyline Blvd/Hwy 84 intersection (SkyLonda) and (2) at gate CM02 (Methuselah Tree trailhead), 0.7 mile farther north. Limited parking on west side of road near preserve gate. (3) Skeggs Point Caltrans Vista Point 1 mile farther north, on east side of Skyline Blvd. Park at Skeggs Point, go 100 yards north and cross road to preserve entrance at gate CM01. (4) Limited parking at gate CM04 on Skyline Blvd. On Star Hill Road, (1) at gate CM08, from off-road parking go downhill to trails on preserve's west side.

A Loop Trip to Sandstone Formation, Vista Point, and a Shady Valley

Try old logging roads and a new trail for an overview of this varied preserve's northern trails.

Distance: 4.4-mile loop

Time: 2 hours

Elevation Change: 300' gain

From the Skeggs Point entrance at CM01 take the wide trail on the right (not the gated paved road on the left) which veers uphill and around a sharp bend. At this bend the road splits, its two branches being old logging roads that now serve as trails. Stay left on the upper road, the Tafoni Trail, for this trip. The lower road, the El Corte de Madera Creek Trail, on which you will return, turns right to follow the creek.

On the Tafoni Trail you continue around a hillside for 0.9 mile, skirting the north side of a ridge and rising gently to reach a multiple-trail junction in a wide clearing—one trail goes sharply to your left and southeast toward the Methuselah trailhead; the middle trail, the Fir Trail, bears slightly right (west) to the vista point, and the third trail, the Tafoni Trail on which you have been traveling, goes right (northwest) to the Sandstone Formation.

For views of the Coastside and ocean, take the Fir Trail for 0.1 mile to a fork. There you take the trail on the right, signed VISTA POINT, to the end of a ridge. Through the rapidly encroaching trees on the slope below, you can see the rolling grasslands running down to the Coast. Here is a good place to picnic and rest in the shade of some young Douglas firs, with chaparral, tan oaks, and madrones bordering the wide trail that circles the vista point.

Return the way you came, rejoining the Fir Trail, to reach the multiple-trail junction you passed earlier, and bear left on the Tafoni Trail toward the Sandstone Formation, which gives the trail its name. After only 0.1 mile, you find a narrow footpath on your right (for hikers only) that leads down to the handsome viewing platform near the outcrops. From this point you can see the picturesque cliffs jutting up some 50 feet above the wooded hillside. Excellent diagrams explain the processes that produce these unusual formations. Rainwater and carbon dioxide from the air combine to form a weak acid which slowly erodes the calcium carbonate cement binding the individual sand grains in sandstone. Over many years this weathering process has produced the honeycomb surface on the rocks and created some picturesque columnar structures. Climbing on these rocks can damage the formation, so examine them with your eyes, not your hands or feet.

For a longer trip along this ridge, retrace your steps on the narrow footpath to the Tafoni Trail you left and bear right (northwest) downhill on it for 0.8 mile under oaks and firs to the El Corte de Madera Creek Trail junction. You bear right (north) on it; the other segment of this trail goes sharply left downhill and west. On the El Corte de Madera Creek Trail you trend gently downhill (east) along a forested hillside past numerous burned-out redwood stumps, some of them remnants of giant trees that stood right across what is now the trail. Walking through a former tree

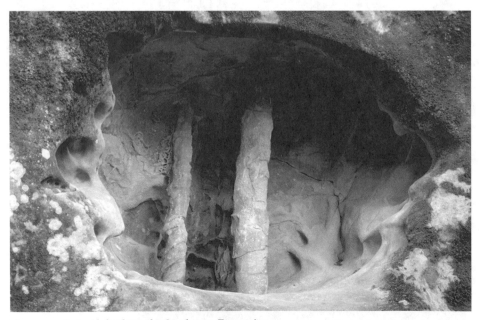

A narrow footpath leads to the Sandstone Formation

trunk gives you a sense of the tree's former girth. Young redwoods are taking over in the tan oak forest, and the trail winds among them down the nose of the ridge surmounted by the Sandstone Formation.

Now descending north along the course of a small creek, which is dry most of the year, you pass through a thriving thicket of young redwoods and quickly reach the upper part of the preserve's main creek, El Corte de Madera. Here is probably the site of one of the earliest sawmills in the canyon, a water-powered mill operated by Ambrose Saunders in the 1860s. In most years this creek still trickles in late August and moisture-loving plants thrive here—brilliant red-blossomed monkey flowers heuchera, redwood sorrel, and in late summer, six-foot-tall elk clover (aralia) topped with a puff of delicate white flowers.

You now turn right uphill (east) toward the preserve entrance. Young redwoods grow in this valley, but as you ascend the old logging road, the continuation of the El Corte de Madera Creek Trail, note the immense stumps of the ancient forest, some with huckleberry bushes sprouting like glistening green top knots. Tall Douglas firs grow here today, but the young redwoods are thriving. As you pass the last redwood, you begin to hear the noise of Skyline Boulevard traffic. When you reach the junction with the Tafoni Trail on which you started, turn left and proceed a short distance to gate CM01.

SEE MAP ON PAGE 170

WESTWARD HO!

Find the reason for the Resolution Trail's name.

Distance: 5.5-mile loop

Time: 3 hours

Elevation Change: 480' loss

For this delightful trip leave the Skeggs Point parking area and enter the preserve at CM01 on the Tafoni Trail. Rounding this ridge and heading a bit south, you come to a fork where the Tafoni Trail goes off left (south) and uphill and the El Corte de Madera Trail continues right and slightly downhill.

Bending south and then west you contour under high canopies of madrone, tan oak, and some old redwoods, most of them fire-scarred and many multi-trunked. Occasional shiny-leaved huckleberry shrubs and spring blooming iris grace the trailside, but the forest understory is relatively open. The well-graded trail is a pleasure to follow, thanks to many volunteers and the rangers who built retaining walls, put in drain pipes and deftly lined the trailside with sandstone rock. If you look uphill as you round a nose of the ridge, you can see a huge sandstone outcrop, a smaller version of the ones you visited in A Loop Trip to Sandstone Formation, Vista Point, and a Shady Valley.

When you come to the foot of a wide ravine, the El Corte de Madera Trail turns abruptly right (west), rounds the shoulder of a ridge and drops down to a trail junction in a small clearing. Now you turn left (south) onto the Resolution Trail, leaving the creek and its namesake trail. However, you can hear the creek in the canyon below, especially after heavy rains, as it gathers volume and turns south on its way to join San Gregorio Creek beyond the preserve boundary and south of La Honda Road.

You climb gradually up a west-facing ridge beside some of the largest redwoods on the preserve. At times some are merely burned-out shells of ancient giants; others are still alive, nurse trees for sprouts that have grown to several feet in diameter. The best trees are downhill from the trail and in ravines where water is more plentiful.

But where is the reason for the trail's name? In a stand of mahogany-barked madrone at the head of a small gulch is the site of a 1953 airplane crash. The plane, en route to San Francisco, was named the Resolution after one of Captain Cook's four ships that explored the Pacific. All aboard were lost.

Beyond this point the trail continues gradually uphill, bends into a ravine where dense stands of tall firs and redwoods flourish, then reaches a west-facing chaparral thicket. Rising above the chaparral is a small forest of chinquapin trees that thrive in a sandstone belt found at this elevation on both sides of the Skyline corridor. Note their dark green leaves with golden undersides and in the fall the prickly seedpods scattered along the trail.

 Shortly you nip into conifer woods again and then emerge in a wide clearing at the junction with the Fir Trail. Take this trail left (northeast) and follow it past the junction with the trail to the vista point and on to the multi-trail junction you met in A Loop Trip to Sandstone Formation, Vista Point, and a Shady Valley. Here you can pick up the Tafoni Trail, on which you can visit the Sandstone Formation, or head northeast on the Fir Trail back to gate CM01 and the Skeggs Point parking area.

MEANDERING THE METHUSELAH

Traverse the preserve from east to west on the edge of steep ravines in a thriving redwood/fir forest.

Distance: 7.0 round trip; 3.5 to CM08 or 4.0 to CM07 with shuttle

Time: 4 hours round trip

Elevation Change: 800' loss, (200' gain climbing Star Hill Road)

Enter the preserve at gate CM02 on the west side of Skyline Boulevard opposite the ancient redwood known as Methuselah. Take the wide trail on the right that skirts the preserve's east periphery and in less than 0.1 mile bear left on the Methuselah Trail. This wide, multi-use trail, named for the venerable redwood, trends downhill, passing the Timberview and the Manzanita trails on the left. The authors hiked this on a fall day when the only sounds were the wind whispering softly through beautiful, second-growth trees, squirrels squawking from the treetops, and woodpeckers hammering holes for acorns in the bark.

Beyond the Manzanita Trail junction you round a sharp bend in the Methuselah Trail and turn due south. In a wide ravine crowded with pampas grass you cross a culvert over a tributary of El Corte de Madera Creek. After several more bends in the trail you cross the stream again in a ravine filled with tan oaks and madrones and little fern gardens beside the trail.

If you glance over the almost-vertical edge of this trail into the tree-filled ravine, you wonder how the lofty trees can keep erect. An occasional tree lying crosswise over the trail lends credence to your conjecture.

After passing the Fir Trail on the right, you head west into a very dense second or third-growth forest. When the trail narrows beyond the Giant Salamander Trail junction, it lies on a southwest-facing slope where filtered sunlight glancing through the trees feels welcome on a cool fall day.

Now on a new, narrower, and very pretty trail cut into the steep hillside, you descend quickly to the banks of El Corte de Madera Creek. No bridge spans the creek at this writing. Evidence of recent storms is everywhere—young redwoods lying across the creek canyon like jack-straws and downed logs littering the creek bed. However, at low water in the fall you can hop across the stream on big boulders and zigzag up the steep-sided canyon toward the South Leaf Trail junction. You could meander south along the creek canyon on this trail for about a mile to the next gate, CM10, or continue uphill 0.4 mile to the North Leaf Trail junction. Here you could turn north to join the El Corte de Madera Creek Trail and continue on it to the Tafoni or Resolution trails as described in the first two trips, A Loop Trip to Sandstone Formation, Vista Point, and a Shady Valley, and Westward Ho!

If you continue uphill past the North Leaf Trail, it is 0.3 mile to gate CM08 on Star Hill Road. You will pass redwoods hanging precariously on the canyon edge, cross little creeks tumbling down the hillside and then emerge in a madrone, tan oak, and Douglas fir forest at a small MROSD parking area. The authors had spotted a car here, so climbed up to Star Hill Road. However, we found that shuttling cars on this narrow road along a sheer-sided canyon took almost as much time as we would have spent hiking the Methuselah Trail back to CM02 on Skyline Boulevard.

SEE MAP
ON PAGE
120

EXPLORING THE HEADWATERS
OF LAWRENCE CREEK

In the depths of the preserve, find the oldest tree in El Corte's forests.

Distance: 4.0 round trip

Time: 3 hours

Elevation Change: 700′ loss (and subsequent gain)

Starting from gate CM02 across from the Methuselah Tree bear right for 0.1 mile, then pick up the Methuselah Trail, descend to the Timberview Trail junction, and turn left. For the next mile you follow Lawrence Creek down a narrow canyon. Sometimes the trail is above the creek, at others it is at creek level. You can look through the trees and across the gulch to a high, sheer slab of sandstone, more of the same formation you met in A Loop Trip to Sandstone Formation, Vista Point, and a Shady Valley, and Meandering the Methuselah. After half a mile the creek

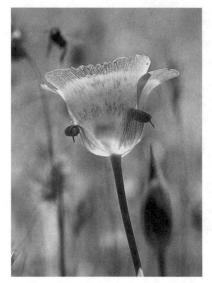

Mariposa lily

drops into a deep, tree-studded, side canyon, but your trail stays high on the east-facing ridge.

After crossing a little tributary you come to the Crosscut Trail junction and turn left on it, pass a cut-off to the Gordon Mill Trail and enter open woodland. Tall, young redwoods are reaching for the sunlight where once loggers may have piled huge trees before hauling them out to the mills. On the narrow Crosscut Trail you are now on the edge of a deep canyon and can see across the treetops to the opposite ridge. Clumps of Douglas iris, young tan oak trees, invasive pampas grass and young Douglas firs crowd the relatively level, narrow trail for almost one-half mile.

When you come to the wide Timberview Trail, turn left and descend 0.2 mile to the left turn-off for the Old Growth Redwood. Bear left in a small clearing and a few yards farther find the venerable giant off to your right. This tree is close to 12 feet in diameter and its bark is lighter than most redwoods. Note the cuts where loggers tried and failed to insert spring boards for holding the long boards on which to stand while cutting down the tree. Walk around the massive trunk, note its fire-scarred cavities, and try to estimate its girth.

Return to the Timberview Trail, turn right on it, pass the Crosscut Trail junction and go 0.3 miles in a more open forest of madrones and toyons to a left turnoff for the Manzanita Trail. Take this narrow trail northward, climbing through lovely tan oak woods and a few burnt-out redwood skeletons to a sharp right turn. Here you begin a stretch of chaparral and find the first manzanita bushes of the trip. They thrive on this west-facing ridge, which can be hot in summer. Other chaparral plants are here—prickly pickeringia with magenta flowers and tiny-leaved chamise with inconspicuous, creamy blossoms. There is a fine stand of chinquapin trees, identified by green leaves with golden undersides, which bear 2-inch round, prickly brown seed pods. You will find them scattered on the trail in fall. The authors also noted a few specimens of the small, crinkly-leaved, gray-green leather oak.

The trail is worn down to bare sandstone here and eroded in long furrows that make unsteady going for hikers as well as for bicyclists. The trail surface improves when you enter the pretty, shiny-leaved, mahogany-barked madrone forest. Then, when you make the right turn onto the Methuselah Trail, you are in a redwood/Douglas fir forest and on your way to gate CM02.

A LOOP TRIP INTO THE PRESERVE'S SOUTHERN CANYONS

A long, challenging loop trip on the main haul road down the steep canyon of the main tributary of El Corte de Madera Creek.

Distance: 9-mile loop

Time: 5 to 6 hours

Elevation Change: 1600' loss

From gate CM03 on the west side of Skyline Boulevard, 3.0 miles north of Highway 84, start down the Gordon Mill Trail, an old timber haul road. This day-long trip follows the broad, well-compacted old logging road for 2.6 miles down the steep canyonside above the creek. After 1.4 miles down this trail, you pass a road going left, downhill, the leg of your return trip.

Handsome second-growth redwoods and firs cover the ridges, in spite of extensive logging over the past century. Continue 1.2 miles on the Gordon Mill Trail in and out of ravines to the creek crossing at the lower end of the preserve. Watch on your left for the Lawrence Creek Trail, which you take for 0.25 mile to the bridge over Lawrence Creek. This tributary of El Corte de Madera Creek is a refreshing sight on a hot day. Its clear waters cascade over mossy rocks and pause in pools above and below the bridge. Thimbleberries and huckleberries grow near its banks, and tiger lilies bloom here in late summer.

At the end of the bridge is the stump of an immense tree 6 feet in diameter, a remnant of the old forest. From the creek crossing you begin a long 2.1-mile climb on the Lawrence Creek Trail up the side of a ridge to the Blue Blossom Trail, a gain in elevation of more than 600 feet. At this junction you could climb another 400 feet to take one of two short routes to gates on Bear Gulch Road or to the Springboard Trail. However, this trip bears left (northwest) and follows the Blue Blossom Trail for about 1.5 miles through pretty, second-growth forest. The shrubs filling openings created by former logging operations are the blue blossom ceanothus, their fragrance and pretty flowers common sights in spring. In this area firs rather than redwoods dominate, some of great size and age.

If you elect to take the Springboard Trail, you will follow an old logging road west and go down into a steep-sided, verdant canyon. The next 1.1 mile is a delightful trip through second-growth forest with a ground cover of sword fern and huckleberry. At little flats along the way you have vistas across nearby canyons.

The Blue Blossom and Springboard trails meet and descend into the canyon to cross a tributary creek where logging activities and grading for roads once disrupted the channel. After 0.4 mile at the Gordon Mill/Steam Donkey junction you reach the larger Lawrence Creek that you followed down the canyon at the start of the trip. Take the Gordon Mill Trail (the Steam Donkey is shorter, but much steeper), jog left, and then right (northwest) on the Gordon Mill Trail, the main haul road. From here it is little less than an hour's trip (1.4 miles) back to the entrance gate, after a day within the enclosing walls of this vast canyon.

La Honda Creek Open Space Preserve

La Honda Creek Open Space Preserve includes 2043 acres of steep forested slopes and hilly grasslands. The preserve takes in a sweep of meadow descending from private Allen Road south along the canyon of La Honda Creek to its intersection with Weeks Creek. The eastern slopes of the preserve are heavily forested; the central and western parts are steeply-rolling grasslands, with the drainage basins of Harrington and San Gregorio creeks in the near view, and the Pacific Ocean far to the west.

This preserve is open only with special permit; the present entrance via Allen Road is through private property and no riding or hiking is permitted on it. Only a few trails on the upper part of the preserve are open at this writing, but a trails plan, which may include a parking area in the southern part of the preserve (the former McDonald "Rocking Martini" Ranch), is being prepared by MROSD.

The loop trip to the meadow takes the visitor to remarkable vistas, flowery grasslands and handsome forests in this preserve. Another trip to a grand old redwood makes a pleasant, 1.4-mile outing with relatively little elevation gain or loss.

MROSD rangers and preserve volunteers faithfully restored the historic red barn with white picket fence on the McDonald Ranch, a famous landmark on Highway 84, La Honda Road. During environmental studies they found a few pallid bats, which are now classified as Sensitive Species.

Jurisdiction: Midpeninsula Regional Open Space District: 650-691-1200

Facilities: Trails for hikers and equestrians

Rules: At this writing the preserve is open by permit only from the MROSD office; no bicycles or dogs permitted; no horse trailers on narrow Allen Road

Maps: MROSD map *La Honda Creek O.S.P*, USGS topos *Woodside* and *La Honda*

How to Get There: On Skyline Blvd. go 2 miles northwest of Skyline Blvd/Hwy 84 intersection and turn south on Bear Gulch Rd. Go 0.5 mile down this narrow, winding road, turn left on private Allen Rd. and go 1 mile to locked gate at preserve boundary. Directions for opening this gate are included in permit. A designated parking place is 0.2 mile beyond gate.

SEE MAP ON PAGE 129

A Trip Down the Meadows for a Bird's-Eye View of the Coastside

Walk out over the meadows to the middle of the preserve and return across the pasture and through the woods on the west side of the preserve.

Distance: 3-mile loop

Time: 1½ hours

Elevation Change: 300' loss

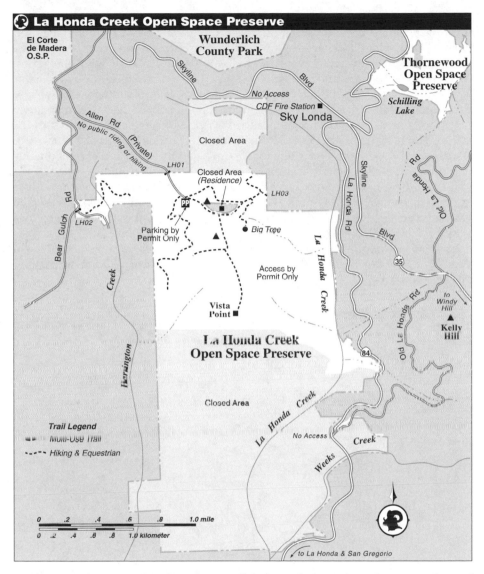

La Honda Creek Open Space Preserve

El Corte
de Madera
O.S.P.

Wunderlich
County Park

Thornewood
Open Space
Preserve

Skyline

Blvd

Schilling
Lake

No Access

CDF Fire Station ■

Sky Londa

Allen Rd (Private)

No public riding or hiking

Closed Area

LH01

Closed Area
(Residence)

LH03

Skyline

La Honda Rd

Bear Gulch Rd

PP

LH02

Parking by
Permit Only

Big Tree

Access by
Permit Only

La Honda Creek

Blvd

35

Old Le Honda Rd

Creek

to
Windy
Hill

Kelly
Hill

Vista
Point ■

La Honda Creek
Open Space Preserve

84

Harrington

Closed Area

La Honda Creek

Trail Legend

— Multi-Use Trail

---- Hiking & Equestrian

No Access

Creek

Weeks

Creek

0   .2   .4   .6   .8   1.0 mile

0   .2   .4   .8   .8   1.0 kilometer

to La Honda & San Gregorio

From the designated parking area walk east on the paved road up a rise through a redwood grove and past a little clearing edged with a few Douglas firs of magnificent proportions. The road soon veers south to a barn and below an enclave of private property. Leave the paved road and go right down a ranch road between the barn and a corral, then go up through a wooden gate to a meadow beyond.

A few steps from the gate along the ranch road one of the dramatic vistas of the coastside ranches and ridges opens up. A sloping pasture is edged on the east by tall, dark oaks, firs, and redwoods. To the south you can see the hills along San Gregorio Creek and forested Butano Ridge. Far west are the gleam of white surf and the blue ocean beyond.

In less than a mile the ranch-road trail enters a patch of forest at the foot of the meadow. Here are a few towering old redwoods passed by in early logging. You emerge quickly into a lower meadow and to more views. In spring these grasslands are bright with wildflowers and the woods are bordered with blue irises. There are no trails here, and you will be stopped by a dense forest on one side, or on the other by a precipitously steep hillside that falls off into the canyon of Harrington Creek. You will find any number of good picnic sites in the meadow.

Retrace your steps to the upper meadow, watching for the path that crosses the pasture about halfway up to the hilltop. Turn left on this path that heads west, descending gradually down a ridge to pick up a service road. You can follow this road downhill for a short distance and then retrace your steps uphill.

This winding road through a pleasant succession of woods and clearings gives you a chance to enjoy the variety of oaks, madrones, firs and redwoods along the way. You can see the 4- and 5-foot stumps of redwoods cut in early logging and compare them with the sizable second growth.

In a half hour you come out on a hillside clearing below a ridge and above a wooded canyon that drains into Harrington Creek. Around a bend are the parking area and your car.

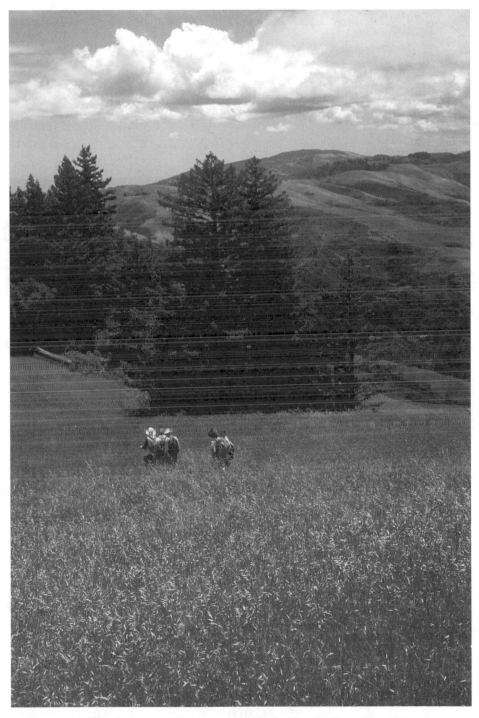

Looking toward Black Mountain from a meadow in La Honda Open Space Preserve

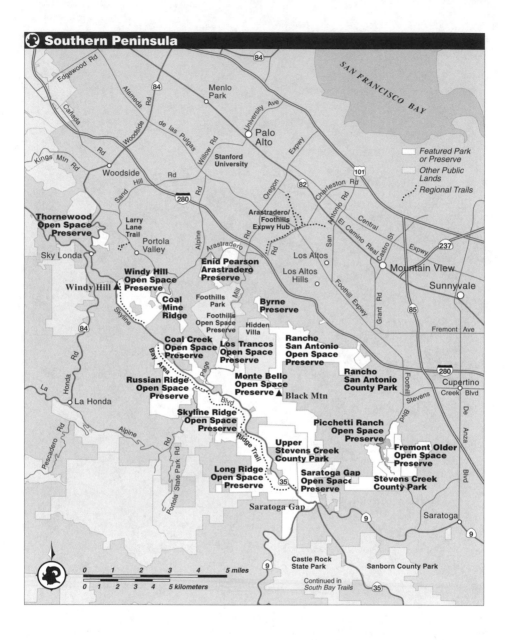

Southern Peninsula

◆ Southern Peninsula ◆

Highway 84 to Saratoga Gap and Highways 9 and 85

A vast complex of public land in parks and preserves now encompasses much of the Skyline area on either side of the crest of the Santa Cruz Mountains from SkyLonda/Highway 84 south to Saratoga Gap/Highway 9. More than 13,520 acres of conifer forests, oak/madrone woodlands, grasslands, canyons, and streamsides are open to trail users.

These public lands and the trails therein now extend east to more than 5400 acres of regional, county and city parks in the foothills and on the urban Bay plain. An additional 14,500 acres of state and county parks lie southwest in the forest parks along Pescadero Creek—Portola Redwoods State Park and Pescadero, Memorial, and Sam McDonald county parks—and on Little Butano Creek, Butano State Park.

A network of trails in these mountainside preserves and parks offers an outstanding variety of trips, from a short outing along the ridges to an invigorating day-long trip into deep canyons. Overnight trips connecting the Bayside with the Coastside are now possible. A hiker can stay at a hostel at Hidden Villa or a backpack camp on Monte Bello Ridge en route from the cities by the Bay to the parks by the ocean. Trail connections now exist via Ward Road, the Skyline-to-the-Sea Trail and the new Basin Trail to the county and state forest preserves. Vacationers can camp in Portola Redwoods State Park and the Pescadero Creek County Park complex and then continue to Big Basin Redwoods and Butano state parks and on to the Coastside via routes along Waddell and Gazos creeks. These links make possible vacation-sized expeditions through the Santa Cruz Mountains from trailheads only a half hour from the Peninsula's urban plain.

Hikers, equestrians, and bicyclists can now follow the Bay Area Ridge Trail for 17 miles along the crest of the Santa Cruz Mountains from Windy Hill to Saratoga Gap. When the 0.7-mile gap in this trail is closed, it will make an unbroken trail along this section of the Southern Peninsula Skyline. South from Saratoga Gap, the Ridge Trail route continues another 6 miles through Santa Clara County parks on the east and Castle Rock State Park on the west.

◆ Mountainside Parks and Preserves ◆
on the Skyline Ridge

Thornewood Open Space Preserve

Thornewood Preserve came to the Midpeninsula Regional Open Space District as a gift. The property, now 109 acres, was developed by Julian and Edna Thorne in the 1920s, and was adjacent to the much larger August Schilling estate. Both properties were part of the Mexican Rancho Cañada de Raimundo, which was purchased by lumberman Dennis Martin in 1846.

The Thornes built a summer house designed in quite unusual style by Gardner Dailey (who also designed the home on the Phleger Estate and the ballroom at Filoli). After Julian's death, Edna maintained the elaborate gardens with the aid of her head groundsman, François Richard, to whom she gave a 2-acre life estate. Mrs. Thorne bequeathed the remainder of the property to the Sierra Club Foundation, stipulating that it should be kept as a "nature preserve." Finding it impossible to maintain, the Sierra Club Foundation donated the property to MROSD in 1978.

By 1982 the District had acquired a part of the adjoining former Schilling property, including a small lake, and had leased the house to a private party. Today, the area outside the leasehold and the life estate are open to the public. An 8-car parking lot and a small picnic area lie just inside the gate, and a short trail leads to Schilling Lake. Occasionally the historic house is open to the public for docent-guided tours, date and time varying. Call MROSD for details.

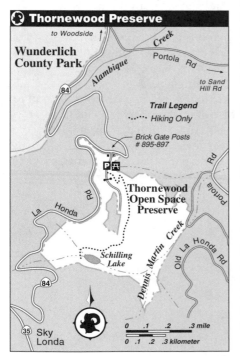

Jurisdiction: Midpeninsula Regional Open Space District: 650-691-1200

Facilities: Trails for hikers, equestrians, and bicyclists

Rules: Open dawn to dusk; dogs on leash

Maps: MROSD map *Thornewood OSP*, USGS *Woodside*

How to Get There: From I-280 take Woodside Rd. (Hwy 84) southwest 4 miles through the town of Woodside. After passing junction with Portola Rd. (on left), Woodside Rd. becomes La Honda Rd. and you continue on it uphill for about a mile to brick gateposts 895 and 897 on your left.

A Trip through the Woods to a Historic Lake

A short, shady trail, just right for children, winds downhill to reach Schilling Lake, a remnant of August Schilling's property.

Distance: 1.4 miles round trip

Time: 40 minutes

Elevation Change: 80' loss

Starting from the small parking lot inside Thornewood's brick gateposts, walk 100 feet south along the driveway (which leads to the private leaseholding) and take the trail on your left. You meander in and out of a thick, second-growth forest and the cleared gardens, abandoned some thirty years ago. The trail winds downhill, sometimes on the remnants of an old road, once part of the Schilling spice king's estate. After 0.7-mile you reach the 1-acre lake, held back by a small dam and once home of some beautiful white swans. Try to imagine this as a centerpiece of Mr. Schilling's extensive gardens, which once featured a redwood temple, a Stonehenge-like pergola and even fake rocks made of wood, wire, and plaster.

On the south side of the lake an old trail leads down to Dennis Martin Road, but goes no farther. When you have enjoyed this woodland setting, return to your car uphill having glimpsed a relic of a former country estate.

Windy Hill Open Space Preserve

This 1308-acre preserve includes the two bald knobs of Windy Hill, the long, grassy ridge extending from the Skyline to the floor of Portola Valley and many forested acres south of a private inholding. The upper grasslands of Windy Hill, familiar landmarks on the Midpeninsula mountains, stand out against the adjacent forested slopes. We watch Windy Hill from the Bay plain as it turns green in spring and as it is occasionally whitened by winter snows. In summer the wind and fog from the ocean sweep over this bare hill to give it the name it has been known by for 75 years or more.

Once part of an early Mexican land grant belonging to Maximo Martinez, known as El Corte de Madera ("the wood-cutting place"), these lands were also used for cattle grazing and hayfields. The Brown Ranch stood on the site of today's picnic area on Skyline Boulevard, and the Orton Ranch was located north at the head of Spring Ridge. Beautiful second growth forests now clothe many slopes and fill the canyons of the preserve.

In 1979 the Peninsula Open Space Trust began a series of land purchases that provided major support for the acquisition of this preserve. Located between clusters of county parks and MROSD preserves north and south along both sides of the Skyline ridge, Windy Hill Open Space Preserve is part of a vast chain of public ridgelands on the Peninsula.

Approximately 15 miles of trails traverse Windy Hill's grassy slopes, climb its steep ridges and follow its stream canyons. From the main entrance on Skyline Boulevard, where a rustic fence encloses a picnic area, you can climb to the summit of Windy Hill for a 360-degree view of ocean, Bay, cities, and distant mountains. Or you can take one of three long ridge trails that descend to Portola Valley, and return on a trail up another ridge. With the addition of the Betsy Crowder and the Meadow trails, two short loop trips are accessible from the Portola Road and Alpine Road entrances.

Fund raising headed by POST brought donations from local citizens to the Windy Hill Endowment Fund to build the 8-mile Windy Hill Loop Trail. These funds also helped construct the Anniversary Trail up and around the Windy Hill knobs. The Windy Hill Loop Trail, one of the longest trips, was laid out and constructed by the volunteers, MROSD staff, and the California Conservation Corps.

Kite-flying on Windy Hill is superb, though the wind will test the sturdiness of your kite. Others who take advantage of the ridgetop breezes include hang gliders

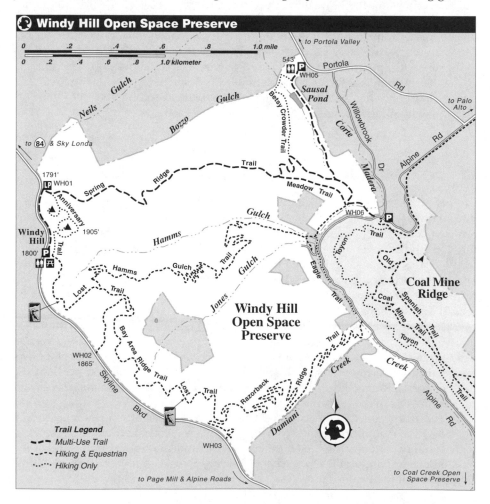

and parasailors and those who operate their non-motorized model gliders on Windy Hill with permits from MROSD.

Jurisdiction: Midpeninsula Regional Open Space District: 650-691-1200

Facilities: Trails for hikers and equestrians; bicyclists on Spring Ridge and Fence-line trails only; picnic area

Rules: Open dawn to dusk; dogs on leash on the Anniversary, Spring Ridge, and Hamm's Gulch trails only

Maps: MROSD brochure *Windy Hill*, USGS topo *Mindego Hill*

How to Get There: (1) Take Woodside/La Honda Rd. (Hwy 84) or Page Mill Rd. to Skyline Blvd. The main entrance is on the east side of Skyline Blvd. 2.3 miles south of La Honda Rd. or 4.9 miles north of Page Mill Rd. Two other entrances north and south of the main entrance are marked by brown pipe gates and hiking stiles. (2) From I-280 take Alpine Rd. south 2.9 miles, turn right (north) on Portola Rd. and go 0.8 miles to preserve entrance on west side of Portola Rd. (WH05); (3) Alpine Rd. entrances: Take Alpine Rd. south past Portola Rd. to corner of Alpine and Willowbrook roads. Park on north side of Alpine Rd. and walk up road to trail entrances on right side: (a) Spring Ridge Trail and Meadow trails entrance (south end) (WH06) and northeast connection to Hamms Gulch Trail, 0.1 mile beyond parking area; (b) Main Hamms Gulch Trail entrance (WH04), 0.3 mile farther at stone gates of Rancho Corte Madera; (c) Razorback Ridge Trail entrance, 0.6 mile still farther up road.

BETSY CROWDER TRAIL LOOP

Through filtered light of oak woodlands, climb to a memorial bench honoring a former MROSD director.

Distance: 1.4-mile loop

Time: ¾ hour

Elevation Change: 200' gain

Walk uphill from the Portola Road parking area (entrance #2) past the gated service road on your left and step into a shady glen from which the trail takes off uphill. En route you will zig-zag gently upward through mixed woodland where toyon bushes and light pink-blossomed buckeye shade blue-flowered hound's-tongue and clumps of low-growing, magenta Indian warriors in early spring. Occasional glimpses south through the trees bring views of the long sweep of Black Mountain and the trace of Page Mill Road climbing toward Skyline Boulevard.

Upon emerging from the forest you are in open grassland, lush green and dotted with wildflowers in spring and tawny gold in summer. Here beneath a fringe of tall live oaks is a bench honoring Betsy Crowder. It overlooks the town of Portola Valley where Betsy lived for many years and where she served on town committees. Portola Valley is in Ward 6 of the Midpeninsula Regional Open Space District, which Betsy represented on its board of directors for 11 years. She was also a co-author of this book.

Betsy hiked to the top of Windy Hill several times a week and was enthusiastic about this new trail. Her tragic death in September 2000 was a great loss to her family, her many friends, and her constituents. It is very fitting that the District chose to name this trail to honor her. You too can pause here to enjoy this beautiful view she loved and worked hard to protect.

Continuing uphill around a few bends, bear left on the Spring Ridge Trail, descend to the Lower Spring Ridge Trail, and turn left again. Shortly you reach Sausal Pond nestled in a grove of trees. With brightly plumed wood ducks in winter and deep-throated frogs croaking in spring, this pond bears special protection. At some future time an observation deck may be constructed. In the meantime, the pond and surrounding banks are off-limits.

Bear right after going through the District gate to return to the parking area.

SUMMIT HIKE
ON THE ANNIVERSARY TRAIL

A short climb to a top-of-the-world view of the Bay Area from Windy Hill's bald knobs.

Distance: 1.4 miles round trip

Time: ¾ hour

Elevation Change: 127′ gain

Leave the left (north) side of the Skyline Boulevard picnic area on the trail that celebrates the 10th anniversary of Windy Hill's purchase. This is an ideal place to

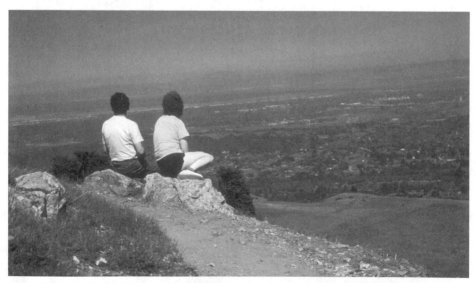

From Windy Hill, the Bay Area lies before you

take your out-of-town visitors, if the day is clear. A climb to the top will orient them with fixes on some Bay Area peaks—Black Mountain, Mt. Hamilton, Mt. Diablo, and Mt. Tamalpais. West lies the Pacific Ocean; north, east, and south are San Francisco Bay and its surrounding cities. The Anniversary Trail continues to the north roadside parking area at the gate (WH01) at the top of the Spring Ridge Trail.

The trip to the summit of Windy Hill is for hikers only, but equestrians and bicyclists can get breathtaking coastal views from the Fence-line Trail, which takes off from the Anniversary Trail less than 0.1 mile north of the picnic area. This route is a broad, unsurfaced, disked 0.3-mile trail that rounds the west shoulder of Windy Hill, and continues north to the top of the Spring Ridge Trail at Skyline Boulevard. This trail and the Anniversary Trail are part of the 3.5 mile Bay Area Ridge Trail route through Windy Hill Open Space Preserve.

SEE MAP
ON PAGE
136

A WINDY HILL LOOP TRIP

A challenging loop traverses two of the preserve's three ridges, a treat not to be missed.

Distance: 8-mile loop; hikers and equestrians only

Time: 4½ hours

Elevation Change: 1120' loss

This spectacular trip starts from the picnic area at the main Skyline Boulevard entrance and follows the route of the Bay Area Ridge Trail south. Take the signed Ridge Trail connector route on the right and contour 0.4 mile around a low knoll to the Lost Trail/Hamms Gulch Trail junction. Bear right there to round a chaparral-covered shoulder of the ridge for 0.2 mile. Here a trail on your right comes in from Skyline. Cross it and step onto an old road renamed the Lost Trail. On this trail, rediscovered by the volunteers who helped build this loop, you go around bends and into hollows below the crest of the Santa Cruz Mountains. Many viewpoint windows open up through the trees to reveal the valley below.

Under madrones and oaks and across rivulets, this trail continues for 1.5 miles to the top of the ridge between Fitzpatrick and Damiani creeks, where a short connector trail ascends to gate on Skyline Boulevard, the south end of the Ridge Trail in this preserve. Here, you turn left, to begin a series of downhill zigzags on the well-graded, 2.3-mile Razorback Ridge Trail. Along the sides of small ravines and out onto shoulders of the ridge, the trail drops steadily downward under a high oak and madrone canopy. You may find deer quietly making their way over the leafy forest floor.

At the lower end of the trail you join a dirt road and cross a bridge to Alpine Road. About 0.3 mile along the road, look for the Eagle Trail beside Corte Madera Creek, which you follow for 0.3 mile downstream. Cool and shaded in summer, it leads to a bridge over Corte Madera Creek at the stone-pillared, gated entrance to Rancho Corte Madera, a private inholding.

Go across the old bridge with the moss-covered stones, then immediately go right and step onto the Hamms Gulch Trail. In a few feet you cross a wooden bridge over Jones Gulch. About 300 feet uphill from this bridge is a foot trail that meanders above Corte Madera Creek to join the Lower Spring Ridge Trail. However, for this trip on the Windy Hill Loop, continue uphill on the Hamms Gulch Trail, built on the alignment of the old Brown Ranch Road. It takes today's trail users through magnificent oak, madrone and fir forests. About a mile up the trail, at a break in the forest, you'll find a bench erected by MROSD rangers. From here you look across the wooded canyon of Hamms Gulch to the grasslands of Spring Ridge.

Continuing uphill, the trail then climbs the south side of Hamms Gulch. On the side of this gulch, immense Douglas firs, some at least 6 feet in diameter, tower over the trail, fortunately having escaped the logging done early in the 20th century. The trail skirts around the trees and out of the forest, and then beyond a few bends you turn right on the trail that leads back to your starting point at the picnic area, the old Brown Ranch site.

SEE MAP
ON PAGE
136

TO THE TOP OF SPRING RIDGE

The round-the-compass views reward you for a vigorous, long ascent to Windy Hill's heights.

Distance: 7 miles round trip on Spring Ridge Trail; 9 miles on loop trip returning via Hamms Gulch Trail (hikers and equestrians only)

Time: 4 hours round trip on Spring Ridge Trail; 5 hours on loop trip

Elevation Change: 1260' gain

The long, grassy ridge rising to Windy Hill's summit provides delightful short trips to large, tree-bordered meadows, and serves as one leg of a long loop trip from the valley floor to the Skyline Ridge and back. The trail follows an old ranch road right up the spine of bald Spring Ridge. The views from this expanse of high grasslands are superb. Start this uphill trip early and carry plenty of water on hot days.

From the main Portola Road entrance take the short trail to a left turn on the Lower Spring Ridge Trail, which goes beside the little reservoir where Sausal Creek is impounded. Or, continue through the shady glade on the Betsy Crowder Trail, making the trip about 0.2 mile shorter. For the less vigorous, the glade is a pleasant site for a picnic under lofty oaks.

At the Spring Ridge/Betsy Crowder trail intersection, your route up the ridge turns right and begins a series of steep rises and short, flat stretches. Curving left, then right, and ever upward, this old road keeps to the open slope. At the edges of wide meadows, clumps of oaks interspersed with maples and spring flowering buckeyes fill the ravines.

After about 1.8 miles, the trail arcs right, then left and levels off a bit—an opportunity to look for bluebird houses on posts in the grasslands. In this area are the springs that gave the ridge its name, and which watered the cattle that grazed here for many years. Uphill is a clump of Monterey cypresses that formerly sheltered the Orton ranchhouse. Only a few old fruit trees and a jumble of fallen logs remain to remind today's trail users of these early settlers. The wide trail curves north above the ranch site, makes a last gentle ascent, and then levels off north of Windy Hill to reach the Skyline Boulevard roadside parking at gate WH01. Here you join the Bay Area Ridge Trail, which runs south through the preserve for 3.5 miles to its present termination at gate WH03.

To return to the valley floor, the shortest route (and the bicyclist route) is back down the Spring Ridge Trail. However, if hikers want a gentler grade and a different way back, they can follow the Anniversary Trail south from here up and over the Windy Hill knobs to the picnic area (see Summit Hike on the Anniversary Trail). From there a 0.6 mile trail leads east to the Windy Hill Loop (see A Windy Hill Loop Trip, above). At the first junction, turn left and drop down into Douglas fir forest on the Hamms Gulch Trail, which you will follow for 2.4 miles back to the valley. About 300 feet before reaching the foot bridge over a small creek, you become aware of the paved driveway across the creek on your right leading to the private residences at Rancho Corte Madera. Then on your left, a foot trail (closed to bicycles), part of the Portola Valley town trails system, meanders above Corte Madera Creek and winds through riparian vegetation to join the south branch of the Spring Ridge Trail. Turn left on it to reach your starting place at the Portola Road entrance. A right turn would take you to Alpine Road and limited roadside parking near the corner of Willowbrook Drive.

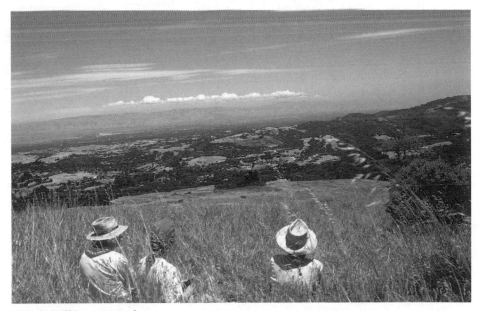

Windy Hill in summer dress

Coal Creek Open Space Preserve and Upper Alpine Road

This crescent-shaped, 493-acre preserve is almost surrounded by other Midpeninsula Regional Open Space Preserves—Russian Ridge west across the Skyline, Monte Bello and Skyline Ridge south, and Windy Hill less than a mile north. Skyline Boulevard forms its west boundary and Upper Alpine Road lies along its south side.

Three lovely meadows lying just below the Skyline ridge are central attractions of this preserve. Their flowery slopes invite springtime outings. Groves of handsome oaks and madrones fringing their grasslands are right for summertime picnics—easy, short walks from Skyline parking, or longer walks up the hill from Upper Alpine Road. Birds, deer, bobcats, and cottontail rabbits flourish in these meadows and forests. Mountain lions have been reported here also.

Two old roads, now part of the preserve's trail system, link these meadows, one in the north and two in the south. Historic Crazy Pete's Road and the Valley View Trail drop down from Skyline Boulevard and traverse oak-and-madrone woodlands above the preserve's steep, forested lower hillsides to end at Upper Alpine Road. This dirt road, closed to motor vehicles, links the two arms of Coal Creek Preserve, and makes a much-needed off-road hiking, riding, and bicycling route between Portola Valley and Skyline.

There was indeed a "Crazy Pete"—Peter O'Shaunessey, a hermit. He was a large man with unkempt beard and hair. He was known as a very strong man who cut trees in this area in the early 1900s. Thought to be a bit "tetched," he spent his last days in the old Agnew Asylum.

Jurisdiction: Midpeninsula Regional Open Space District: 650-691-1200

Facilities: Trails for hikers, equestrians, and bicyclists; dogs on leash

Rules: Open dawn to dusk

Maps: MROSD brochure *South Skyline Region*, USGS topo *Mindego Hill*

How to Get There: Take Woodside/La Honda Rd. (Hwy 84) or Page Mill Rd. to Skyline Blvd. On the east side of Skyline Blvd. are: (1) north entrance at Crazy Petes Rd., 6.1 miles south of Hwy 84, limited parking, stay clear of mailboxes; (2) south entrance at Caltrans Vista Point, 8.9 miles south of Hwy 84, 1.2 mile north of Page Mill Rd. Alternately, (3) take Alpine Rd. from I-280 south for about 6 miles to limited roadside parking at intersection with Willowbrook Rd. No parking at upper gate where road is closed.(4) Take Page Mill Rd. 8 miles south from I-280 to Monte Bello parking lot and take unnamed trail 0.5 mile southwest, paralleling Page Mill Rd., to gate MB05 to reach un-numbered, gated entrance to Upper Alpine Rd. on northwest side of Page Mill Rd.

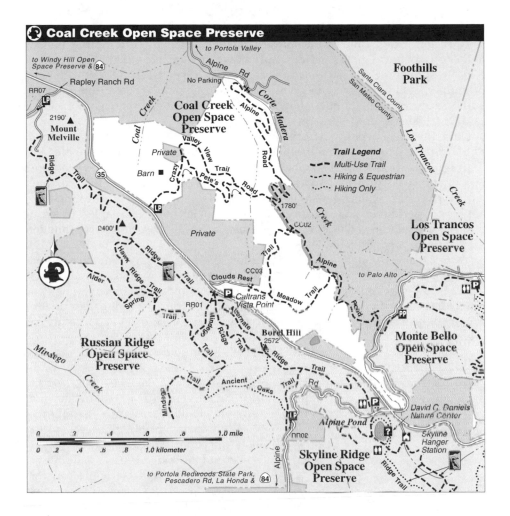

Coal Creek Open Space Preserve

to Windy Hill Open
Space Preserve & 84

to Portola Valley

Foothills
Park

Rapley Ranch Rd

RR07

No Parking

Alpine Rd

Santa Clara County
San Mateo County

Coal Creek

2190'
Mount
Melville

Coal Creek
Open Space
Preserve

Alpine

Corte Madera

Los Trancos

Valley

View

Private

Road

Trail Legend

Creek

Ridge Trail

Barn

35

Crazy

Trail

Pete's

Road

Multi-Use Trail

Hiking & Equestrian

Hiking Only

1780'

Los Trancos
Open Space
Preserve

2400'

Private

Creek

CC02

Ridge

Hawk Ridge Trail

Alder

Trail

Clouds Rest

CC03

Trail

Alpine

Meadow

Trail

Road

to Palo Alto

Monte Bello
Open Space
Preserve

Spring

Trail

RR01

Caltrans
Vista Point

Alternate

Minder

Ridge

Trail

Russian Ridge
Open Space
Preserve

Minsego

Creek

Minder

Trail

Ridge

Trail

Borel Hill
2572'

Ridge

Trail

Ancient

Oaks

Trail

Rd

David C. Daniels
Nature Center

0   .2   .4   .6   .8   1.0 mile

0   .2   .4   .6   .8   1.0 kilometer

to Portola Redwoods State Park,
Pescadero Rd, La Honda & 84

Alpine Pond

2000'

Alpine

Skyline Ridge
Open Space
Preserve

Skyline
Hanger
Station

Ridge Trail

OVER THE MEADOW
AND THROUGH THE WOODS

SEE MAP
ABOVE

Traverse the preserve's southernmost meadow and a historic road to a leafy streamside and a sunny knoll. Bicyclists enjoy making a loop through the preserve trails before returning down Upper Alpine Road to the valley.

Distance: 4-mile loop

Time: 2 hours

Elevation Change: 400' gain

Starting from the Caltrans Vista Point on Skyline Boulevard, walk north along the road 200 yards to the first driveway on the right. Take this unpaved road, the

Cloud's Rest Trail, downhill past one private driveway to the preserve entrance at MROSD gate CC03. Under wide-spreading live-oak trees you reach a trail junction at the top of a broad grassy meadow surmounted by a grove of immense madrone trees. In springtime this meadow is a beautiful swath of green, flecked with blues of lupines, gold of poppies, and pinks of checker bloom. (On an autumn day the authors saw a four-point buck standing in this meadow. Although such a sight is rare, you often see does along preserve trails.)

From the trail junction at the top of the meadow, the Cloud's Rest Trail descends to the left, the return route on this loop trip. Now, however, you take the Meadow Trail right (east) and slightly uphill through a forest of moss-covered madrones and gnarled oaks growing among large sandstone outcrops. Then the trail veers left (northeast) and emerges in another large ridgetop meadow surrounded by oaks, both deciduous and evergreen, Douglas firs and big-leaf maples. In spring big, yellow-blossomed daisies called mule ears brighten these grasslands, and late into summer poppies bloom here.

After 0.8 mile through woods and meadows you reach Upper Alpine Road just below the culvert that carries a small creek under the road. You are now about half a mile below Page Mill Road. Turn left, downhill, on unpaved, Upper Alpine Road following the west edge of Corte Madera Creek Canyon. The trail passes under a canopy of deciduous black oaks where you find shade in summer and brightly colored leaves in fall.

About 0.5 mile down the canyon on the left is the gate to Coal Creek Preserve's middle entrance. Note it for the return trip, but go 0.2 mile farther, watching for the gate uphill on your left, marked with an MROSD sign. Leave Upper Alpine Road here and step over the stile to this historic road, now used as a trail. In 200 yards you cross a bridge over a boulder-strewn creek. Ferns, moss and other moisture-loving plants line the banks of pools on either side of this bridge.

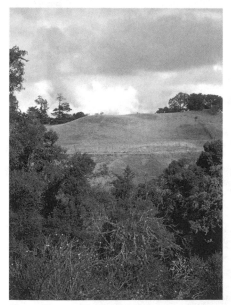

Beyond the bridge, beneath wide-spreading madrones is a veritable thimbleberry terrace extending to a Y-shaped trail junction. Here Crazy Pete's Road arcs left and the Valley View Trail goes right. This trip takes the Valley View Trail and returns on Crazy Pete's Road. In woods of live oak and madrone, the trail narrows and curves around the mountain, with views north and east over the canyon of Corte Madera Creek. In about 15 minutes you come to a little knoll in a clearing that catches the sun in midday.

Gaining altitude now, the 0.5-mile trail becomes a narrow, uneven path trending left through a miniature forest of long-leaved, lavender-flowered yerba santa. Shortly before reaching a gate you swing left on Crazy Pete's Road for the return leg of your journey.

From Upper Alpine Road

This 0.7-mile service road climbs through oak woodlands where vistas, framed by the trees, open up to the east. Passing an open hillside, where a few private homes sit outside the preserve, you now descend around a big curve and into the shade of the madrone woods. At the Y-shaped junction you meet the Valley View Trail again, and turn right to cross the bridge and rejoin Upper Alpine Road.

To finish this loop trip, first bear right for 0.2 mile to the next trail entrance at gate CC02. Go through the gate and begin a steady climb to the high grasslands on the Cloud's Rest Trail. This trail may have been a construction road for the high-tension wire tower you pass here. Beside the trail in spring, blue irises and purple lupines bloom, and later wild roses flower.

At the Meadow Trail junction swing right, go through gate CC03 and return uphill through the woods to your car at the Vista Point. From here, looking beyond the meadows and forests of your hike, you see the Midpeninsula cities below, less than 10 miles from the many preserves along the Skyline ridge greenbelt.

A SHORT TRIP
TO A PROTECTED MEADOW

Another route to Coal Creek's trails and sheltered grasslands above the urban scene.

Distance: 2.5 miles round trip to knoll

Time: 1 hour round trip to meadow; 1.25 hours
round trip to knoll

Elevation Change: 200' loss to meadow; 370' loss to knoll

With a sketch book, your favorite flower guide or bird book, and a snack in your daypack, start at the northern entrance to Coal Creek Preserve, 0.5 mile north of the Vista Point. There is limited parking where Crazy Pete's Road intersects Skyline Boulevard.

Walk along Crazy Petes Road less than 0.5 mile to a point on your left where you can see a big old barn (closed to the public) in a sloping meadow. One of only a few extant barns, this one serves as a storage shed for MROSD rangers. In spring, poppies, blue-eyed grass, and tall lupines fill this meadow. Here too, are the headwaters of Coal Creek, which flows down a steep canyon to join Corte Madera Creek on the west side of Upper Alpine Road outside the preserve boundary.

You can walk 0.25 mile farther along Crazy Pete's Road and continue to the protected knoll on the Valley View Trail, described in the first trip, Over the Meadow and Through the Woods, where the only sounds are those of birds in the trees, or possibly deer in the forest.

AN ALTERNATE ROUTE TO SKYLINE ON HISTORIC UPPER ALPINE ROAD

Follow a tree-shaded route beside the canyon of Corte Madera Creek. This section of Alpine Road, now closed to motorized vehicles, is a quiet, winding way up a wooded mountainside where no traffic intrudes.

Distance: 2.5 miles one way

Time: 1¾ hours on foot

Elevation Change: 1000′ gain

Since there is room for only two cars at the southern gate to Upper Alpine Road, this trip entails a 2.5-mile walk or bike ride uphill on paved Upper Alpine Road to reach the gate at the unpaved section. Hikers may prefer to park on Skyline Boulevard and do the trip as a continuation of the Over the Meadow and Through the Woods trip, described above, by continuing beyond gate CC02 on Upper Alpine Road for 1 mile downhill, making a 3.8-mile round trip.

Alpine Road gets its name not from the heights of the Santa Cruz Mountains, which are not really alpine, but from a pine tree, *El Pino*, (probably a Douglas fir) which grew beside the Pescadero Trail to the coast. The area near the intersection of the present Alpine Road and Portola State Park Road (3.1 miles southwest of Skyline Boulevard), called "El Pino" by Spanish Californians, became "Alpine." The name was first attached to the road west of Skyline, built in 1879. The part of the road you are traversing, built in 1894, was for some time called the Martinez grade, after the owner of Rancho Corte de Madera.

Before you start uphill, you have a scenic drive up Corte Madera canyon, as Alpine Road leaves the open valley. The road beside the creek makes it way beside the maples, alders, and bays that shade its winding course. Wood ferns clothe its steep banks. When the maples turn golden, this is an enchanting drive.

On the opposite side of the road from the creek, the sheer canyon wall rises to Coal Mine Ridge, where you may glimpse thin veins of coal along the road cuts. Low-grade coal was once mined from this ridge.

About 3 miles from the Alpine/Portola Road intersection, just past Joaquin Road, you come to a fork in the road where a heavy metal gate bars vehicular traffic. Go through the stile on the right and start up unpaved Alpine Road. San Mateo County owns and maintains this road, but it runs through some lands owned by MROSD and private lands border its east side.

At the first bend you cross the creek running through a culvert. Frequent landslides on the road a bit higher up produce some interesting loop trails around them. This wide trail with an easy gradient is popular for bicycle riding.

Whether you take this road in winter after the first rains freshen the foliage and the cold turns leaves to gold, in the spring with a burst of pale new leaves and flowers along the way, or at some less dramatic time of year, this historic road offers a good workout. The uphill route, being slower, allows time to savor the ambience of tall trees meeting overhead and new views opening up at each turn.

In late fall or early winter, you will find that the shrubby willows that line the creek are yellow. The tall maples along the creek are golden, and other maples make bright splashes of color here and there on the hillsides where they mark springs that give them the moisture they need.

From the canyon the road climbs to a flat on a ridge covered with deciduous black oaks. Under the umbrella of this grove the autumn light takes on a golden hue from the yellow of their leaves. Many deer inhabit these woods, as you can see from their tracks on the road. In fall and winter, bucks, does, and the fawns born the preceding spring stay together, and you can see the hoof prints of these family groups where they cross the road to the creek below.

From this flat the road continues up the ridge on an easy grade. In late fall and early winter madrones on the hills are heavy with red berries, and thick-clustered toyon berries are accented against their dark-green leaves. Black-headed Oregon juncos feast on wild cherries hanging below shiny leaves.

MROSD's Coal Creek Open Space Preserve borders Upper Alpine Road to the west almost up to the Page Mill Road intersection. Trails from Upper Alpine Road into Coal Creek Preserve, described in the first two trips in this section, make good loop trips from the Alpine Road trailhead, especially favored by bicyclists. You can extend your trip in Monte Bello Open Space Preserve by taking the unnamed trail across Page Mill Road at gate MB05. See the chapter on Monte Bello Preserve for possibilities. If you take the trip to the pond, you will find a charming spot for a picnic before retracing your route down this historic road.

Los Trancos Open Space Preserve

There is an enticing variety of trails over meadows and into canyons in this 274-acre preserve. A self-guided fault trail explains earthquake phenomena, and a hike out to the far end of the preserve offers magnificent Bay views. As a joint project of the Midpeninsula Regional Open Space District and Foothill College, geologists interpret for you the evidence of earthquake activity along a self-guided trail through an area changed by the 1906 earthquake and earlier ones.

Docents lead walks along the San Andreas Fault Trail on a regular schedule, another good way to learn about the effects of fault movement. After you have completed one of these explanatory trips, walk up to the western ridge of the parking area and look straight down the rift valleys. You will sense the awesome force of the constant movement of the segments of the earth's skin as they float on top of the deeper mantle of semi-molten rock.

Jurisdiction: Midpeninsula Regional Open Space District: 650-691-1200

Facilities: Self-guiding earthquake-fault trail and trails for hikers and equestrians

Rules: Open dawn to dusk; no dogs; all trails for hikers only, except the Page Mill Trail, open to equestrians also

Maps: MROSD brochure *San Andreas Fault Trail*, USGS topo *Mindego Hill*

How to Get There: From I-280, take Page Mill Rd. south for 7 miles and park at preserve entrance on right.

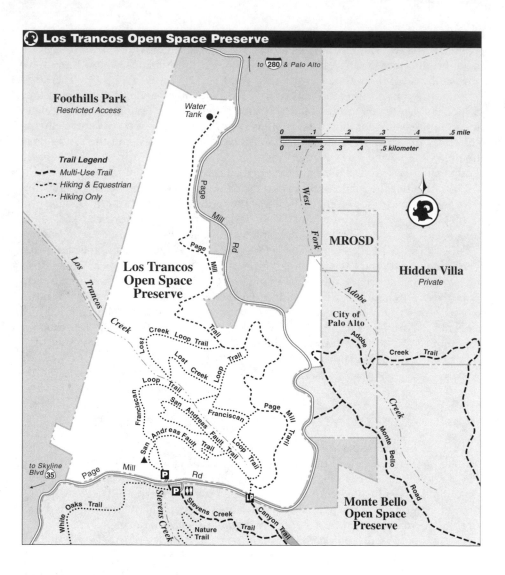

Los Trancos Open Space Preserve

to [280] & Palo Alto

Foothills Park
Restricted Access

Water
Tank

0   .1   .2   .3   .4   .5 mile
0   .1   .2   .3   .4   .5 kilometer

Trail Legend
Multi-Use Trail
Hiking & Equestrian
Hiking Only

West   Fork

MROSD

Los Trancos
Open Space
Preserve

Page   Mill   Rd

Los   Trancos   Creek

Hidden Villa
Private

Adobe

City of
Palo Alto

Adobe   Creek   Trail

Lost   Creek   Loop   Trail

Lost   Creek   Loop   Trail

Loop   Trail

Franciscan   Loop   Trail

San   Andreas   Fault   Trail

Franciscan

Page   Mill   Trail

Creek

Monte   Bello   Road

San   Andreas   Fault   Trail

to Skyline
Blvd [35]

Page   Mill   Rd

P

P

White   Oaks   Trail

Stevens   Creek

Stevens   Creek

Nature
Trail

LP

Canyon   Trail

Trail

Monte Bello
Open Space
Preserve

SAN ANDREAS FAULT TRAIL

Distance: 1.5-mile loop

Time: 1+ hour

Elevation Change: 240' loss

A self-guided trail through a section of the fault zone shows you many signs of the violent movements of the earth in quakes of past centuries. With the District's information-packed brochure in hand, follow the yellow markers and learn all about plate movements, sag ponds, benches, and scarps. Though it is only a short walk, you will want to spend at least an hour on this fascinating loop trail learning how the grinding action along the fault line affects the land.

On the docent-led trips you will have an informative, two-hour tour of the nine stations that explain the physical effects of one of the world's longest and most active faults.

LOOP TRIP ON FRANCISCAN AND LOST CREEK TRAILS

Descending into the cool, shady forest of the preserve's north-facing slope, this trip combines the Franciscan and Lost Creek Loop trails.

Distance: 2.4-mile loop

Time: 1½ hours

Elevation Change: 400' loss

Start from the parking lot on the San Andreas Fault Trail, and then turn left onto the Franciscan Loop Trail. As you cross the meadow on a clear day, you can see straight up to the Crystal Springs Lakes filling the San Andreas Fault Zone. Your trail soon descends into the woods under massive canyon oaks. In the fall, deciduous oaks and big-leaf maples brighten the forest as their leaves turn golden.

You round the hill to cross a bridge over Los Trancos Creek, and then a short climb brings you to an open flat and a trail junction. Here you leave the Franciscan Loop Trail and begin the Lost Creek Loop. Keep to the left and go up a little rise through the woods. At the top of the rise the trail turns down to follow a ridge into the canyon of Los Trancos Creek.

Here and there firs tower above the oaks and you can see a scattering of these tall trees across the canyon as the trail descends toward Los Trancos Creek, mossy and fern-lined. Wild currant bushes show their pink blossoms very early in spring; later, mission bells, false Solomon's seal, star flower, trillium, and wood fern grace the hillside.

As the creek drops into a narrow gorge, the trail veers away, traversing the hillside to follow a minor tributary. In the shade of large bays and oaks your trail climbs to a ridgetop. For a short stretch you join the Page Mill Trail on its way to the north meadow, then you turn right (west) on the Lost Creek Loop Trail, zigzag left and right again up to the flat where it completes its loop.

From the flat take the Franciscan Trail. Bear left then veer right, following the trail down into a glade of bay trees. As you circle a low hill, you pass a scattering of great craggy limestone outcrops and some ancient oaks that probably lost limbs in the violent shaking of the 1906 earthquake.

Ascending gradually to more open country, you reach the grasslands near the start of your trip and turn left on the Fault Trail to return to the parking lot. From early spring to summer this upper meadow is a bright exuberance of flowers. By fall the meadow has dried, leaving pale beige, gauzy-textured grasses with accents of dark seed pods from the small lavender and pink flowers of dwarf flax.

PAGE MILL TRAIL TO THE NORTH MEADOW

SEE MAP ON PAGE 148

An easy trail along open countryside parallels Page Mill Road.

Distance: 4.2 miles round trip

Time: 2 hours

Elevation Change: 400' loss

On the north side of Page Mill Road, east of the main parking lot and across from Monte Bello Preserve's Canyon Trail, is a stile for hiker and equestrian access to this trail. Immediately turn right on this 2+-mile trail, which keeps high above the canyon but below Page Mill Road. The trail turns briefly down into the woods, where you can examine a most remarkable stand of huge, ancient bay laurel trees, many with multiple trunks. These trees provide deep and welcome shade on a hot day.

Curving right around a hill east of the Lost Creek Loop Trail junction, the trail comes out of the trees and emerges onto a series of rolling, grassy meadows that overlook the Bay. Canyon oaks and madrones rim these hilltop meadows, their dark foliage contrasting with the new light green grass in spring and the golden dry grass of summer and fall. Remains of an old orchard dot the hillside. Just short of gate LT01 opening onto Page Mill Road, you turn sharp left (south) and cross a little depression before bending right (west) past one and then another junction of the Lost Creek Loop Trail.

At the second junction you turn right (due north) continuing to the farthest north edge of the preserve. On this 0.5-mile leg of the Page Mill Trail look for just the right spot to enjoy the view and watch hawks sail on the updrafts. While you won't see the small meadow creatures—mice, gophers, and ground squirrels—that the hawks are searching for, you can see their myriad holes riddling the meadows.

In the northwest you will see the distant, dark shape of Mt. Tamalpais in Marin County. After taking in the exhilarating vistas and enjoying your knapsack lunch in the sun, retrace your steps at your leisure.

✦ Monte Bello and Saratoga Gap ✦ Open Space Preserves and Upper Stevens Creek County Park

These 5625 acres of open space preserves and county park encompass most of Stevens Creek Canyon from Page Mill Road to Saratoga Gap and from Skyline Boulevard on the west to Monte Bello Ridge on the east. This aggregation of woodlands, streams, and grasslands is a magnificent near-wilderness treasure close to Peninsula cities. Trails into the vast canyon of upper Stevens Creek invite you to explore its depths and to climb the heights of Monte Bello Ridge.

Monte Bello Open Space Preserve includes 3239 acres of the source and upper reaches of Stevens Creek, the west flanks of Black Mountain, and some of the densely forested east side of the Skyline ridge. One of the first preserves acquired by the Midpeninsula Regional Open Space District, Monte Bello is just across Skyline Boulevard from Skyline Ridge and Long Ridge open space preserves and immediately southeast of Los Trancos and Coal Creek preserves and Palo Alto's Foothills Park. On the north side of Monte Bello Road the preserve adjoins Rancho San Antonio Open Space Preserve. Monte Bello's 15 miles of trails serve as links between the parks and preserves north and south along the Skyline ridge, those east near urban areas, and those west to the Coastside.

The Black Mountain Backpack Camp, available by reservation from MROSD, is just one-half hour from Bayside cities. It has 1 group and 4 single campsites; water is available but must be purified.

Upper Stevens Creek County Park includes 1095 acres that lie along the Skyline between Monte Bello and Saratoga Gap open space preserves. Dense woods of old-growth Douglas fir, madrone, and big-leaf maple cover its steep, rugged terrain. Two long trails, the Grizzly Flat and Charcoal Road/Table Mountain trails, each with two alignments, rise through the park from Stevens Creek to the Skyline and link with trails in the adjoining Long Ridge Preserve to the west and Saratoga Gap Open Space Preserve to the south.

Saratoga Gap Open Space Preserve's 1291 acres extend northwest from Saratoga Gap on the east flank of the Skyline ridge and both north and south of Highway 9. The Saratoga Gap Trail, a 1.7-mile segment of the Bay Area Ridge Trail, and a short section of Charcoal Road all cross the preserve. Notable along the Saratoga Gap Trail are great outcrops of lichen-covered, wind- and rain-carved sandstone. The preserve's steep wooded hillsides indented by stream canyons are a cool environment for summer hiking.

Jurisdictions: Midpeninsula Regional Open Space District: 650-691-1200, and Santa Clara County: 408-255-3741

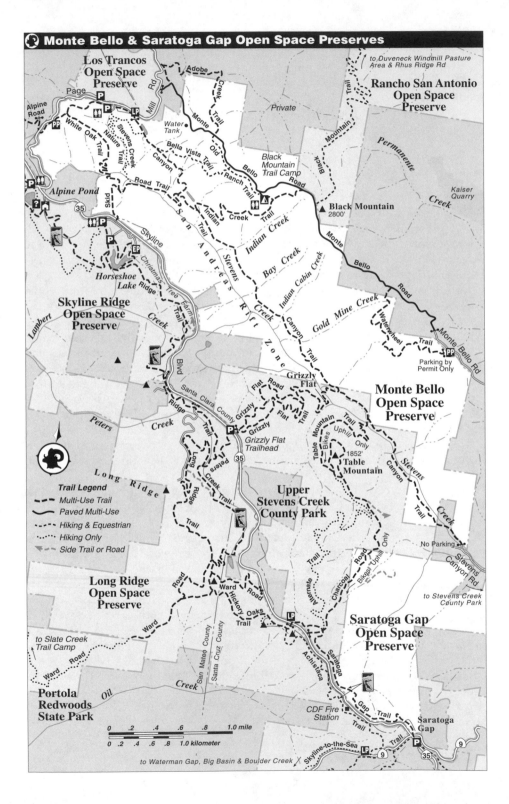

Monte Bello & Saratoga Gap Open Space Preserves

Facilities: Trails for hikers, equestrians, and bicyclists; a nature trail for hiking only, accessible for an eighth mile to physically limited; most other trails open to equestrians and bicyclists; restroom at Page Mill Road parking area, wheelchair accessible; equestrian parking by reservation at special parking area on Page Mill Road

Rules: Open dawn to dusk; no dogs allowed; no bicycles or horses on Nature Trail

Maps: MROSD brochures, *South Skyline Region Open Space Preserves*, *Monte Bello OSP* and *Long Ridge/Saratoga Gap OSP*, Santa Clara County *Upper Stevens Creek Park*, and USGS topos *Mindego Hill* and *Cupertino*

How to Get There: There are 5 access points: (1) At Monte Bello O.S.P. main entrance on south side of Page Mill Rd. 7 miles south of I-280; (2) on east side of Skyline Blvd. 0.7 mile southeast of Page Mill Rd., limited roadside parking; (3) at Grizzly Flat in Upper Stevens Creek Park 3.1 miles from either Page Mill Rd. or Hwy 9; (4) at Charcoal Rd. on east side of Skyline Blvd. 1.5 miles north of Hwy 9 and 4.7 miles south of Page Mill Rd., and (5) at Saratoga Gap on southeast corner of intersection of Hwy 9 and 35 (Skyline Blvd).

Monte Bello Open Space Preserve

STEVENS CREEK NATURE TRAIL

Explore the headwaters of Stevens Creek to see ladybug wintering sites, creekside vegetation, and the manifestations of movement along the San Andreas Fault Zone.

Distance: 3-mile loop

Time: 1¾ hours

Elevation Change: 450′ loss

More than the usual walking time is listed, to allow leisure to experience all the sights, sounds, and smells of this delightful walk down the canyon by this lovely creek. Spring-fed, it flows year-round, unusual for these dry hills and most welcome in summer and fall.

Four marked stations on the route tell salient facts about the linear valleys, sag ponds, and pressure ridges created when stress along the San Andreas Fault was released by earthquakes. Other stations describe the intricate process of wood decomposition by beetles and ants, and the life cycle of the ladybug. Several rustic benches along this route offer vantage points from which to enjoy the views.

From the parking area head out to the viewpoint above the canyon. Here, on a bench commemorating Frances Brenner, a former Palo Alto City Council member who did much to preserve these open-space lands, you can sit and appreciate the vastness of the near-wilderness below. Spread out before you is the watershed of Stevens Creek, along which in fall the gold of big-leaf maples marks the course of the creek down the canyon. Firs of great height grow thickly on the eastern side of the canyon and oaks of immense breadth flourish on the warmer west-facing hills.

The Nature Trail starts from the right side of the entrance trail and zigzags down into the creek canyon. At the first trail junction the 0.7-mile Skid Road Trail takes off right (southwest) and uphill on a pleasant grade to Skyline Boulevard. Directly across the Skyline a stile leads to hiking and riding trails in the 2143-acre Skyline Ridge Open Space Preserve. However, the Nature Trail Loop bears left (east) and after the last creek crossing, it meets the Canyon Trail, turns left (northwest) to complete the loop, passing oak-topped knolls, sag ponds, and former walnut orchards.

If you want to learn more about this area's natural history, call the MROSD office for days and times of docent-led hikes.

LOOP TRIP TO BLACK MOUNTAIN ON INDIAN CREEK AND BELLA VISTA TRAILS

A steep climb to Black Mountain rewards the hardy with spectacular views and wildflowers in season. Finish the loop on the well-designed Bella Vista Trail through the grasslands.

Distance: 4.5-mile loop

Time: 2 hours

Elevation Change: 840′ gain

Note: this is a loop which can be started on either leg, but the steep Indian Creek Trail, not recommended for the downhill leg, offers excellent views southeast down the creek canyon. However, taking the Bella Vista Trail both ways is a gentler, easier route.

Bring your wildflower guide and binoculars and choose a cool day or an early start. The Indian Creek Trail up the ridge has little shade for much of its length, so it can be very hot. From Page Mill Road parking area take the Canyon Trail toward Saratoga Gap. In 0.2 mile you pass the Bella Vista Trail, but continue another mile and turn left on the Indian Creek Trail. This old ranch road is shaded by oak trees at the start, but soon the trees are widely spaced, with only an occasional one for shade when you pause for breath. Then, for the rest of the trip to the top, the trail passes through treeless chaparral and grasslands, great for cool, winter hiking days.

As you pause on your climb, look west at the series of mountain ridges stretching to the ocean. In ever-paler hues of blue and purple, their tops seem like small waves on the horizon. At times, the fog hangs in the valleys between the ridges; often fog blankets them. To the south you can see all the way to Mt. Umunhum, and to the north to San Bruno Mountain and Mt. Tamalpais.

In spring a brilliant succession of flowers blooms through the grass. In early summer yellow and black butterflies flutter about the purple blossoms of the shrubby, sticky-leaved yerba santa. On the open hillsides are patches of chia, its whorls of lavender flowers forming little globes on stiff stems. Its fine seeds were a delicacy of the Indian diet, ground for their pinole (seed cakes) and considered medicinally valuable.

Near the summit a poplar tree by the road marks an old spring and the cut-off trail on the left to the backpack camp a short distance uphill in the trees.

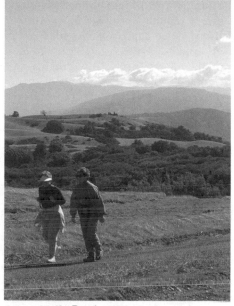

Monte Bello Road on Black Mountain

If you continue 0.2 mile on the Indian Creek Trail, you come to Monte Bello Road. Here is the site where once stood the old red barn of the mountaintop cattle ranch and the houses that belonged to the Morrell family. This road was the old route from Cupertino to Page Mill Road. It starts at Stevens Canyon Road, and winds up the northeast side of Monte Bello Ridge. No longer open to through traffic, but open to hikers, equestrians, and bicyclists, it follows the ridgetop, then makes a short descent to Page Mill Road. Closed to the public auto traffic, it serves primarily as a fire road.

This road makes a breath taking, top-of-the-world walk, bicycle ride, or horseback ride over the high grasslands above Santa Clara Valley. In late June the deep magenta blossoms of farewell-to-spring that carpet the hilltop and the songs of meadowlarks in the grass are rewards for your climb. In fall you may encounter large herds of deer that congregate in this area.

The backpack camp is a good place to have lunch and, if you have time, to explore along the road to the southeast. In about 0.5 mile you reach the 2800-foot summit of Black Mountain, where an airway communication beacon and telephone relay towers stand. A hikers- and equestrians-only, 4-mile trail north down the mountainside connects with the Duveneck Windmill Pasture Area of Rancho San Antonio Open Space Preserve. See the trip in Duveneck Windmill Pasture Area, page 208.

Retrace your steps to the MROSD backpack camp, where there is water to be filtered, a pay phone, and a portable toilet. With advance reservations, you can spend the night at this camp under the stars.

To return to the preserve entrance on Page Mill Road, continue straight ahead (northwest) on Monte Bello Road or take the parallel Old Ranch Trail on your left. This trail, with steadier footing than continuing on Monte Bello Road, zigzags downhill on a moderate grade through steep grasslands. In 0.4 mile it meets the Bella Vista Trail in a gentle swale. You turn left (west) on it for the great views that its name implies. (Taking the Bella Vista Trail last on this loop trip makes for a safer descent that on the loose rock surface of the Indian Creek Trail.) In June brilliant lemon-yellow mariposa lilies fill small meadows. At the Canyon Trail junction bear right and continue on it 0.3 mile to Page Mill Road, or after 0.2 mile take the foot trail 0.4 mile through the old orchard and over the ridgetop to the parking area.

For an interesting addition to this loop trip, from the Bella Vista/Old Ranch Trail junction go north and continue on the Old Ranch Trail 0.5 mile, cross graveled Monte Bello Road, look to your right and pick up the Adobe Creek Trail, a patrol road. Take this trail for a 1.4-mile loop north above the canyon of Adobe Creek. In spring you will see the tall candles of buckeye trees blooming; by fall the blossoms and leaves are gone and fist-sized nuts hang from the branch tips. Early summer brings bright orange monkey flowers. On the authors' last trip there the meadows were adorned with numerous clumps of large, yellow-flowered mule-ears.

As the trail makes a wide curve west, you have a spectacular view of the forested and chaparral-covered canyon of Adobe Creek. Here is the Hidden Villa Ranch, described in the Duveneck Windmill Pasture Area of this book, page 206. Farther to the north and east lies the Santa Clara Valley, with the huge hangar of Moffett Field a conspicuous landmark. This side hike is particularly good on a hot day because it is north-facing and shaded. Dropping down some 500 feet, you cross the upper end of the west fork of Adobe Creek in a delightfully cool canyon.

Climbing again, you pass under power lines and find some rocky outcrops uphill from Monte Bello Road. These would make a good picnic spot. Look for a red-tailed hawk's nest of sticks and twigs on the power poles. Return southeast up Monte Bello Road to reach the Bella Vista Trail on your right, and continue as described above.

FROM SARATOGA GAP
TO MONTE BELLO PRESERVE

Follow the San Andreas Rift Zone from Saratoga Gap to Page Mill Road. (After dropping down to Stevens Creek, it leads up the quiet valley where the creek originates.)

Distance: 7.6 miles one way

Time: 5-6 hours

Elevation Change: 1400′ loss to Stevens Canyon; 800′ gain to Page Mill Road

This long trail, best done with a car shuttle, can be taken in reverse, but by starting at Saratoga Gap, the trip's highest point, you walk the steep grade of Charcoal Road going downhill. For a car shuttle, leave one car at the Page Mill entrance and take another to the Saratoga Gap entrance. Bicyclists planning to do this trip must begin at the Page Mill Road end, because the Charcoal Road segment is open to uphill bicycle traffic only.

From the parking area at Saratoga Gap, cross Highway 9 to the northeast corner of the intersection, where you'll find the signed entrance to Saratoga Gap preserve. Here too, is a Bay Area Ridge Trail sign marking the beginning of a continuous 12.6-mile trip northwest through four MROSD preserves and a county park. A stile in the wooden fence leads to the trail, which at first closely parallels Skyline Boulevard through a mixed woodland of firs, madrones, bays, and oaks. These lands, too steep even for grazing, have remained virtually as they were before the coming of the Spaniards.

After 1.7 miles through a fragrant forest, the trail emerges in a clearing where the old Charcoal Road comes in from Skyline Boulevard. Across this opening, another 0.3 mile trail takes off west through the woods to reach Skyline Boulevard opposite the Hickory Oaks Trail in Long Ridge Open Space Preserve.

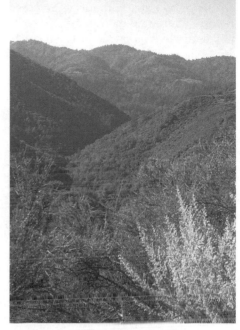

Stevens Creek Canyon

From the east side of this clearing, a narrow path for hikers only, known as the Alternate Trail, approximately parallels Charcoal Road on its west side, then joins it at the north end of Table Mountain. This delightful, narrow trail starts to the left about 100 feet down Charcoal Road and meanders through a woodland of black oaks, live oaks, and madrones with spring wildflowers dotting the trailside. Then the trail passes through a section of dense chaparral—fragrant sage, magenta-pink-blossomed pickeringia, some chinquapin, and even the small, prickly-leaved leather oak—which now covers the rocky soil following a hot fire. The views open up north across a deep canyon and east toward Black Mountain.

Then the Alternate Trail doubles back south, crosses to the east side of the ridge, and emerges on a south-facing slope with views southeast of Mt. Copernicus and Mt. Hamilton. You descend steeply through a mature fir forest, cross two little creeks, and follow the second one on its east side up to Table Mountain. Here the bedraggled remnants of a tree farm are being replaced by healthy madrones and young firs. In a clearing the foot trail joins the wide Table Mountain Trail.

In about 0.1 mile, the Table Mountain Trail to Stevens Canyon ducks into the trees on the left (this section of the trail is multi-use, quite narrow, eroded, and replete with switchbacks). You follow this trail with equestrians and bicyclists going uphill through meadows graced by iris, blue and cream-colored, into the deep shade of tall firs, and across a creek that tumbles into a steep ravine.

Soon you can hear Stevens Creek below in the canyon; go around a couple of switchbacks and you will see it. When the creek is running full in spring, it is a challenge to cross without getting wet. In this remote canyon, you can believe reports that a few mountain lions still survive here. On the far side a small flat makes an inviting picnic place where you can lunch to the sounds of the creek.

If hikers and equestrians had taken the Charcoal Road Trail from the ridgetop clearing, they would have stayed right on the broad old farm road, built long ago for cutting cordwood to make charcoal and for hauling it out of the forest. This road leading north, downhill, into an oak woodland is a one-way trail for bicyclists; they must ride uphill only. After a steep descent of more than a mile, you pass an old road to the right and veer left on the Table Mountain Trail. At Table Mountain you would join the narrow, multi-use trail, down to Stevens Canyon described above.

After crossing Stevens Creek and starting uphill on the Canyon Trail you cross a tributary, and begin to climb away from the creek. In less than 0.5 mile the Canyon Trail passes the Grizzly Flat Trail taking off to the left. This trip continues straight and follows the former ranch road for 3.1 miles, all the way to Page Mill Road. However, if you climb to the heights of this park on the Grizzly Flat Trail in Upper Stevens Creek Park, you can return to Saratoga Gap on trails through Long Ridge Open Space Preserve. The tree-canopied Canyon Trail route crosses the little watercourses that furrow Monte Bello Ridge—Gold Mine, Indian Cabin, Bay, and Indian creeks. The canyon gradually widens into more open, grassy slopes and a few meadows shaded by valley oaks. The Canyon Trail passes the Indian Creek Trail, which leads right to Monte Bello Ridge.

Shortly past this trail intersection look for the left turnoff to the Stevens Creek Nature Trail. From this trail there is another route, the Skid Road Trail, to Skyline Boulevard, 1.3 miles away. This trail comes out across the road from Skyline Ridge Open Space Preserve and is described in the Hike to Grizzly Flat, page 159. This trail offers another possibility of returning to Saratoga Gap on trails through Skyline and Long Ridge open space preserves.

Continuing on the Canyon Trail, you pass the Bella Vista Trail on the right and go through an area of sag ponds, which provide evidence that you are walking in the San Andreas Fault Zone. Over thousands of years, repeated earth movements along the fault have created both the benches that interrupt watercourses and the small, linear ponds—two signs of an active fault.

The knolls rising west of the trail beckon you to clamber up for a view of your hike along the earthquake valley to Saratoga Gap, where you started. Beyond, you see the trough of the San Andreas Fault lying west of Loma Prieta, where the 7.1 magnitude 1989 earthquake was centered. Mt. Umunhum, with its square tower remaining from World War II defenses, is conspicuous on the horizon.

As you near Page Mill Road, there are remnants of former ranching—orchards and old fences. And then, after a day spent in the remote canyons and forests of Stevens Creek's headwaters, you are at the preserve entrance on a busy route from here to the Santa Clara Valley.

WHITE OAK TRAIL ALTERNATE TO UPPER CANYON TRAIL

As you return up the Canyon Trail, you can take a pleasant alternate to the west to return to the parking lot at Page Mill Road.

Just after passing the Indian Creek Trail turn left on the trail to the Stevens Creek Nature Trail. (Horses and bicycles are not permitted on parts of the Nature Trail, but should continue west for 0.9 mile to the junction of the Skid Road and White Oak trails). Take the White Oak Trail right (north) uphill through the grasslands. This narrow trail is named for the white oaks that dot its hillsides, and as you pause to catch your breath, look west and south for a different view of the Skyline Ridge.

After 1.2 miles you are at a junction with the trail coming in from the Upper Alpine Road Trail at gate MB05. Near this point is the equestrian permit parking lot at gate MB04. Turn right here and take the 0.3-mile trail back to the Monte Bello parking lot.

Upper Stevens Creek County Park

HIKE TO GRIZZLY FLAT

An old jeep road descends 2 miles through woods to a stately fir forest and a delightful creekside picnic spot in Upper Stevens Creek County Park.

Distance: 4 miles round trip

Time: 2½ hours

Elevation Change: 900' loss

Follow directions to the Grizzly Flat parking area, access point (3) on page 153 and go through the opening in the fence. Two trails leave from this park entrance. The broad jeep road on the left is the well-used and better-graded route. If you take the right-hand trail, which has recently been cleared, you will find some steep pitches and occasional rough footing. However, it is slightly shorter and provides variety, especially on the uphill trip.

Taking the left-hand trail, you descend through oak and madrone woods. About halfway down, the steep grassy slopes of Monte Bello Ridge come into view on the far side of the canyon.

Black oaks and canyon oaks form dense woodland here, but as you descend farther into the canyon you see increasing numbers of Douglas firs. Near the creek you find yourself in a forest of large firs and maples. Although some wood cutting has occurred in the past in the upper part of this park, the lower canyon's great firs, 5 or 6 feet in diameter, are a fragment of virgin forest. Big-leaf maples filter the light

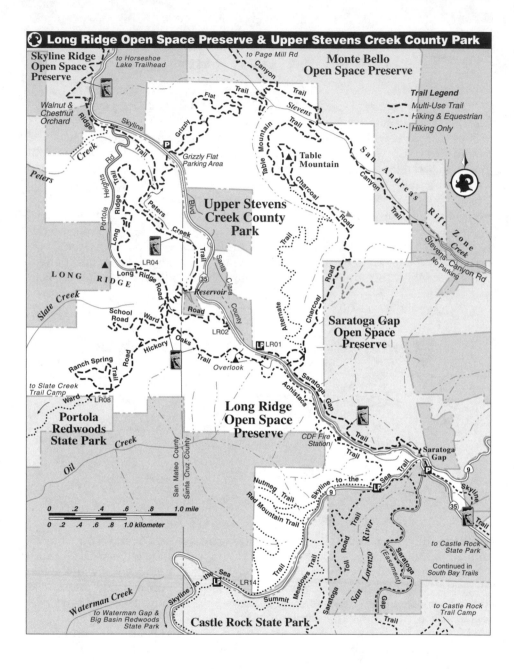

Long Ridge Open Space Preserve & Upper Stevens Creek County Park

at the bottom of the canyon, and a mosaic of the large, deeply lobed leaves of colts-foot edges the stream. Here you will find choice sites for a picnic. The meadow above the creek is a ladybug wintering site and presently closed for rehabilitation.

If you veer left at Grizzly Flat, a narrow path around a thimbleberry thicket takes you to a crossing over Stevens Creek. Several sandy flats under maples and tanks edge clear pools in the creek protected by a high south wall clothed with five-finger ferns. This trail continues 0.4 mile uphill on many switchbacks to meet the Canyon Trail in Monte Bello Open Space Preserve.

For an 8-mile loop trip starting on the west side of the Grizzly Flat parking area in Long Ridge Open Space Preserve, follow its trails southeast, crossing Skyline Boulevard to pick up Charcoal Road and follow it down to the Canyon Trail, then climb back uphill on this Grizzly Flat Trail.

This cool creekside is a fine destination for an early supper expedition in summer, but allow plenty of time for your return trip before dusk. At a leisurely pace hikers may take an hour and a half to get back up to Skyline Boulevard, a delightful trip in the shade of the hills. As you climb out of the canyon in the early evening, you will want to pause often to look out between the dark firs at tawny Monte Bello Ridge glowing in the setting sun.

Russian Ridge Open Space Preserve

Russian Ridge Open Space Preserve's 1580 acres lie along the west side of Skyline Boulevard for about 3 miles north from the Page Mill/Alpine Road intersection through the Mt. Melville area and extend southwest into the deep canyons of Alpine and Mindego creeks. Trails run along the ridgetop parallel to Skyline Boulevard, surprising routes lead through beautiful wooded canyons and old ranch roads descend the west slopes. Spectacular views east to San Francisco Bay and the Diablo Range and west to the ocean over an expanse of ridges greet the visitor to Russian Ridge. Strong winds that bring clear skies can also carry dense fog, especially in summer.

Jurisdiction: Midpeninsula Regional Open Space District: 650-691-1200

Facilities: Trails for hikers, equestrians, and bicyclists

Rules: Open dawn to dusk; no dogs permitted

Maps: Map on page 162 MROSD brochure *South Skyline Region*, USGS topo *Mindego Hill*

How to Get There: Take Hwy 84 from Woodside, Page Mill Rd. from Palo Alto, or Hwy 9 from Saratoga to three preserve entrances: (1) at Skyline Blvd/Alpine Rd. intersection, with parking on northeast corner, (2) at Caltrans Vista Point 1 mile north of this intersection, and (3) at Rapley Ranch Rd. 0.5 mile north of vista point with roadside parking on west side of Skyline Blvd.

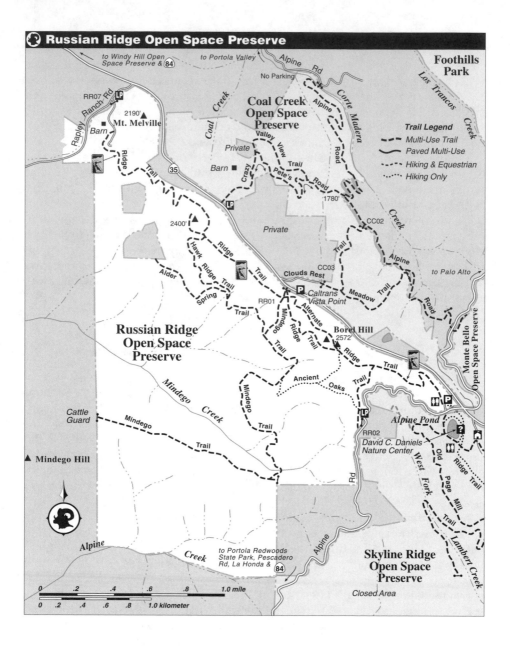

Russian Ridge Open Space Preserve

to Windy Hill Open Space Preserve & 84
to Portola Valley
Alpine Rd
No Parking
Alpine
Corte Madera
Foothills Park
Los Trancos Creek

RR07 Rd LP
Rapley Ranch Rd
2190' Mt. Melville
Barn
Ridge Trail
35

Coal Creek Open Space Preserve
Coal Creek
Valley View Trail
Private
Barn Crazy
Pete's
Road Road
1780'

Trail Legend
～ Multi-Use Trail
━ Paved Multi-Use
--- Hiking & Equestrian
···· Hiking Only

CC02
Creek
2400'
Hawk Ridge Trail
Alder
Spring
Ridge Trail
CC03
Clouds Rest
Trail
CC02
Alpine
Meadow Trail
to Palo Alto

Russian Ridge Open Space Preserve
Trail
RR01
Caltrans Vista Point
Mindego Ridge
Alternate
Borel Hill
2572'
Trail
Ridge
Trail
P

Mindego Creek
Mindego
Trail
Mindego
Ancient
Oaks
Trail
Alpine Pond
LP
RR02
David C. Daniels Nature Center

Cattle Guard
Mindego
Trail
Mindego Trail

▲ Mindego Hill

Monte Bello Open Space Preserve

West Fork
Old Page Mill Trail
Ridge Trail
Lambert Creek

Alpine
Creek
to Portola Redwoods State Park, Pescadero Rd, La Honda & 84
Alpine Rd

Skyline Ridge Open Space Preserve
Closed Area

0 .2 .4 .6 .8 1.0 mile
0 .2 .4 .6 .8 1.0 kilometer

A Bay Area Ridge Trail Trip for Those Clear Days When You Can See Forever

A trail along Russian Ridge for the length of the preserve has views out to the Pacific Ocean across ranchlands and forests little changed since American settlers moved to California over 150 years ago.

Distance: 6.4 miles round trip

Time: 3¼ hours

Elevation Change: 300′ gain

From the Russian Ridge parking area at the northwest corner of Skyline Boulevard and Alpine Road, take the trail that climbs the ridge to the northwest. After a long switchback you pass a trail that leads left (south) to a trailhead on Alpine Road. However, continuing along the Bay Area Ridge Trail route, go 0.2 mile to another junction where you can go right to the summit of Borel Hill (2572′) or take the left fork, which winds along the west-facing slopes with canyon and ocean views. On either trail in early spring, poppies, red maids, Johnny-jump-ups, and lupines are in bloom and, by April, a profusion of goldfields covers these grasslands.

Few spots can beat this ridge for views that take in the Peninsula from Bay to ocean. If you take the trail to Borel Hill on a clear day in winter, with binoculars you can see the snow-capped Sierra Nevada through the gap of Niles Canyon to the northeast and the Farallon Islands to the west. On a still, fogless evening in early summer when daylight lingers, this is a spectacular supper picnic site. Among the scattered rock outcrops are many places to spread out an evening meal and watch the sunset over the Pacific Ocean.

The left-hand trail follows a gentle meander along the west side of the ridge, passing a junction where a trail leads south to the Ancient Oaks Trail (see Ancient Oaks Trail Loop, page 165). However, the Ridge Trail curves north into the head of a swale, then bends west past sandstone outcrops that frame views of the grasslands, wooded creek canyons, and forested ridges south and west.

Whichever Ridge Trail route you take, you reach the saddle near the Caltrans Vista Point entrance to the preserve. To complete this Russian Ridge segment of the Bay Area Ridge Trail, you briefly follow the Mindego Ridge Trail left (south) and then continue right (north) on the Ridge Trail. You are on a trail that gradually ascends the west side of the ridge. To the west stretch ranchlands, creek canyons, and ridges, and the ocean lies beyond. In the morning light mists often hide the ocean, but late in the day the ocean waters glisten as they reflect the light of the late afternoon sun.

Southwest before you is Mindego Hill. In spring its green bulk stands out against dark ridges beyond. Mindego Hill is of volcanic origin, probably formed more than 135 million years ago. At that time it was submerged below the ocean as part of a range of mountains at the edge of the Pacific Plate. These mountains, now known as the Santa Cruz Mountains, have been moving northwest along the San Andreas Fault. In today's time frame, this trip traverses the eroded, worn-down remnants of these mountains little changed over the last century of cattle ranching.

Continuing 0.5 mile along the Ridge Trail toward a group of radio antennas, you come to a junction, where the 0.6-mile Hawk Ridge Trail leads left (west) and then south, downhill. You can take this trail for a shorter return to your starting point (see below). On the northward Ridge Trail route, you wind in and out of lovely woods with views alternating east and west. Surprisingly, a wooden deck appears beside the trail, inviting a sheltered lunch stop. Just beyond are some intriguing sculptures emplaced by a former owner. Enjoy these amenities, but respect the private residence by staying on the trail.

Winding down the ridge, the trail passes the site of an ancient barn (recently removed) near the Rapley Ranch Road gate. Cross the stile, turn right on the gravel-surfaced road and go 0.1 mile out to Skyline Boulevard. Plans to extend the Ridge Trail 0.7 mile north to Windy Hill Open Space Preserve are in process at this writing. If you have arranged a car shuttle, you can end your trip here. Otherwise for variety, return to the Hawk Ridge Trail junction and take the Hawk Ridge and Alder Spring trails back to the Mindego Ridge Trail. Turn left (north) on it and retrace your route to your starting point.

SEE MAP
ON PAGE
162

DOWN TO MINDEGO CREEK AND TO THE SLOPES OF MINDEGO HILL

Follow an old ranch road southwest in and out of canyons to reach one of Mindego Creek's main branches and to approach Mindego Hill.

Distance: 6 miles round trip

Time: 3½ hours

Elevation Change: 400' loss

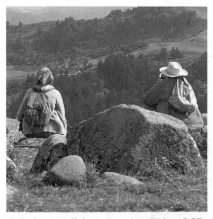

Park at the Caltrans Vista Point, cross Skyline Boulevard and go through the gate onto the old ranch road that heads downhill. It passes both trails described in the previous trip, and turns southeast. It descends through grasslands and soon turns into a canyon shaded by oaks, madrones, and Douglas firs. In half an hour you emerge into open pasture again, looking out across forests toward Mindego Hill's truncated summit.

Groves of buckeyes and oaks bordering the grassland below the road are tempting sites for a picnic stop or a welcome pause on

Mindego Hill from Russian Ridge OSP

the trip back up. Look for the intersection of the Ancient Oaks Trail uphill on your left. It is described in the next trip.

A few minutes' walk farther down the trail brings you to a little flat beside a tributary of Mindego Creek. On one side of the flat pasturelands furrowed by a century of grazing cattle rise steeply. On the other side, huge canyon oaks and tall laurels edge the creek, making a cool lunch spot for a hot day or a good place to turn around for a shortened trip. But to continue, cross the creek and go up over a little ridge and down to another branch of the creek. From here you make a brief climb to another ridge overlooking the canyon of Alpine Creek and the ridges to the south. A private road on the left, where public access is prohibited, leads out to Alpine Road. However, you follow the road northwest on the narrow ridge toward Mindego Hill.

Immense canyon live oaks line one side of the road. A mile walk along the ridge brings you to the fenced boundary of the preserve on the lower slopes of Mindego Hill. Turn back at this private property-line fence to retrace your steps to the Skyline.

ANCIENT OAKS TRAIL LOOP

A shady hikers' trail winds through enormous canyon live oaks to emerge in grasslands with views of the world.

Distance: 2.5 miles round trip

Time: 1¼ hours

Elevation Change: 175' gain

Park at the roadside pullout on Alpine Road, 0.8 mile down Alpine Road from Skyline Boulevard, head uphill, cross the patrol road and go west following the hikers-only Ancient Oaks Trail. From here it is 0.7 mile to the Mindego Ridge Trail. The Ancient Oaks Trail rises across slopes with a superb view of Butano Ridge to the southwest. Shortly you pass a trail junction, but bear left here for 0.3 mile to a stand of huge oaks. These trees have multiple trunks rising from massive boles. Did they sprout from the stumps of ancient trees after a long-ago fire?

In the grove you reach an unnamed hikers-only trail on the right, on which you will return later. However continue left past more gnarled oaks, following the grassland border and maintaining splendid views even to the ocean on a clear day. Many young firs are growing among the oaks, probably seeded from large firs in the canyons below.

The trail goes down through the trees to the Mindego Ridge Trail, a patrol road for all users, where in winter the roaring of Mindego Creek fills the air. If the trail is muddy, you will see the tracks of deer, coyotes, foxes, and bobcats, which use human trails when they can. Walking northeast (right) on the Mindego Ridge Trail, you pass the Alder Spring Trail on your left, part of a loop in the previous trip. You can see Skyline Boulevard near the Caltrans Vista Point ahead, and you turn right (south) uphill on the Ridge Trail.

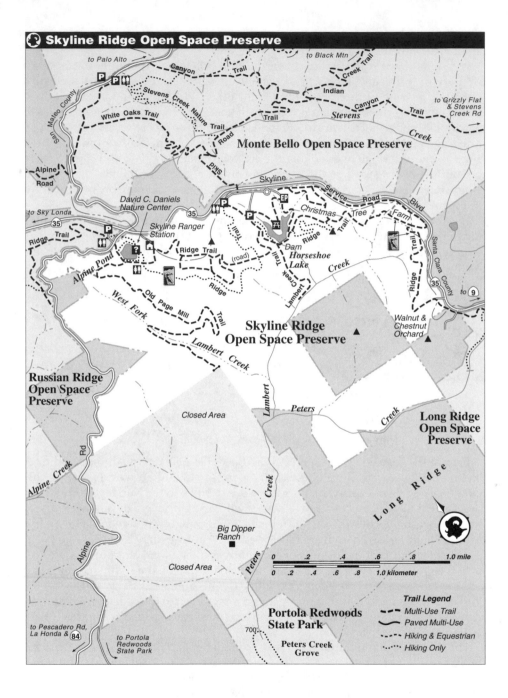

Skyline Ridge Open Space Preserve

to Palo Alto

Canyon Trail

Creek Trail

to Black Mtn

Stevens Creek Nature Trail

Indian

White Oaks Trail

Trail

Canyon

to Grizzly Flat & Stevens Creek Rd

Trail

Stevens

Monte Bello Open Space Preserve

Alpine Road

Skid

Road

Skyline

Creek

David C. Daniels Nature Center

to Sky Londa

35

Service

Road

Blvd

35

Christmas

Tree

Farm

Skyline Ranger Station

Ridge Trail

Ridge Trail

Santa Clara County

Ridge Trail

?

Dam

Horseshoe Lake

Creek

35

to 9

Alpine Pond

Ridge

(road)

Lambert Creek

Old Page Mill Trail

Ridge

Walnut & Chestnut Orchard

West Fork

Skyline Ridge Open Space Preserve

Russian Ridge Open Space Preserve

Lambert Creek

Lambert

Peters

Creek

Long Ridge Open Space Preserve

Closed Area

Alpine Creek Rd

Creek

L o n g   R i d g e

Alpine

Big Dipper Ranch

Closed Area

Peters

| 0 | .2 | .4 | .6 | .8 | 1.0 mile |
| 0 | .2 | .4 | .6 | .8 | 1.0 kilometer |

to Pescadero Rd, La Honda & 84

to Portola Redwoods State Park

700

Portola Redwoods State Park

Peters Creek Creek Grove

Trail Legend
- – – Multi-Use Trail
- Paved Multi-Use
- ·–·– Hiking & Equestrian
- ····· Hiking Only

As you start uphill, take the foot trail which bears right, rather than the patrol road on the left, and curve across the southwest-facing grassy slope. After 0.5 mile, you pass an unnamed trail on your right. Mark this for your return trip, but continue straight a short distance, and then angle sharp left onto the patrol road to crest 2572-foot Borel Hill for the spectacular views described in the first trip.

Retrace your steps from the Borel Hill summit to the Ridge Trail route on which you came, and turn left on the aforementioned unnamed, hikers-only, 0.3-mile trail, which descends a grassy hillside and then enters a lovely oak forest. You soon reach the Ancient Oaks Trail, on which you go left (south) to your starting point at Alpine Road.

A 2.1-mile variation of this trip starts from the Alpine Road/Skyline Boulevard parking area, goes north on the Bay Area Ridge Trail route, takes the first trail on the left, for hikers only, intersects the Ancient Oaks Trail in about 0.3 mile, turns right (north), turns right again on the next trail and then takes the Bay Area Ridge Trail route right (south) back to the parking area—a delightful, late afternoon outing to watch the sun set over the Pacific.

Skyline Ridge Open Space Preserve

Skyline Ridge Open Space Preserve lies along the western crest of the Santa Cruz Mountains in the heart of thousands of acres of public open space. Russian Ridge, Coal Creek, Monte Bello, and Long Ridge open space preserves adjoin Skyline Ridge Preserve. From its highest point, one can see south and west to the nearby forests of Castle Rock and Portola Redwoods state parks and Pescadero Creek County Park.

Skyline Ridge Preserve is rich in history, varied in landscape, and easily accessible to a million Peninsula residents. Skyline Ridge's 2143 acres also include two small reservoirs that lie in the valleys flanking a high central 2493-foot unnamed knoll. Rolling grasslands cover the preserve's more exposed heights and evergreen forests clothe its steep lower slopes.

Native Americans gathered acorns from oak forests and ground them on bedrock grinding stones that have been found here. As early as 1850, settlers built ranchhouses and raised cattle, hogs, horses, and hay along the crest of the Skyline ridge. In 1868 William Page built a road across the northwest corner of the preserve to link his mill in present-day Portola Redwoods State Park with the embarcadero in Palo Alto.

The most famous previous owner of the land was Governor James "Sunny Jim" Rolph, who used the modest farmhouse at Skyline Ranch as an occasional summer capital in the 1930s. Today a chestnut orchard and a small Christmas tree farm occupy several acres on the east and south sides of the preserve.

Parking areas in the north and center of the preserve provide access to 10 miles of trail, including two short trails for the physically limited. From the north parking area at Alpine Road and Skyline Boulevard, the Bay Area Ridge Trail heads 3 miles south through the preserve. From here also, one can quickly reach Alpine Pond, where the Daniels Nature Center features environmental exhibits and a viewing deck above the water. The nature center, built by private donations and contributions from POST, is open on Sundays from April through mid-November and staffed by volunteer docents. School groups can use the center by reservation. A short trail for the physically limited circles the pond and another trail follows Old Page Mill Road to the boundary of the preserve. The main entrance 0.75 mile south along Skyline Boulevard offers ample parking for all visitors, including a horse trailer area and a disabled parking lot near Horseshoe Lake. Starting from here are trails to the lake and to a few picnic tables above it, a trail into the canyon of Lambert Creek, and connections to the Bay Area Ridge Trail.

Jurisdiction: Midpeninsula Regional Open Space District: 650-691-1200

Facilities: Picnic area, Nature Center, and observation deck; 2 small lakes; miles of trails for hikers, bicyclists, equestrians, and the physically limited

Rules: Open dawn to dusk; no dogs

Maps: MROSD brochure *Skyline Ridge OSP*, USGS topo *Mindego Hill*

How to Get There: Take Hwy 84 from Woodside, Page Mill Rd. from Palo Alto, or Hwy 9 from Saratoga to two preserve entrances: (1) On northwest corner of Skyline Blvd/Alpine Rd. intersection. Park here for trail entrances: (a) through an immense underpass leading to Alpine Pond for hikers and wheelchairs only, (b) 400' down Alpine Rd. on left for bicyclists and equestrians, and (c) northwest uphill to Ridge Trail in Russian Ridge Preserve. (2) On Skyline Blvd. 0.75 mile southeast of this intersection.

SEE MAP ON PAGE 166

A TRIP DOWN HISTORIC OLD PAGE MILL ROAD

Hike down to the western arm of Lambert Creek on the early logging route to Page's Mill.

Distance: 3.6 miles round trip

Time: 1½ hours

Elevation Change: 650' loss

From the preserve's north entrance at the corner of Skyline Boulevard and Alpine Road walk 400 feet down Alpine Road to the trail entrance on the left. Take this multi-use trail, which passes west of Alpine Pond, to its intersection with paved Old Page Mill Road. Turn right here, heading downhill (northwest) under tall old firs and past some sculptured sandstone outcrops. You are soon in a clearing with splendid views southeast over a succession of forested ridges.

At this clearing the now unpaved road arcs left, winding around the forested east side of the canyon of intermittent West Lambert Creek. On the way it crosses Lambert Creek tributaries cascading over sandstone boulders on the steep mountainside. About a mile downhill the road goes through some chaparral on a south-facing slope. Blooming at road's edge in summer are yellow bush poppies and magenta chaparral-peas. Around a sharp switchback look to your left to see the site of the former Glass Ranch, said to be a stagecoach stop on this route over the mountains to the Bay. No buildings remain today.

Back into the tall Douglas fir forest, you negotiate several more switchbacks to reach a bridge over the creek near the preserve boundary. Old Page Mill Road, long closed to the public, continues on to present-day Portola Redwoods State Park, where William Page milled logs that he transported up this canyon and on to Palo Alto's embarcadero. At this writing, you can cross the bridge and continue another 0.5 mile along the east-facing hillside. After heavy rains MROSD built retaining walls and repaired the trail tread. Plans to extend this trail to Portola Redwoods State Park are under way.

To begin your upward trip, retrace your same route uphill on Old Page Mill Road. When you reach the junction with trails circling Alpine Pond, you can turn right and then left to reach the Nature Center. Nearby is a bedrock mortar used by Native Americans to grind acorns.

If you continue around the pond, the ranger office is a bit right, uphill on the site of the former ranch buildings. Or take the trail around the pond's east side to enjoy its blue waters rimmed with reeds. Then follow the path through the underpass to the parking area.

A Loop Around Alpine Pond

A trail circling the pond leads to the Daniels Nature Center and to observation points from which to enjoy birds, fish, frogs, and insects.

Distance: 0.5 mile loop

Time: ¼ hour

Elevation Change: Nearly level

From the preserve's north entrance at the corner of Skyline Boulevard and Alpine Road, hikers and wheelchair users take the trail through the underpass. About 100 feet inside the preserve take the trail to the right and follow it through a meadow, which is filled with yellow buttercup blossoms in spring. At breaks in the lake's cattail-and-willow border on your left are several places where visitors can get close to the water and look for fish, frogs, and waterskeeters.

You can watch for red-wing blackbirds, barn swallows, and marsh wrens from the shore, and look for raccoon and deer tracks in the mud at lakeside. Later you may want to picnic in the meadow or sit by the lake in the shade of tall willows.

After 0.3 mile around the pond you reach the Daniels Nature Center described above, and on weekdays you can relax on the deck while viewing the pond.

On a floating observation platform built over the pond or from the deck of the nature center, you can get a closer look at the aquatic life—fish and turtles are often visible. You may see a northern harrier hawk as it monitors the marshy lakeshore for unsuspecting frogs; other avian visitors are an occasional belted kingfisher and a great blue heron.

THE BAY AREA RIDGE TRAIL

Follow a segment of the Bay Area Ridge Trail down the length of the preserve.

Distance: 6 miles round trip

Time: 3¼ hours

Elevation Change: 250′ gain to Vista Point; 90′ loss to south end of preserve

This trail, formerly the Skyline Trail and now renamed a part of the Bay Area Ridge Trail, follows two alternatives from Alpine Pond to Horseshoe Lake. Bicyclists and equestrians take the high road over the preserve's central knoll; hikers contour around its southwest face on a lower alignment. Then, all can continue to the southeast end of the preserve on a multi-use trail. On the first segment after Horseshoe Lake, hikers may take a slightly longer, woodsy trail up and over a high ridge before rejoining bicyclists and equestrians on the rest of the route to the southeast end of the preserve.

Starting from the preserve's north parking area, hikers take either the underpass trail to the east side of Alpine Pond or the bicyclist/equestrian route from the trail entrance 400 feet south along Alpine Road. Both routes converge on Old Page Mill Road beyond Alpine Pond.

From there bicyclists and equestrians go uphill, (east) pass former ranch buildings and take the old farm road going off to the left. They continue on it over the top of the preserve's summit and down to Horseshoe Lake (an elevation gain of 200′ and loss of 400′ in 1.4 miles).

Hikers veer off south beyond the pond on a foot trail through a mature canyon-oak forest. Following an easy contour uphill, this trail traverses terraces where former owners of the preserve grew hay and pastured horses. It passes the low shed where other owners slaughtered hogs raised on this site. Then, as the trail gradually ascends the sloping grasslands above the canyon of Lambert Creek, the views extend to miles and miles of forested ridges and rolling grasslands. Through a notch in the west the coast is visible on clear days.

As you reach the summit of the hiker's trip at an overlook chiseled out of a sandstone outcrop, you can look across to Butano Ridge, the prominent buttress above the Pescadero Creek canyon where Portola Redwoods State Park and Pescadero Creek County Park are situated. Beyond this long, high ridge lies Butano State Park.

Continue around the steep sides of the preserve's central knoll into heads of little ravines and out onto its rugged, imposing brow. You pass through stretches of dense chaparral and then into little oak and madrone woods. This trail, with a southwest exposure, is best taken on a sunny winter day or in the cool hours of a summer day.

Rounding the southernmost point of the ridge, you turn northeast and descend quickly to intersect the graveled farm road, the bicyclist/equestrian route that leads to Horseshoe Lake. Cross the farm road and dip into a forest of oak, bay and

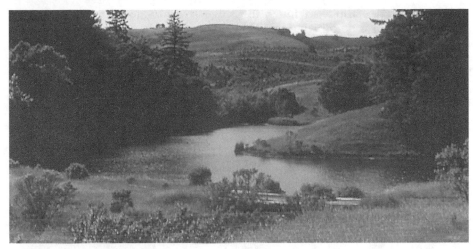

Horseshoe Lake

buckeye trees on a gently graded foot trail. Back into ravines where intermittent streams flow in rainy winters, you amble downhill past moss-covered tree trunks and sandstone outcrops. When you emerge on southeast-facing grassy slopes ablaze with orange poppies and blue lupines in spring, you can see east over the canyon of Stevens Creek to Monte Bello Ridge. Just before entering the parking area, take the 0.3-mile multi-use trail that cuts diagonally across the meadow to the shores of Horseshoe Lake, a two-armed reservoir that impounds the waters of East Lambert Creek.

Now, hikers, equestrians, and bicyclists follow the same Bay Area Ridge Trail route across the dam and uphill around the east side of Horseshoe Lake. At the first trail junction, don't take the trail that keeps close to the lake's edge. Instead, take either the multi-use, former farm road straight ahead (east) or the hikers-only trail right (south). The wide, multi-use trail goes into the forest and proceeds 0.3 mile southeast under a high canopy of evergreen branches. The 0.6-mile, hikers-only route ascends on many switchbacks along the west side of a steep-sided ridge to reach a small plateau shaded by mature Douglas firs. Almost immediately the hikers' trail drops down the east side of the ridge, makes a few traverses and shortly joins the multi-use route.

From this junction the graveled farm road winds around small knolls, crosses gullies and passes the small Christmas tree farm. There the formal plantings, set out in straight rows across the hillside, contrast markedly with the casual elegance of white oaks dotting the grasslands. Then you leave the farm road and follow a section of the old Summit Road through cool oak woodland. After 0.5 mile, you veer right onto a beautiful trail that traverses the fern-clad banks of a tributary of Lambert Creek. Gradually you climb to a walnut and chestnut orchard on a little knoll overlooking the southeast end of the preserve. If you come here in November, you can buy freshly harvested chestnuts from the orchard's former owners.

Then you take a 1-mile section of the Ridge Trail between this hilltop orchard and the Peters Creek bridge in Long Ridge Open Space Preserve. From there the Ridge Trail continues on a 3.8-mile leg to Saratoga Gap.

Unless you have a car shuttle waiting at one of the Long Ridge entrances or at Saratoga Gap, turn around here to complete your 6-mile round trip from the north entrance of Skyline Ridge Open Space Preserve. For variety, hikers can return on the bicyclist/equestrian route over the top of the preserve's central knoll.

LOOP HIKE AROUND THE SHORES OF HORSESHOE LAKE

A short downhill trip from the ridge takes you to vistas of a forested canyon and to picnic sites beside the lake.

Distance: 1.5 mile loop

Time: ¾ hour

Elevation Change: 115′ loss

From the preserve's entrance on Skyline Boulevard, 0.75 mile southeast of Alpine Road, pick up the trail heading downhill into a valley surmounted on the west by the steep flanks of the preserve's summit. As you descend through this upper watershed of East Lambert Creek, the U-shaped lake comes into view, wrapped around a tree-topped knoll.

In 0.5 mile from the parking area you are at the south end of the lake, where you walk across the earthen dam on a farm road, then take a trail along the lake's marshy southeast rim. In the quiet of early morning or late on a summer day, you may catch sight of the deer, raccoons, or foxes that inhabit the woods and meadows of this preserve. At any time of day you can watch the birds swooping down to the lake for insects. In winter a variety of migrating ducks rest at the lake.

Continuing on the path around the lake, you pass through a copse of moss-draped buckeyes and around the elbow of the east arm of the lake. Just before reaching the equestrian parking area, a footpath curves south. Take this path to reach a grove of hickory oaks on a knoll high above the lake. Here is a delightful, shady place to enjoy your daypack refreshments.

Then follow the trail north around the other arm of the lake, making a gentle descent to the main trail from the parking area.

MEANDER ALONG LAMBERT CREEK

A downhill saunter means an uphill return.

Distance: 1.4 miles round trip

Time: 1 hour

Elevation Change: 450′ loss

This short trip is perfect for a late afternoon outing. With a backpack supper you can amble along the creek's west bank until you find an appropriate picnic site.

Leave the Horseshoe Lake area just west of the bridge over the lake's outlet and turn due south on a wide track. For the first half mile you descend under oak, bay, and fir trees that completely overarch the trail. Fern-draped banks, accented with showy, long-leaved, creamy-white and blue iris, extend high on the uphill side.

After 0.5 mile you step into a clearing beyond which the trail makes a wide curve east. Here is a marshy reed-choked area where you can hear, but not see, Lambert Creek. As the trail swings west, it comes a bit closer to the creek, but this marks the end of the trail. A large fallen tree in the clearing makes a seat for enjoying a snack or picnic.

The preserve closes at dusk; allow enough time to regain the 450-foot elevation loss and get to your car before the gates are locked.

Long Ridge Open Space Preserve

Long Ridge Preserve extends along the heights of the Santa Cruz Mountains for 4.1 miles just west of Skyline Boulevard and southeast along Highway 9 for another 1.5 miles. Its 1985 acres of wooded hillside and open grasslands offer breathtaking views west to the Pacific on a clear day. Sometimes fog shrouds the ocean and hangs in the canyons of the Santa Cruz Mountains. However, whatever the weather, a trip over these uncluttered lands will be a refreshing experience.

The preserve's unspoiled mountainsides fall away from the ridge in successive flanks of rounded shoulders and gentle valleys. Craggy rocks stand like sentinels on sloping grasslands. Firs, oaks, and madrones cover the eastern slopes, and magnificent spreading canyon oaks, known also as hickory oaks, stand in clumps along its upper hillsides. This evergreen oak, pruned high by generations of grazing cattle, is also known as the maul oak, so named by the early settlers who used its wood for mauls and other tool handles.

The headwaters of Peters, Slate, and Oil creeks rise in the heights of the preserve and descend westward through its wooded canyons, each joining Pescadero Creek in Portola Redwoods State Park at the base of prominent Butano Ridge you see to the southwest.

Fourteen miles of trail lead through pretty creek canyons, up to and across its high grasslands. A 3.8-mile segment of the Bay Area Ridge Trail traverses the preserve connecting Long Ridge to Saratoga Gap in the south and to Skyline Ridge Open Space Preserve to the north. The Hickory Oaks and Ward Road Trail connect to Portola Redwoods State Park. The Hickory Oaks and Grizzly Flat trails connect to trails in Upper Stevens Canyon that join the Canyon Trail in Monte Bello OSP.

Trails along Highway 9 southwest of Saratoga Gap form a short segment of the Skyline-to-the-Sea Trail which links to the new hikers and equestrians Achistaca Trail.

Jurisdiction: Midpeninsula Regional Open Space District: 650-691-1200

Facilities: 10 miles of trail, most open to hikers, equestrians, and bicyclists

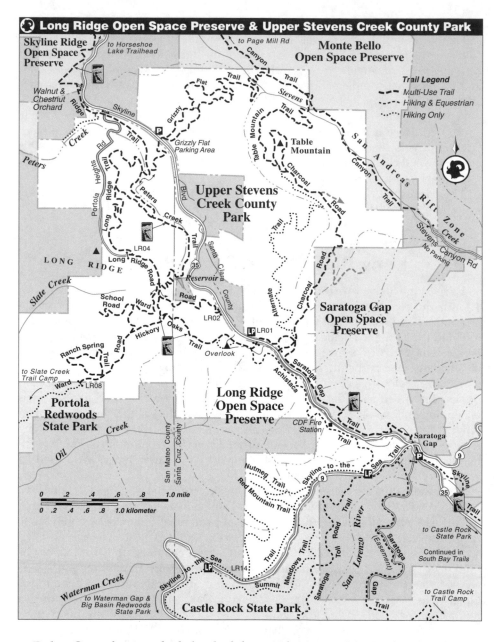

Long Ridge Open Space Preserve & Upper Stevens Creek County Park

Rules: Open dawn to dusk; leashed dogs with permits (obtained at Grizzly Flat entrance) allowed on Peters Creek Trail, Long Ridge Trail, and firebreak that parallels Skyline Boulevard

Maps: MROSD *South Skyline Region*, Portola Redwoods State Park brochure *Portola Redwoods State Park*, USGS topo *Mindego Hill*

How to Get There: Grizzly Flat Entrance: Take Skyline Blvd. south from Page Mill Rd. 3 miles or north from Saratoga Gap 3.6 miles to parking on west side.

Hickory Oaks Entrance Gate LR01: Take Skyline Blvd. south from Page Mill Rd., pass the Grizzly Flat entrance and continue 2 miles to roadside pull-outs at MROSD gate on west side of highway or go north from Saratoga Gap 1.6 miles to roadside parking on east side of highway. Achistaca Trail Entrance gate: take Hwy 9.25 mile southwest of Saratoga Gap to parking on north side of road.

OVER THE BRIDGE AND THROUGH THE WOODS TO LONG RIDGE VIEWS

Experience thousands of acres of uncluttered open space from the preserve's high ridges.

Distance: 5.0 miles round trip on Long Ridge Road and Long Ridge Trail; 5.1 miles round trip via the cross-trail midway along the ridge; 4.7 miles via Peters Creek valley

Time: 2½ hours

Elevation Change: 300′ loss (and subsequent gain)

The trail from Grizzly Flat descends 0.4 mile across a grassy slope, passes the north leg of the Bay Area Ridge Trail and enters a little canyon where Peters Creek winds through the woods. When you cross the bridge over this creek, you will see on your right the Long Ridge Trail turning uphill (north). Note this trail, which you can take on the return trip. However, continue now 0.4 mile along the Peters Creek Trail upstream as it passes through a narrow, steep canyon. Huge moss-covered boulders lie in the creek bed; laurels, firs, and oaks meet overhead, and ferns line the banks.

You soon emerge from the canyon into a sunny valley where the trail rises gently and the creek disappears beneath tall willows. An apple orchard, part of an old farm, grows between the willow-bordered creek and the hillside to the west. The trees are thriving in spite of neglect, and you may find a few apples in the fall—those out of reach of the resident deer.

Watch on the west side of the valley for a sign marking a sharp right turn uphill. Here is a trail through the woods leading 0.4 mile toward Long Ridge's summit on which you could return. Instead, you continue on the Peters Creek Trail through the valley. Early settlers on their way to Saratoga Gap used this old road, shaded by tall oaks and maples. In 0.7 mile you turn right and cross the little dam that holds back the waters of Peters Creek. After following a 0.5-mile zigzag route uphill, you reach the 4-way junction with Long Ridge Road and Ward Road. If you turn left, south, you would reach the Hickory Oak forest, described in the Hickory Oaks trip, following, or the cut-off for the trip to Portola Redwoods State Park.

However, this trip turns right (north) on Long Ridge Road. You are now out in open grasslands looking over a succession of forested ridges extending to the coast. Wend your way north for 0.5 mile on this wide road that undulates up and down past sandstone outcrops punctuating the steep hillside. Grassy hills fall away precipitously from the crest of the ridge and clumps of spreading canyon oaks dot the hilltop. From here you can orient yourself to the ridges and canyons before you, much of which are in the public parklands that you can explore with the help of this book.

Due west in the great redwood canyon of Pescadero Creek is Portola Redwoods State Park. Its east boundary adjoins this preserve, reached via the Ward Road Trail (see the Hickory Oaks trip, following). Downstream are Pescadero Creek County Park and adjoining Memorial and Sam McDonald county parks. You can see the long flank of Butano Ridge that forms the western boundary of Pescadero Park.

When you arrive at the gated junction (LR04) with the private road (on your left) and Long Ridge Road, look for a stone bench dedicated in May 1996 to commemorate author Wallace Stegner, a strong supporter of open space and wilderness preservation. Wallace and Mary Stegner were part of a group who preserved and then sold the former Long Ridge Ranch to MROSD.

After remembering Stegner for his many contributions, continue due north for 0.8 mile. At times great canyon oaks and firs cast heavy shade. Then the trail rises to a clearing at the junction with the cross-trail you met on the Peters Creek Trail south. You could take this pretty 0.4-mile route downhill to rejoin the Peters Creek Trail in the valley and turn left on it to reach the Grizzly Flat parking area.

However, the Long Ridge Trail continues north before it climbs to a wide swing west. Then it circles right through the forest and descends rather abruptly to join the Peters Creek Trail near the bridge. In 20 minutes you will be back at the creek. Turn left to cross the creek and climb the short hill back to the preserve entrance.

HICKORY OAKS AND SIDE-TRIP TO TABLE ROCK

An impressive walk for visitors and locals alike.

Distance: 0.8 mile round trip + 0.2 mile round trip to rock

Time: ¾ hour

Elevation Change: 100' gain

Go over the stile at the gated fire road and go uphill on the old ranch road. In 100 yards the Hickory Oaks Trail turns right under the wide-spreading trees for which the trail is named. From their massive, clear trunks, some up to 5 feet in diameter, grow huge horizontal and often contorted limbs. This oak, *Quercus chrysolepis*, also called canyon, gold cup, and maul oak, has fine-grained hardwood, which early settlers prized for wagon wheels and farm implements.

Beyond the grove and uphill to the left (west) a side trail leads to a park-like meadow, rimmed with handsome trees and dotted with great, sandstone outcrops. One table-like rock is said to have been a sacrificial altar for Indian tribes. At the winter solstice the setting sun shines directly through a vertical crack in this same rock. Linger here perched on a bench to enjoy the western panorama of successive forested ridges creased by wooded canyons—an uncluttered pastoral scene.

Returning to the road from the north side of the meadow, you rejoin the wide Hickory Oaks Trail. To the left this trail climbs over rolling pasturelands that fall off to the forested canyons below. From this junction you can retrace your steps or continue on to Long Ridge Road, as described in the trip to Long Ridge. Or you can follow the Hickory Oaks Trail west through meadows and woodlands to Ward Road and into Portola Redwoods State Park and its forested canyons. See Downhill to Portola Redwoods State Park, following.

On your return note the gated entrance to the Achistaca Trail which leads to Highway 9.

DOWNHILL TO PORTOLA REDWOODS STATE PARK

Two historic sites and a lovely creek walk make this a memorable trip. With a car shuttle waiting at the state park, this is an easy trip.

Distance: 7 miles one way to Portola Redwoods State Park office

Time: 3¾ hours

Elevation Change: 800' loss

Starting from the Hickory Oaks entrance on Skyline Boulevard, take the Hickory Oaks Trail northwest along the route described in the Hickory Oaks trip above to the Long Ridge Road junction. Here you turn left (west), go 0.3 mile and arc southwest on Ward Road to begin your descent along this wide old ranch road.

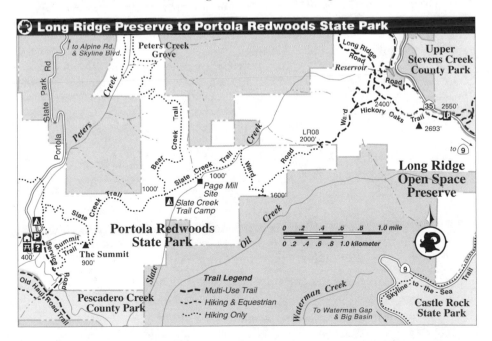

At first, you amble along through broad grasslands gloriously green in spring, golden in summer and fall. Off to the east is the ridge where Highway 9 winds its curving way down along the west boundary of Castle Rock State Park, the approximate route of the Skyline-to-the-Sea Trail. To the southeast are the deep, lush, canyons of Oil and Waterman creeks, sometimes clothed in mist, sometimes so clear that individual trees are discernible.

Descending steadily, you reach a broad plateau where the 0.9-mile Ranch Spring Trail circles the site of a ranch owned by the Panigetti family, from whom MROSD bought land in 1990. The loop trail swings around the plateau and into woods of black oak and Douglas fir, passes an old spring and returns to the main trail. At this remote ranch site you could pause on its sunny, south-facing grasslands to admire the views and to explore the pretty flat enclosed by venerable trees.

After another mile beside banks clothed with creeping manzanita bushes and lavender-flowered yerba santa, you reach the gate of Portola Redwoods State Park, beyond which bicyclists and horses are not permitted. Hikers walk around the gate and continue downhill, winding around the southeast-facing slope. After passing a forsaken farm site on the left, you enter the shade of an evergreen forest, and go up a little rise. Look here on your right for the marked trail to Slate Creek and the Portola Redwoods.

Along this circuitous trail are old redwood logs, cut into three- to ten-foot lengths, evidence of an abandoned logging and shingle-making operation. After descending steps cut into the steep hillside, you cross Slate Creek to follow it uphill through the cool redwood forest. This is an excellent, well-graded trail—a pleasure to walk on.

In less than 0.5 mile you'll find a large rustic sign declaring that William Page had a mill at this site, although there are no logs, buildings, or old wagons to verify the fact. This was his second mill; the other was on Peters Creek downstream from the destination of the Peters Creek Loop Trail, one of the Portola Redwoods State Park trips in this book. A lunch stop here will give you time to ponder how Page hauled his lumber out of this canyon.

Shortly you pass the Slate Creek Trail Camp at the junction with the Peters Creek Loop Trail and continue 1.3 miles to the Slate Creek and Summit trails junction. Take either trail for a 1+ mile trip to the park visitor center, where your friends await your arrival.

SEE MAP
ON PAGE
174

THE BAY AREA RIDGE TRAIL

Take a link in the 400-mile regional trail that circles the Bay on its ridgetops.

Distance: 3.8 miles one-way, multi-use on Peters Creek route; 4.2 miles one-way multi-use on Long Ridge Road route; 4.2 miles one-way, hikers, equestrians from Hwy 9 on Achistaca Trail

Time: 2 hours one-way, multi-use trail; 2¼ hours one-way, hikers, equestrians

Elevation Change: 150' gain

Combining parts of the trips to Long Ridge and to Hickory Oaks, this multi-use segment of the Ridge Trail route traverses the entire preserve. The trip starts on the Hickory Oaks Trail and turns uphill (north) on Long Ridge Road for 0.3 mile to its junction with the Peters Creek Trail. Here on a high ridge you can choose to take Long Ridge Road through the grasslands up and around the preserve's west side or to turn east on the Peters Creek Trail and switchback through oaks and madrones down to the Peters Creek reservoir, then follow the creek downstream through dense forest and past the apple orchard in a tight valley.

Just before the Peters Creek bridge, both routes converge, cross the creek and in 0.1 mile bear left (north) at the Grizzly Flat Trail junction. This 1-mile segment of the Ridge Trail parallels the east side of Peters Creek, then crosses two private roads and enters Skyline Ridge Open Space Preserve near an old chestnut orchard (see page 170).

NORTHWARD ON THE ACHISTACA TRAIL

A walk in the woods with splendid views west.

Distance: 1.7 miles one way

Time: ¾ hour

Elevation Change: Relatively level

Hikers and equestrians begin this trip from the small parking area just 0.25 mile southwest of Saratoga Gap at a pullout on the north side of the road. More parking is nearby at the junction at Saratoga Gap. Bicyclists can take the Ridge Trail route on the east side of Skyline Boulevard, from Saratoga Gap.

This newest trail for hikers and equestrians in Long Ridge is relatively level and meanders northwest along the route of an old road used by early settlers. Almost entirely under the shade of venerable oaks, it passes beside large sandstone cliffs and below the CDF fire station. From a wide, sloping, grassy meadow there are spectacular views over successive forested ridges to the heights of Butano Ridge and through a notch in the mountains out to sea.

At the junction with the Hickory Oaks Trail, you can continue north or pause for awhile in another sloping meadow.

The Achistaca Trail makes a pleasant, easy 3.4-mile round trip for those not taking the complete Bay Area Ridge Trail route through Long Ridge Open Space Preserve. Or combine it with a return trip to Saratoga Gap on the east side of Skyline Boulevard.

◆ City Parks and Trails in the Foothills ◆ of the Southern Peninsula

Town of Portola Valley

Portola Valley lies along the San Andreas Fault in the foothills of the Santa Cruz Mountains. These lands were part of a Mexican land grant, Rancho Corte de Madera (meaning cutting of timber), later divided into agricultural ranches acquired by Anglos in the late 1800s. By the end of World War II, further subdivisions divided the larger properties and the area rapidly became suburban.

Some of the subdivisions included horse trails in their design, but by 1964, with the incorporation of Portola Valley, most of the land was private, fenced, and inaccessible to hikers or equestrians. The town adopted a Trails Plan in 1969, and as new properties subdivide, their designs must implement trails. The MROSD purchases of the Windy Hill and Coal Creek open space preserves, comprising 1801 acres mostly within the town limits, gave residents easy access to trails in wooded, hilly open space.

Portola Valley has many trails that are open to the public, and maps of these are available at Town Hall, 775 Portola Road. These include trails in the Portola Valley Ranch subdivision, close to Windy Hill, trails along Alpine Road and Portola roads, and the Larry Lane Trail in the Hayfields subdivision. All the town trails are well marked by sign posts that bear the name of the trail you are using, its length, and the distance to the next junction on the trail. Some posts bear the name of the donor and an honoree. The generosity of the donors and the work of volunteers made these helpful trail signs possible.

Remember, when using Portola Valley town trails, you are going through private property. Although the trails are unfenced, it is your responsibility to stay on the trail and to comply with trail rules. Hard-working volunteers spend weekends constructing and maintaining these trails.

Following are three trips on the town trails and a long loop trip through the valley and into Menlo Park.

Jurisdiction: Town of Portola Valley: 650-851-1700

Facilities: Trails for hikers and equestrians; trailside benches

Rules: Open dawn to dusk; hikers only on Toyon Trail; dogs on leash allowed on upper Old Spanish Trail; no bicycles

Maps: Map on page 182 Available from Portola Valley Town Hall, USGS topo *Mindego Hill*

How to Get There: From I-280 take Alpine Rd. exit south. Continue on Alpine Rd. past Portola Rd. junction to intersection of Willowbrook Dr., where there is limited parking on north side of Alpine Rd.

A LOOP TRIP ON COAL MINE RIDGE

SEE MAP ON PAGE 182

A delightful trip at any time, this loop tours a flowery garden in spring.

Distance: short loop: 3.1 miles; long loop: 4.6 miles

Time: 1½ hours, short loop; 2½ hours long loop

Elevation Change: 400' gain

The Old Spanish Trail for hikers and equestrians starts up through the woods opposite the parking area at Willowbrook Drive. When you reach a junction where the Toyon Trail turns right, take a few steps farther and bear right, uphill, on the Old Spanish Trail, under oaks and past small meadows. As you come out of the woods, the Old Spanish Trail turns right, paralleling the service road going uphill. Before reaching the water tank, the trail crosses the road and continues across the meadow to the left of the big water tank. Just beyond the water tank you bear left, and step onto the Coal Mine Trail, which continues across the meadow to the left of the big water tank. On the opposite ridge you can see the homes of Portola Valley Ranch, whose owners dedicated this private land as an open space easement to the town.

Beyond the water tank, the Coal Mine Trail goes into the woods and continues left past a connector to the Toyon Trail, your return route. The Coal Mine Trail zigzags southeast uphill under oaks and bays to an opening in the trees where you will find the Vernal Pool, perhaps a sag pond, a sign of past earthquakes and land movements. Stay on the trail to avoid disturbing the pond plants at its edges. By summer the water may have evaporated, yet the plants have adapted to the dry summers and they return each year. Another half hour through the woods takes you to the high point of the trip—a long meadow known as Ridge Rest. In spring

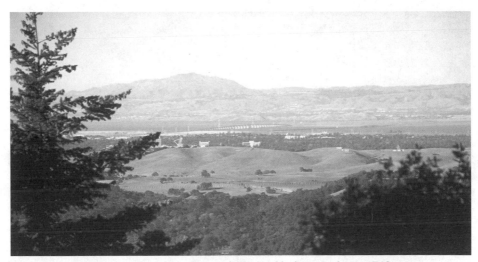

Looking across Portola Valley to the Bay and Mt. Diablo from Coal Mine Ridge

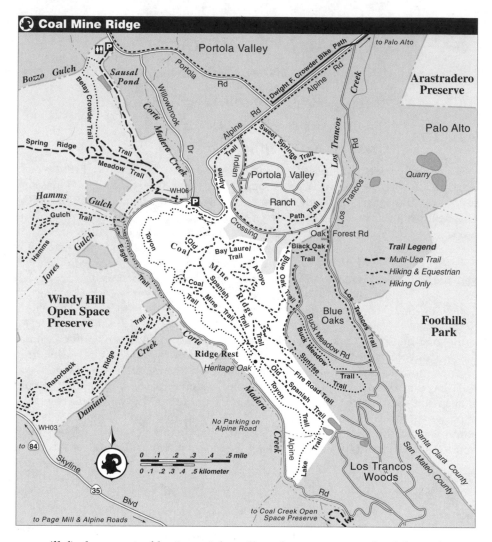

you will find a carpet of lupine, pink mallow, forget-me-nots, dandelions, butter-cups, cowslips, and poppies in this ridgetop meadow.

From this meadow you can see the Bay and across to the eastern foothills (unless it's smoggy). In the foreground to the southeast the brush-covered ridge of Foothills Park on the far side of Los Trancos Creek rises to join Monte Bello Ridge.

As you enter this meadow, look for the junction with the Toyon Trail on your right. Pass it and continue a few steps farther on your left to an ancient, wide-spreading live oak, known as the Old Heritage Tree. Here is a good, shady resting place on a downed log beside the trail.

In 2004 the Blue Oaks section of Portola Valley developed a 3.1-mile loop on the Old Spanish and Toyon Trails that extends to the heights of Los Trancos Woods. If you take this loop, continue uphill on the Old Spanish Trail, keeping on the east side of the ridge. A few eucalyptus trees, remnants of an old forest, drop their shaggy bark along the trail, and lush cow's parsnip and toyon bushes edge the trail. As you mount higher on the ridge, you pass a reservoir and ponds on your right and soon reach the junction with the Lake Trail. In the shade of great oaks you bear right on this well graded, narrow trail, for hikers only.

At the next junction turn right onto the upper section of the Toyon Trail that descends up and down small hillocks along the west side of the ridge, almost always under the shade of oaks, mahogany-barked madrones, and bay trees. Openings in the forest provide peeks of the heavily wooded flanks of Windy Hill Open Space Preserve. Farther south only a few dwellings interrupt the rich green blanket that clothes the ridges and canyons of the Corte Madera Creek watershed.

When you reach the crossover trail to the Old Spanish and Coal Mine trails, bear left and continue down the 2.25-mile Toyon Trail. This narrow trail for hikers only, cut into the steep side of the ridge, descends through an oak forest on a very gentle grade down into the canyon of Corte Madera Creek.

In about a mile along the Toyon Trail you come to a junction where a short connector to the lower water-tank meadow on the Coal Mine and Old Spanish trails take off right. Continue straight ahead. You soon cross two wooden-plank bridges over little streams. Though the streams run only after a rain, there is moisture enough for a garden of maidenhair ferns lining their banks. The trail continues past a couple of sunny chaparral-covered slopes, then turns back into the woods of oaks, bays, and buckeyes. Benches along the way invite you to sit and enjoy the view of grassy Windy Hill through the trees and the heavily forested ridges across the canyon. As you listen to the calls of birds, you may also hear the sounds of Corte Madera Creek below. Then continue downhill to the short trail that descends to the parking area at Willowbrook Road near the creek.

SEE MAP ON PAGE 182

A Hike or Horseback Ride into History

Follow in the footsteps of explorers and early settlers.

Distance: 5-mile loop

Time: 2½ hours

Elevation Change: 360' gain

Start up the Old Spanish Trail as in the Loop Trip on Coal Mine Ridge, but keep left (east) where the Coal Mine Trail goes uphill past the water tank. Your route on an unsurfaced service road goes through an oak glade on a gentle grade, and then turns up through chaparral and oak woodland. In 0.5 mile you reach the hilltop meadow and meet the Coal Mine and Toyon trails. After a pause to catch your breath (or in spring to admire the flowers in the meadow), start down the Arroyo Trail, which heads down switchbacks on the east side of the ridge under spreading canyon oaks. You cross grasslands, and go through a eucalyptus grove before descending through oak-madrone woods along a fern-clad north slope to reach a bridge across a tributary of Los Trancos Creek.

Shortly beyond the bridge, the trail forks. Bear left and continue along the hillside for 0.5 mile to the gravel-surfaced Bay Laurel service road. Cross it, turn left, uphill, on the trail beside the road, and go 0.25 mile to an intersection where you rejoin the Old Spanish Trail. Turn downhill here and retrace your steps back to Willowbrook Drive.

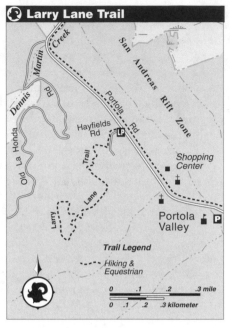

THE LARRY LANE TRAIL

A trail to remember the founder of Sunset Magazine and avid equestrian.

This 1.75-mile loop trail climbs 500 feet from the floor of the valley halfway to Skyline Boulevard to a vista point. This public riding and hiking trail is dedicated to Laurence W. Lane, who loved to ride these hills with his family and friends. Lane promoted horse trails, mostly along roads built in the Westridge subdivision, which a homeowners' association maintains.

The trail begins at Hayfields Road where there is limited parking at the first roadside pullout a block above Portola Road. On switchbacks the trail climbs past some homes along the way, so trail users should stay on the trail at all times except at trailside rest areas. As the trail emerges from the woods, it splits east and west, and then the branches meet on a traverse at the top of the hill. Here a magnificent oak spreads its ancient limbs over the trail. Benches along the way give you a rest on your climb and a place to enjoy the mountainside scene. Locked gates in the upper part of the trail lead into Woodside Trails Club paths for equestrians only.

"The Loop"—Through Portola Valley, Woodside and Menlo Park

A roadside trail of nearly 12 miles goes past the community of Ladera, through Portola Valley and along the outskirts of Woodside and into Menlo Park. It includes off-the-road paved paths, unsurfaced horse and hiking trails and continuous bike lanes on road shoulders.

Jurisdiction: San Mateo County, Town of Portola Valley, Town of Woodside, City of Menlo Park

Maps: *Tour of Historic Portola Valley*, USGS topos *Palo Alto* and *Mindego Hill*

How To Get There: From I-280 take Alpine Rd exit, go north toward Palo Alto to parking areas at trail access points: (1) beside Alpine Rd south of Santa Cruz

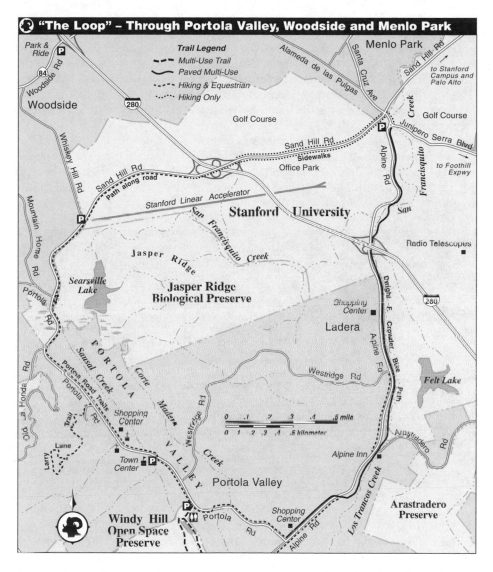

"The Loop" – Through Portola Valley, Woodside and Menlo Park

Trail Legend
- – – Multi-Use Trail
- Paved Multi-Use
- – – – Hiking & Equestrian
- ······· Hiking Only

Ave/Junipero Serra Blvd intersection; (2) near San Francisquito Creek bridge opposite entrance to Portola Valley Training Center; (3) Town Center in Portola Valley and many other entrances along the way.

Distance: 12–mile loop; many convenient entry points allow trips of different lengths.

Time: 6 hours—hikers; 1–2 hours—bicyclists and equestrians.

Elevation Change: Gentle grade

San Mateo County built the first two miles of trail in 1969 under a federal program to encourage trail building in urban areas. At this writing, the first section described here is under re-construction as part of road widening. Until the project is finished, watch for trail re-route signs or begin the trip about 1 mile south at entrance (2) across from the Portola Valley Training Center.

(1) This trail leaves from Alpine Road just south of the Santa Cruz/Junipero Serra Boulevard intersection, skirts the Stanford Golf Course and curves onto the old road fronting a small settlement formerly known as Stanford Weekend Acres. (2) Opposite the P.V. Training Center (rear entrance to the Stanford Linear Accelerator), the trail leaves the road and crosses a bridge over San Francisquito Creek on the old road alignment.

San Francisquito Creek drains the area from the Phleger Estate and Huddart County Park to the San Mateo County boundary. Just upstream from the bridge the smaller Los Trancos Creek joins San Francisquito Creek. As the path comes back to Alpine Road it goes under I-280 and dips down toward the creek, where it has its own underpass below the freeway on-ramp.

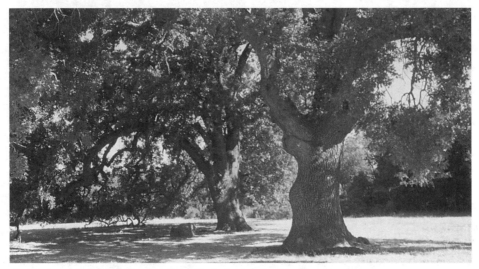

Ancient valley oaks in Dorothy Ford Park along "The Loop"

The trail passes the Ladera community and a swim and tennis club, then enters the Portola Valley town limits and becomes the Dwight F. Crowder Memorial Bicycle Path. This trail was built in 1971 with memorial funds to honor a Portola Valley geologist, conservationist, and bicycling enthusiast who worked long and successfully to get the trails plan adopted in newly incorporated Portola Valley. The path veers away from the road to skirt a meadow shaded by immense valley oaks, the memorial Dorothy Ford Park, which adjoins Kelley Park, where Alpine Little League plays baseball in the spring.

Again the path comes close to the road, but is shielded from it by trees and tall chaparral. This sunny stretch is welcome on winter walks. Crossing Arastradero Road, along which horse trails lead to Palo Alto and Los Altos Hills, you come to California's oldest roadhouse, the Alpine Inn. Formerly called Rossotti's, it is now a registered historical landmark. The bronze plaque embedded in a boulder by the entrance tells that the structure was built in the 1850s as a gambling retreat and a meeting place for Mexican Californios. It was strategically located on the earliest trail used by rancheros and American settlers crossing to the coast. It has continued to serve as a roadhouse and saloon to this day.

Once past the adjoining soccer field, you head straight toward the mountains. The weather on the dark-forested Skyline ridge ahead often gives early warning of changing weather in the valley—gathering clouds signal impending rain, blue haze heralds a smoggy day ahead and fog flows indicate cooler temperatures from the coast.

At Los Trancos Woods Road the horse path continues straight while the paved path crosses to the other side of Alpine Road. By the redwood at the path's edge is a historical marker noting the home of Maximo Martinez, who in the 1830s received the grant of Rancho Corte de Madera, the first in San Mateo County. Three generations of Martinezes lived here in the house which remained until 1940. The path continues along Alpine Road to its intersection with Portola Road, where it ends in a charming little park planted by the Town of Portola Valley. Furnished with benches and graced by a fanciful iron deer, this park is a good place to picnic or rest before continuing.

An unpaved footpath and equestrian trail continues around "The Loop." Go west from the park at the corner of Alpine and Portola roads on the trail along the northeast side of Portola Road. After passing playing fields and orchards, the trail crosses the road at the stone gatehouse of the former Willow Brook Farm. Built in 1912 of wood faced with stones from Corte Madera Creek, this is the only structure left of the estate which with its mansion once dominated the valley.

Here Portola Valley widens and before you fields and orchards spread across the valley floor and unbroken views encompass the sweep of the Santa Cruz Mountains. Going through the valley on foot allows you to appreciate the charm of this quiet rural scene. Right below your feet, nevertheless, is one of the most active earthquake faults in the country. Because of this seismic hazard, much of the valley floor is still planted to hay and fruit trees or used for riding rings. In the great earthquake of 1906, the land displacement in some places nearby was as much as 8 feet.

Farther on is the little Portola Valley schoolhouse, built in 1912. An interesting example of the mission-revival style popular in the early 20th century, it is now a historical landmark. The more modern buildings next to it, built as a school before earthquake hazards were fully recognized, currently house the Town Center, library, and meeting rooms, and now are about to be re-constructed.

At the Village Square Shopping Center the path returns to the northeast side of the road. Beyond is the charming California mission-style Church of Our Lady of the Wayside. Built in 1912, it is a favorite subject of local art classes. For the next mile the trail follows along the fences of tree farms, orchards, and estates.

Where Portola Road turns north at Old La Honda Road, you can see Searsville Marsh. Bordered by willows and cattails, it is a favorite resting place for ducks and other migrating waterfowl. Beyond the marsh Portola Road turns west but the path continues straight ahead along Sand Hill Road. On the northwest side of this junction the historic marker notes the lumberman's village that once stood here. John Sears, the first settler, arrived here in 1832. His hotel, store, school, and dwellings were removed as the water rose behind the new dam which created the lake now known as Searsville.

From here to the junction of Whiskey Hill Road the path follows the fence of Stanford University's Jasper Ridge Biological Preserve and Research Center (within which is Searsville Lake). Somewhat removed from the road and its traffic, the path goes gently up and down through the trees.

There is no formal off-road path on Sand Hill Road between Whiskey Hill Road and I-280. Many hikers and joggers use the unpaved road shoulder. It is a favorite stretch for bicyclists because the wide bike lanes are uninterrupted by side roads.

The mile-long linear accelerator lies on the south side of the road beginning opposite the Whiskey Hill Road junction. Rising beyond is the rocky promontory of Jasper Ridge, a protected treasure of unique flora and fauna. (See Appendix III for docent-led walks through the preserve.)

In summer and fall dark-green valley oaks accent the pale gold fields of oat grass on both sides of the road. This once-common kind of grassland scene, cherished by Californians, is fast disappearing. On the north side of Sand Hill Road, an equestrian center leases acreage for riding events. On the south side former Christmas-tree farms are defunct, with native species slowly taking over. Crossing the I-280 interchange is a hazard for bicyclists and pedestrians, and should not be attempted by equestrians.

From I-280 to Santa Cruz Avenue you walk or ride on paved paths over knolls where office buildings and their parking lots are interspersed with open fields and stately oaks. The sidewalks on both sides of Sand Hill Road from the freeway to Santa Cruz Avenue are good cool-weather walks, with vistas of the rolling foothills and their forested mountain backdrop.

At the Santa Cruz Avenue/Sand Hill Road intersection, you pass the entrance to the Hewlett Foundation and the former Buck Estate, willed to Stanford University. Until the Sand Hill reconstruction project is finished in 2005, follow the signs that indicate temporary routes through this busy intersection to the continuation of the trail along Alpine Road.

Whether taken in short sections or in its entirety, this easily accessible and varied loop trip is an asset to Peninsula hikers, bicyclists, and equestrians. It is a favorite among cyclists whose phalanx formations sweep through on their daily noontime rides.

Enid Pearson Arastradero Preserve

For a glimpse of the rolling grasslands and magnificent oaks of foothill ranchlands, visit this city of Palo Alto preserve. In the spring of 2004 Enid Pearson's name was added to this preserve in appreciation of her efforts to buy the land for Palo Alto. Most of its 609 acres are located on the south side of Arastradero Road between Alpine and Page Mill roads, but 176 acres lie on the north side of Arastradero Road. The preserve is open daily to the general public. It adjoins two large open-space areas—Palo Alto's Foothills Park on the south and Stanford lands west of I-280 on the north, although neither is accessible from the preserve.

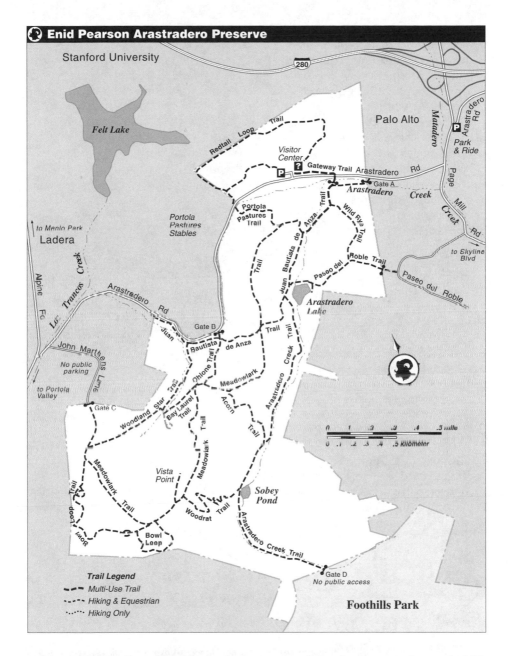

Enid Pearson Arastradero Preserve

Stanford University

Felt Lake

Palo Alto

Park & Ride

to Menlo Park

Ladera

Visitor Center

Gateway Trail

Arastradero Rd

Gate A

Arastradero Creek

to Skyline Blvd

Portola Pastures Stables

Portola Pastures Trail

Wild Rye Trail

Roble Trail

Paseo del Roble

Paseo del Roble

Redtail Loop Trail

Juan Bautista de Anza Trail

Arastradero Lake

Arastradero Rd

Gate B

Juan Bautista de Anza Trail

Arastradero Creek Trail

No public parking

to Portola Valley

Gate C

Woodland Star Trail

Bay Laurel Trail

Ohlone Trail

Meadowlark Trail

Acorn Trail

John Martens Lane

Alpine Rd

Las Trancos Creek

Meadowlark Trail

Bowl Loop Trail

Vista Point

Meadowlark Trail

Woodrat Trail

Sobey Pond

Arastradero Creek Trail

Bowl Loop

Gate D
No public access

Foothills Park

Trail Legend
- – ▪ – Multi-Use Trail
- ▪ ▪ ▪ Hiking & Equestrian
- ▪▪▪▪▪ Hiking Only

More than 7 miles of trails, mostly former ranch roads, traverse the gentle hills and valleys of the preserve. Just minutes away from midpeninsula cities, it is easy to find quiet and solitude on a hike to nearby Arastradero Lake or to the oak-studded ridge at the south end of the preserve. Equestrians especially, use the Juan Bautista de Anza Trail to make connections between Portola Valley and Los Altos Hills trails. A proposal for a trail from Arastradero Preserve up through Foothills

Park to Los Trancos Open Space Preserve has yet to be implemented.

Arastradero Preserve is managed by Acterra (formerly the Bay Area Action group) in a cooperative arrangement with the city of Palo Alto. Since 1997 this group has made improvements to the trail system, controlled the spread of non-native plants, and conducted environmental education programs and habitat restoration projects. If you see groups of people planting native trees, repairing trails, or removing non-native, noxious thistle and teasel, consider joining one of many groups that are caring for this fine preserve.

Jurisdiction: City of Palo Alto: 650-329-2423

Facilities: Trails for hikers, equestrians, and bicyclists; interpretive facility under construction; restroom

Hikers descend the Anza Trail in Arastradero

Rules: Open 8 A.M. until dusk; dogs permitted on leash only; no boating or swimming in the lake; no hunting or camping; some trails closed after heavy rains

Maps: city of Palo Alto *Arastradero Preserve* and USGS topo *Palo Alto*

How to Get There: From I-280 take Page Mill Rd. south, turn right on Arastradero Rd. and go 0.5 mile to preserve parking lot on north side of road. Take a graveled path, the Gateway Trail, east from parking area and cross Arastradero Rd. to reach the preserve's larger area. The stile to the north side of the preserve leaves directly from this parking area.

SEE MAP ON PAGE 189

HIKE ALONG ARASTRADERO CREEK TO THE LAKE AND UP THE CANYON TO ITS HEADWATERS

Try this hike in the early morning when ducks are paddling on the lake and birds are singing in the willows by the creek.

Distance: 4 miles round trip

Time: 2 hours

Elevation Change: 300' gain

Start on the Juan Bautista de Anza Trail, which leaves the preserve entrance beside Arastradero Creek. In late winter and in spring this can be a rushing stream, but by summer it is reduced to a trickle. The huge tree stumps on the far side of the creek are remnants of giant eucalyptus that bordered an old ranch road, damaged during a serious fire here in 1985.

Beyond the creek crossing, a well-worn trail climbs up a short hill where brilliant orange poppies and blue lupines bloom profusely in spring. Stately white oaks with wide-spreading limbs dot the grasslands. As you approach the lake, the Paseo del Roble Trail takes off left, and almost immediately you come to the tree-shaded, reed-bordered lake. The slanting light of the morning sun streams through the trees, picking up the iridescent green of mallard ducks and the glossy shoulder patches of red-wing blackbirds.

To continue upstream along Arastradero Creek, bear left (southeast) on the Arastadero Creek Trail and follow its willow-bordered course. Dense stands of trees clothe the hillsides east of the creek. Occasional oaks and some stands of buckeyes offer shade on the grassy slope west of the trail, and in spring flowers bloom in abundance. A haze of magenta clarkia covers the hillside in late June. As the creek bends east, so does the trail. As you pass the Acorn Trail on your right, note it for an alternate return route.

In less than 0.2 mile you come to marshy Sobey Pond, once used for watering cattle. Here the Woodrat Trail takes off right uphill, but you continue a bit farther in the ever-narrowing, moist canyon. Soon the trail ends, and your route becomes a utility service road that terminates at Gate D, just 2 miles from the start of this trip.

You can retrace your steps to the preserve entrance by the same route, or use the Woodrat or Acorn trail cutoffs to reach the Meadowlark Trail and descend on it to the Juan Bautista de Anza Trail and your starting point.

SEE MAP
ON PAGE
189

SAMPLE-ALL-THE-TRAILS LOOP

From creekside to topside this trip offers wide views and a stop in a quiet, wooded dell.

Distance: 4-mile loop

Time: 2¼ hours

Elevation Change: 400' gain

Begin on the Juan Bautista de Anza Trail as in the Hike along Arastradero Preserve, pass the cut-off to the lake and follow this trail (a gravel surfaced road) through wide meadows, which in spring are filled with flowers. Shortly you meet the Meadowlark Trail and turn left (uphill) on it. Out on top of the rolling grasslands you may see red-tailed hawks, black-shouldered kites, or northern harriers in their endless sky patrol for rodents and snakes. An occasional great blue heron wings overhead on its way to fish in the lake.

Passing the Acorn and Woodrat trails and still climbing, you soon reach the crest of the hill where a short trail on the right goes out to a fine vista point. Beyond here the trail levels off, passes several exits to the Bowl Loop, a favorite hilly, mountain bicycle course, and bends north to end at a gated road. However, just beyond the north end of the Bowl Loop, this trip goes right (northeast) on the narrow Woodland Star Trail. On it you descend past fields of oat grass dotted with ancient oaks and accented with bright flowers through spring and early summer. Under a light forest cover of mature buckeye trees, you drop down to a grassy valley beside a little watercourse, and a remote dell.

From this quiet place cross the creek on a wooden bridge to the Bay Laurel Trail, pick up the Ohlone Trail, and traverse a tree-shaded hillside where ferns and horsetails thrive and in spring deep-pink shooting stars bloom.

In a few minutes you reach the wide central plateau of the preserve. Bear right on the de Anza Trail with views of the northern cities by the Bay's shore. On this plateau you may hear the meadowlark's call, even before you meet the Meadowlark Trail. Turn left on this trail and walk down the plateau on a compacted dirt trail across broad fields of oat grass dotted with monarch valley and live oaks. Note the protected plantings of new oak seedlings surrounding these large, mature trees.

At the junction where the Portola Pastures Trail goes left, you go right on the Meadowlark Trail. To the north is the private property, where barns and buildings were lost in the same 1985 fire that destroyed the eucalyptus trees, and that is now being held by POST for future inclusion in this preserve.

Bear left on the de Anza Trail, cross the creek and wend your way 0.25 mile back to the preserve entrance.

THE REDTAIL LOOP TRAIL

A brisk climb to the trip's highest point brings views of Stanford land, Felt Lake, and the western foothills.

Distance: 1.37-mile loop

Time: 45 minutes

Elevation Change: 140' gain

Leave the north side of the preserve west of the interpretive facility and cross the stile to the trail on your right. Immediately you climb up a steep southwest-facing hillside, then level off briefly before mounting the next uphill stretch. As you rise, the views open up toward the east and south. After yet another upward pitch, you arrive at the trip's summit and a chance to look around the compass. Off to the southeast is the long flank of Black Mountain atop Monte Bello Ridge. The crest of the Santa Cruz Mountains is punctuated by the prominent high points of Borel Hill, Mt. Melville, and Windy Hill, a familiar, treasured back-drop of the mid-peninsula and the site of many popular open space preserves.

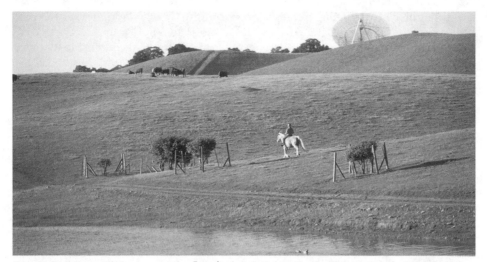

The Redtail Loop offers views of the Stanford dish, horses, and grazing cattle beside Felt Lake

Ambling gently downhill you follow the fence-line that separates Stanford land south of I-280 from this preserve. You circle around an oak-filled ravine, continuing downward past a long row of mature eucalyptus trees that frame the view of Felt Lake on Stanford lands where you may see wind-surfers skimming across the water. In the spring the red-shouldered blackbirds ceaselessly fly in and out of nests in the eucs, trilling their spritely song. As you head southeast, note the horse trail leading to the barns and corrals of a private stable. It's possible to cross Arastradero Road from the stables and take the Portola Pastures Trail to the preserve's many trails.

The Redtail Loop Trail turns due east and meanders through the meadows above Arastradero Road for about a third of a mile to the parking area and main gate. In spring you will see that the busy blackbirds are finding nesting materials and food in a shrubby ravine just north of your trail. Meanwhile, redtail hawks patrol the sky, also looking for a meal for nestlings.

Foothills Park

The 15 miles of trail through the woodlands, grasslands, and chaparral-covered hills of this park are restricted to residents of the city of Palo Alto and their accompanied guests.

The park, as stated in its brochure, "preserves 1400 acres of serenity and beauty on the fringes of a vast metropolitan area. Quiet oak-woodland, rolling grassland, rugged fields of chaparral, and cool hollows studded with ferns and scented with bay comprise a diverse and inspiring natural scene. Superb vistas punctuate the park's picturesque setting between baylands and redwood forests."

Foothills Park is popular with Palo Alto residents, whose frequent visits number in the hundreds of thousands each year. Understandably, it arouses some envious thoughts in those living in neighboring communities, who may visit the park only as guests. However, the park, to quote the Palo Alto Municipal Code, "has been established as a nature preserve in order to conserve for the residents of the City the natural features and scenic values within the City boundaries, to protect and maintain the ecology of the area . . . The fire hazard in Foothills Park is extreme and the population load in Foothills Park must be restricted and said park must be subject to reasonable closing hours and open only to residents of the city of Palo Alto. . . "

Jurisdiction: City of Palo Alto (Residents Only): 650-329-2261

Maps: USGS topo *Mindego Hill* and maps available at park entrance

How to Get There: From I-280 take Page Mill Rd. south about 3 miles to park entrance on the right.

The Arastradero/Foothill Expressway Hub

Three paved paths radiate out from this busy intersection to quiet rural scenes. Though school children and commuters hurry along these convenient routes, you can enjoy a leisurely stroll on each and find creeks and beautiful trees along the way. Combining two of these trails provides an off-the-road route from Los Altos Hills or Los Altos to Palo Alto.

In addition, the Arastradero Bike Path leads to on-road bike lanes and intermittent foot paths to Arastradero Preserve and its many trails, lakes, and South Bay views.

Jurisdiction: City of Palo Alto (and city of Los Altos for the Los Altos Bike Path)

Facilities: Paved paths for pedestrians and bicyclists

Rules: Open daylight hours; no motorcycles

Maps: USGS topos *Palo Alto* and *Mountain View*

How to Get There: From El Camino Real or Foothill Expressway in Palo Alto, take Arastradero Road to Gunn High School. Parking limited during school hours.

VARIAN/BOL PARK PATH

On the west side of Gunn High School a path winds gently north along a wide, abandoned railroad easement, reaching charming, secluded Bol Park and Hanover Street in Stanford Industrial Park. Tree-shaded paths that skirt the east side of Bol Park and Gunn High School offer alternate routes.

Distance: 2.8 miles round trip

Time: 1½ hours

Elevation Change: Level

Starting from Arastradero Road in front of Gunn High School, go west around the corner to Miranda Way. Take the path that follows the school's western edge,

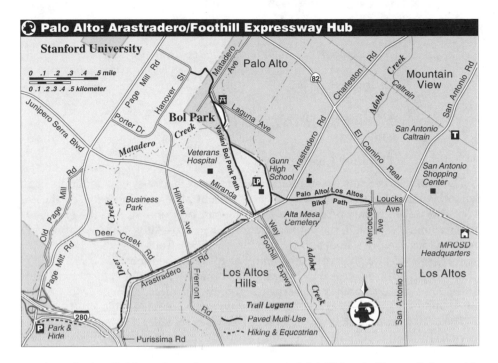

Palo Alto: Arastradero/Foothill Expressway Hub

passing playing fields and tennis courts on your right. This winding path in a wide old railroad easement is the former route of the Southern Pacific Railroad and the Peninsular Electric Railway on their runs to Los Gatos and San Jose. Though houses, industry, and heavy traffic are now nearby, the city of Palo Alto has used this easement in a way that retains the feel of the open countryside that the early trains used to travel through.

Views to the west are dominated by ever-changing light patterns on the Peninsula foothills. Crossing the sturdy wooden bridge over Matadero Creek, you come down into the green lawns of Bol Park. Magnificent oaks, benches, and playground equipment invite you to stop in this little park dedicated to Cornelis Bol. Tree-bordered Matadero Creek, which runs the length of the park on its east side, and the gentle rise known as Roble Ridge on the west side shelter this peaceful dell.

On leaving the park, cross Matadero Avenue and continue on the path to Hanover Street, three blocks ahead. Many pedestrians and bicyclists take this pathway to their jobs in the adjacent industrial park.

When you return, you can take the path along the east side of Bol Park and admire the big valley oaks there and on Roble Ridge. *Los robles* is the Spanish name for the deciduous valley oaks, while *encina* is Spanish word for live oak.

Then you can take the path skirting the school's east side or return the way you came. In either case you can look up to Black Mountain, magnificent in every season. A crystal-clear day reveals every canyon and ridge on its flank; a stormy one finds big billowy clouds hanging on its upper slopes.

Back at the Miranda Way entrance, you turn left at the corner to the Gunn High School entrance, your starting point.

PALO ALTO/LOS ALTOS BIKE PATH

A wide, paved path winds through the landscaped right of way for the city of San Francisco's Hetch Hetchy aqueduct. This is a good path for a winter stroll in midday.

Distance: 1.5 miles round trip

Time: ¾ hour

Elevation Change: Level

The path starts from Arastradero Road opposite and just east of Gunn High School. A sign, BIKE PATH, LOS ALTOS, marks the entrance. Passing between the old trees and well-kept lawns of Alta Mesa Cemetery on the right and the expansive playing fields on the left, the path continues toward Los Altos. Much used by children on their way to school and by families on short strolls near their homes, this path also serves as a shortcut for commuters going to their jobs.

You cross Adobe Creek, which forms the boundary between Palo Alto and Los Altos. The path meanders past backyard gardens as an occasional apricot tree, a lonely remnant from Los Altos' former vast orchards, stands beside it.

The path ends at a cross street, although city streets will take you the short distance to El Camino Real or San Antonio Road. Turn around at the cross street and retrace your steps to Gunn High School.

ARASTRADERO BIKE PATH

A third walk and bike ride follows Arastradero Road westward along the route of the Spanish timber haulers on a paved path to Purisima Road in Los Altos Hills.

Distance: 3.5 miles round trip

Time: 1¾ hours

Elevation Change: 100' gain

This path follows the route of one of the earliest roads on the Peninsula. Its name recalls the days when the Spanish hauled trees, cut in the forests of present-day Portola Valley, down this route to build the Santa Clara Mission. *Arrastradero* (the correct Spanish spelling uses a double *r*) signifies a place where something is dragged along. Cars now speed along Arastradero on a divided road, but now there is a place for those on foot or bike. And indeed, it is well-used, especially during lunch breaks.

For 1.5 miles from the expressway the path goes past landscaped industrial buildings, an occasional vineyard, and parking lots on the north side of the road. However, beyond the industrial park, the path is routed away from Arastradero Road into the ravine beside the creek, where there is a peaceful scene of grassy hills, valley oaks, and grazing horses. This is a short, pleasant walk for the rainy season, when it is good to have paving underfoot.

When the path emerges from the creekside, it ends at Purissima Road. However, bicyclists can veer right, go under the freeway and continue for about 0.5 mile to Page Mill Road. There you can turn left, go another 0.25 mile and turn right on the western leg of Arastradero Road. In less than 0.5 mile you arrive at Arastradero Preserve, the City of Palo Alto's 609-acre open space preserve with many trails, a lake and pond, and splendid views of the Skyline and Bay.

There is an off-road path for equestrians and hikers on the south side of Arastradero Road a bit beyond its emergence from under the freeway, but in the authors' view, it is not safe to get to the path at this writing.

Foothills Open Space Preserve

Clinging to the east side of upper Page Mill Road in Palo Alto is the 211-acre Foothills Open Space Preserve, one of the first purchases made by the newly created Midpeninsula Regional Open Space District 32 years ago.

Jurisdiction: MROSD: 650-691-1200
Facilities: 0.5 mile of trail
Rules: Open Dawn to dusk; multiple-use; dogs allowed on leash
Maps: USGS topo *Mindego Hill*
How to Get There: From I-280 take Page Mill Road south for about 6 miles, park at roadside pullouts.

Parking for this tiny preserve is indicated by split-rail fencing and small District signs. Walk a short distance downhill to get a glorious view over the southern Santa Clara Valley and the Diablo Range. In winter, Mt. Hamilton sometimes sports a blanket of snow; in summer, its Lick Observatory buildings glisten in the sun. Below you lie the headwaters of Adobe Creek, which flows to the Palo Alto Baylands.

Town of Los Altos Hills

Ranching families, who planted orchards on its sunny slopes and rode horseback through its wooded canyons, settled Los Altos Hills. By the time the town was incorporated in 1956 there were many existing horse trails, which the town fathers kept as a nucleus for the extensive trail system still growing today. Presently Los Altos Hills has about 95 miles of trails owned and maintained by the town. Nearly all that have been built since incorporation were acquired through the development process. As large properties were subdivided, trail routes were required to be set aside and trails constructed.

A glance at the town's Pathways Map shows that most of the trails run beside roads. However, on closer inspection some quite long routes run along the backs of properties, following drainage patterns or linking the town's two large open space preserves, Byrne and Juan Prado Mesa preserves.

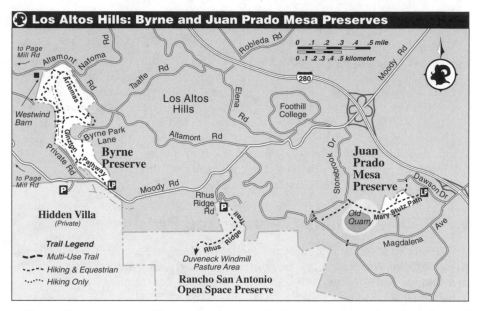

Byrne Preserve, now 79 acres, was named after an early settler, Col. Bernard Byrne, whose son donated the bulk of the land to the Nature Conservancy. In turn the conservancy gave the land to the town of Los Altos Hills in 1967, and Col. Byrne's daughter then donated another 25 acres.

The adjoining Westwind Barn was built in the 1940s to house Morgan and Arabian horses. A subsequent owner, Countess Bessenyey, raised Hungarian thoroughbred horses there, and in 1975 the Town acquired the property. Now the Friends of Westwind run the barn as a cooperative stabling facility.

Juan Prado Mesa Preserve, 13 acres in size, named for the original owner of the Rancho San Antonio land grant, was created in 1970 as part of the Dawson subdivision.

All of Los Altos Hills' pathways are open to the public, suitable mainly for hiking and horseback riding, but remember you are going through private property. Be courteous and respect residents' privacy. Described here are two walks you can take in this community, so completely subdivided, yet remarkably rural.

Jurisdiction: Town of Los Altos Hills: 650-941-7222

Maps: *Los Altos Hills Pathways*, USGS topos *Mindego Hill* and *Cupertino*

Facilities: Paths for hikers, equestrians, and bicyclists

Rules: Observe common sense and courtesy; bicyclists should yield to other users, and must stay on hard-surfaced roads and paths

How to Get There: From I-280 take Magdalena Ave. south 0.2 mile to the first street on your right, Dawson Dr. Turn right and go 0.3 mile to the bottom of hill. Park on roadside, taking care not to block driveways or mailboxes.

SEE MAP ON PAGE 198

JUAN PRADO MESA PRESERVE

From a wooded neighborhood, climb to rolling grasslands.

Distance: 1 mile round trip

Time: ½ hour

Elevation Change: 120′ gain

Start westward along a shady path marked by a wooden post, walking between two houses where you must remember to respect the privacy of residents. Soon you are on an old roadbed running through the small canyon of an intermittent creek, shaded by live oaks, buckeyes, small redwoods, and some black walnuts. There is so much foliage that the adjacent houses on the hills above you are invisible, although human activities are sometimes audible.

When you come out of the woods onto grasslands, you find the creek henceforth confined in a trench as it emerges from the pond of a 43-acre rock quarry, now a residential neighborhood. The path skirts this quarry on the northeast and winds uphill across former grazing lands to Stonebrook Drive.

About halfway to Stonebrook Drive there is an opening in the fence that runs behind the homes and gardens close to the quarry. One can walk through the opening onto a paved path that descends to the streetside paths that connect to lower Stonebrook Drive. Beyond here no off-road path exists at this writing. Town maps indicate streets that one could use to reach Rhus Ridge Road and the trail to the Windmill Pasture parking area.

SEE MAP ON PAGE 198

ARTEMAS GINZTON PATHWAY

Find a secret path that leads to glorious Bay views.

Distance: 2.2 miles round trip

Time: 1½ hours

Elevation Change: 330′ gain

The Artemas Ginzton pathway was named in 1991 in honor of Los Altos Hills' premiere trails advocate, the person most responsible for including trails in the original design of the town at incorporation. Mrs. Ginzton and the Town Pathways Committee laid out a number of the town pathways. Later, she devoted her energies to Santa Clara County when she served on its Trails and Pathways Committee.

From I-280 take El Monte exit west, go 0.5 mile, and then turn left (southwest) on Moody Road. After 2.2 miles look for a pathway sign on the right-hand bank and park at roadside pullout on opposite side of road. Starting northwest up the hill from Moody Road, the Artemas Ginzton Pathway parallels the road in an open, bay-tree forest. The hillside is full of springs that nourish the riparian vegetation in this intermittent branch of Adobe Creek. In May two species of brodiaea bloom, as well as apricot monkey flower and white yarrow.

After 0.3 mile you come to a four-way junction where the left route goes down a private road to Moody Road. The right-hand path, on which you will return, goes to Byrne Park Lane, and the path you take goes straight ahead to Westwind/Altamont. At 0.6 mile from where you started, you pass a bridge over the small creek on your left. This trail leads eventually to Page Mill Road. However, you keep to the right (east) toward Westwind/Altamont. You will pass another rather indistinct trail on your left, heading uphill to the Byrne Preserve, but your trip continues east. Pass open grasslands and then houses, skirt left by a vineyard, and then go through a horse gate into 79-acre Byrne Preserve.

Here you can walk up through grasslands dotted with oaks to a 788-foot knoll to take in the 360° view. Looking clockwise from Windy Hill in the north, your eye follows landmarks from Montara Mountain to San Bruno Mountain, past San Francisco to Mt. Diablo in the East Bay and along the Diablo Range to Mt. Hamilton. Closer at hand Hoover Tower at Stanford University peeks up over grassy knolls, and the developed parts of San Mateo and Santa Clara counties spread before you.

In Byrne Preserve you are 1.1 miles from Moody Road. On your return trip retrace your route through the horse gate and continue straight onto Byrne Park Lane, following a roadside path to its cul-de-sac. A somewhat indistinct and very steep path leads down through the grasslands to a canyon trail which you follow to the four-way junction you passed on your way up. Take the left-hand route back to Moody Road, where creek dogwood's inconspicuous but very fragrant flowers bloom in May.

There are other adventures to be found in Los Altos Hills, so buy their Pathways Map and explore further on your own. On the other side of Moody Road is the entrance to Hidden Villa, a private, nonprofit farm and environmental center, where hiking and equestrian trails lead to Monte Bello and Rancho San Antonio open space preserves. See pages 153, and below.

◆ Open Space Preserves and a County Park ◆ in Los Altos, Cupertino, and Saratoga Foothills

This splendid foothill retreat consists of a 165-acre Santa Clara County park and a neighboring, 3800-acre Midpeninsula Regional Open Space District preserve. A diversity of trail environments, from spreading oaks and cool creeksides of the valley floor to dry chaparral and oak-madrone forests on the slopes of Black Mountain, makes this a place of endless interest. With the 1993 addition of the former quarry ridge lands, the Duveneck Windmill Pasture and the Preserve are linked by a 2.1-mile trail along the preserve's northern ridge.

Most of these lands were part of Rancho San Antonio, a Mexican land grant deeded to Juan Prado Mesa in 1839, whose boundaries ran from Adobe Creek to Stevens Creek. Richard Henry Dana owned these lands for a brief period. In 1860 the Grant brothers purchased much of the land included in the preserve site for a

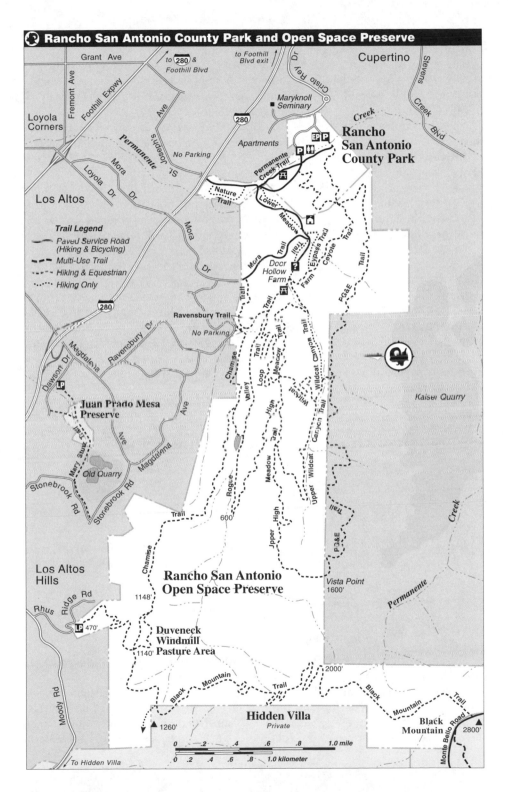

Rancho San Antonio County Park and Open Space Preserve

Grant Ave

to 280 &
Foothill Blvd

to Foothill
Blvd exit

Cupertino

Fremont Ave

Foothill Expwy

Ave

St. Joseph's

No Parking

Maryknoll
Seminary

Cristo Rey Dr

Stevens

Creek

Creek Blvd

Loyola
Corners

Permanente

280

Apartments

EP P

P

Rancho
San Antonio
County Park

Los Altos

Mora Dr

Loyola Dr

Permanente
Creek Trail

Nature
Trail

Lower

Meadow

Trail

Rancho
San Antonio
County Park

Mora Dr

Door
Hollow
Farm

Mora

Trail

Bypass Trail

Farm

Coyote

Trail

PG&E

Trail

Trail Legend

Paved Service Road
(Hiking & Bicycling)

Multi-Use Trail

Hiking & Equestrian

Hiking Only

280

Ravensbury Trail

No Parking

Chamise

Trail

Valley

Loop

Trail

Meadow

Trail

High

Meadow

Trail

Wildcat

Wildcat Canyon Trail

Upper Wildcat Canyon Trail

PG&E Trail

Kaiser Quarry

Dawson Dr

Magdalena

Ravensbury Dr

LP

**Juan Prado Mesa
Preserve**

Magdalena Ave

Mary Ave

Old Quarry

Magdalena Rd

Stonebrook Rd

Stonebrook Rd

Trail

600'

Rogue

Meadow

Trail

Upper High

Los Altos
Hills

Ridge Rd

Rhus

LP 470'

1148'

Chamise

Trail

**Rancho San Antonio
Open Space Preserve**

**Duveneck
Windmill
Pasture Area**

1140'

Vista Point
1600'

Permanente

Creek

Moody Rd

1260'

Black Mountain

Trail

2000'

Hidden Villa
Private

Black

Mountain

Black
Mountain

Trail

**Black
Mountain** 2800'

Monte Bello Road

To Hidden Villa

0   .2   .4   .6   .8   1.0 mile

0   .2   .4   .6   .8   1.0 kilometer

cattle ranch. Many of the original ranch buildings remain, adding to the pleasure of walks through the preserve.

The city of Mountain View's Department of Parks and Recreation operates Deer Hollow Farm within Rancho San Antonio Open Space Preserve, using some of the old ranch buildings, and conducts programs for children. MROSD has occasional docent-led tours.

The accessibility and variety of the park and preserve's 23 miles of trails make them some of the most popular on the Peninsula for hikers, runners, and equestrians.

Jurisdiction: Midpeninsula Regional Open Space District: 650-691-1200, and Santa Clara County: 408-355-2200

Facilities: County Park: trails for hikers and equestrians that link to MROSD trails; picnic areas; two meadows for informal activities; a model-airplane flying area; environmental education programs; parking for cars and horse trailers; restrooms. MROSD: trails for hikers and equestrians, Deer Hollow Farm

Rules: Open dawn to dusk; bicycles allowed only on paved path in County Park and on service road to Deer Hollow Farm; no dogs; farm open Tuesday through Sunday, 8 A.M. to 4 P.M.

Maps: MROSD brochure *Rancho San Antonio Park and Open Space Preserve*, Santa Clara County's *Rancho San Antonio*, and USGS topos *Cupertino* and *Mindego Hill*

How to Get There: From I-280 north or south, take Foothill Blvd. south. Immediately turn right on Cristo Rey Dr. and go 1 mile, veer right around traffic circle and turn left to county park entrance. For trips in open space preserve use northwest parking area and take hiking or bicycle path to Deer Hollow Farm and preserve trails.

Rancho San Antonio Open Space Preserve and County Park

SEE MAP
ON PAGE
201

DEER HOLLOW FARM

A walk through Deer Hollow Farm gives children (and adults too) a chance to see farm animals and some of the Grant brothers' barns.

Distance: 2.2 miles round trip

Time: 1½ hours

Elevation Change: Nearly level

The farm buildings go back to the days of the Grant Ranch that thrived here over a hundred years ago. From the cattle chutes visible at the entrance to the preserve, to the barns and outbuildings at the farm, you have an opportunity to see a ranch complex, now rare, but once common in Santa Clara County. The board-and-batten, white-washed redwood construction, and functional design have a classic simplicity that delights the eye and appeals to photographers and painters. The high, airy feed barn at the far end of the farm is a fine example of the uncontrived grace of ranch architecture so characteristic of the county's rural past. The historic Grant Cabin, once inhabited by the foreman for the Grant family, is now restored using historic grant funds. For preserve visitors, the cabin's restored furnishings provide a glimpse of early 20th century life.

Although the Deer Hollow Farm is closed to visitors except for the programs of the Mountain View Parks Department, from the pathway through the farm one can see the goats, pigs, chickens, and other farm creatures. For school-group environmental-education programs run by the city of Mountain View, contact the Department of Parks and Recreation at 650-903-6430.

WILDCAT CANYON, MEADOW RIDGE, ROGUE VALLEY LOOP

SEE MAP ON PAGE 201

A popular loop with hikers and runners along the canyons and over Meadow Ridge.

Distance: 5.6-mile loop

Time: 2½ hours

Elevation Change: 620' gain

Take one of the trails that skirt Deer Hollow Farm on the western hillside to reach the trailhead just beyond the last barn. One, the Coyote Trail, veers left off the preserve's main entrance trail; the other, longer, multi-use bypass trail leaves the PG&E utility service road higher on the ridge. At the junction after the farm, take the Wildcat Canyon Trail (for hikers only) to the left (southwest). You enter a cool, fern-walled, narrow canyon under the arching branches of dark bay trees, a quiet place remote from the suburban world only a mile or so away. After 0.5 mile the canyon widens and the path rises gently to reach a junction with the Upper Wildcat Canyon Trail, on which you turn right (west). Here the PG&E trail joins the Wildcat Canyon Trail and hikers and equestrians follow the Upper Wildcat Canyon Trail to reach the Wildcat Loop Trail and bear right (north).

A few easy switchbacks take you up a sunny, chaparral-covered slope where quail call from the cover of

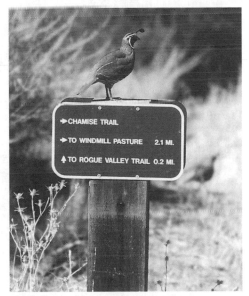

A vigilant quail watches her covey

sagebrush and mountain mahogany beside the path. Soon the path levels off as it reaches Meadow Ridge above. Spring is a time to linger here to enjoy the flowers dotting the rounded grassy hills—bold yellow daisies of mule ears, orange poppies, purple brodiaea, dark-blue lupine, and patches of blue-eyed grass. You will find good views and a number of choices for other hikes/rides in this preserve.

Although you could cut the trip short and return 1.1 miles down the High Meadow Trail from here, to continue this loop, take the Wildcat Loop Trail north 0.9 mile down to Rogue Valley. The shady trail descends on long switchbacks through the woods, a pleasant route for a hot day. Oaks meet overhead and in the dampness of spring maidenhair ferns cover the banks. Each turn offers new glimpses of the valley below.

In a half hour you are down in Rogue Valley, and bearing right (east) you go past the farm to the parking area.

UP ROGUE VALLEY AND BACK OVER THE RIDGE TO UPPER WILDCAT CANYON

SEE MAP ON PAGE 201

Explore the upper valley and the canyons on either side of the ridge.

Distance: 8.0-mile loop

Time: 4 hours

Elevation Change: 600' gain

From the Deer Hollow Farm you have the choice of starting either up Rogue Valley or up Wildcat Canyon. However, from Rogue Valley you have a shady climb to the crest of Meadow Ridge, rather than climbing a sunny south-facing slope.

Going west up the valley by the creek, you soon come to tall bay trees, alders, and maples. A dam impounds the creek to create a small reservoir (dry in summer). Farther upstream beyond the reservoir the maples are even taller, and like the others, they turn satisfyingly golden in fall. In 0.5 mile past the pond you come to a junction with an old ranch road and you make a sharp left onto it, the Upper Rogue Valley Trail, to reach the ridgetop. As you climb the mile up an easy grade, you begin to see across the canyon and beyond to the East Bay hills.

At the ridgetop trail junction the ranch road turns downhill back to the farm, but this trip arcs sharply right, continuing uphill along the Upper High Meadow Trail. You look southwest toward Black Mountain and across Wildcat Canyon to the dark, wooded flank of the ridge between Wildcat and Permanente creeks. In 0.3 mile you come to another junction at the 1000-foot level, where you leave the ridge and the road, which continues to the top of the preserve. Here you bear left along another old ranch road, the Upper Wildcat Canyon Trail, down into the canyon of the same name.

It is an easy descent into the tight canyon of Wildcat Creek. Thick stands of bays and oaks darken this steep canyon, making it a good route on warm summer days.

The creek and the trail beside it drop rapidly for 1.3 miles to a junction with the Wildcat Loop Trail on the south side of the ridge.

Near the junction, in late winter and early spring, the trail is brightened by the tiny, bright yellow blossoms of the uncommon shrub, leatherwood (*Dirca occidentalis*). Masses of this shrub along the canyon have the effect of a sprinkling of flecks of gold against the dark bay laurels. Where the canyon widens there are the pink blooms of wild currant. From the junction it is about 1.5 miles by one of the several routes back to the parking area.

TO THE SHOULDER
OF BLACK MOUNTAIN

A dramatic hike to the 1400-foot heights of the preserve returns down the south side of the ridge. Note: As described, this trip is perfect for sunny winter days, but on hot days, take this trip in reverse: the PG&E trail is in shade most of the way.

Distance: 8.1 miles round trip

Time: 4½ hours

Elevation Change: 1000' gain

Park in the equestrian parking lot in the county park., go 0.5 mile south and take the Coyote Ridge Trail to pick up the High Meadow Trail at the junction with the Wildcat Canyon Trail. A few turns and 1.0 mile up the buckeye-, oak-, and madrone-covered slope you come to the grassy expanse of the ridge, green and flower-covered in spring or golden as the season turns. From these 1000-foot heights turn around to gaze at densely settled Santa Clara Valley. In the other direction are the wooded slopes that rise to Black Mountain's 2800-foot summit.

Continue up the ridgetop past junctions with the Wildcat Canyon Loop trails descending to Rogue Valley and Upper Wildcat Canyon. Your trail up the mountain, the Upper High Meadow Trail, continues around bend after bend as it climbs. Views become more sweeping with each turn in the road. Across Wildcat Canyon you can see the utility service road which you will take on the return trip.

After another mile's climb you leave the grassy slopes as the road makes a sharp turn south into oak woods before circling a knoll at 1400 feet. Crowning the little knoll above the road are a few spreading oaks and a madrone. This is a dramatic place to pause or picnic. You can take in the whole Peninsula from here. Looking far north beyond San Bruno Mountain, you see the unmistakable outline of Mt. Tamalpais in Marin County. Black Mountain's summit, marked with antennas, is just visible above the southern ridge. Southeast lies the Santa Clara Valley.

After another 0.5 mile up the mountain, the trail turns east at the boundary of the preserve. From a commemorative bench under a tall transmission tower, you can enjoy the view. After a snack here you pick up the utility service road, known colloquially as the "PG&E Trail," and start the return trip. From this vantage point you look straight down the wilderness of Wildcat Canyon. The road here is outside the preserve's boundaries, but hikers and equestrians can use it.

Downhill all the way from here, you wind in and out of wooded ravines along the south edge of the preserve passing under five or six towers. The road banks are furrowed by so many deer trails that you know that a great number of these wild creatures live on Black Mountain. However, unless you are here in the early morning or evening you will see only the tracks they make on their way to water in the creeks below. Bobcats and mountain lions share this mountain too, but usually are too shy to make their presence known.

Stay on the utility road for 4 miles back to the county park and your parking place there.

Duveneck Windmill Pasture Area

These 710 acres are part of the Rancho San Antonio Open Space Preserve. The Pasture Area lies immediately west of the original Rancho San Antonio preserve and extends south to the heights of Black Mountain. With the 1993 purchase of the acreage immediately east of the Windmill Pasture Area, there is now trail access to the main Rancho San Antonio Open Space Preserve and Rancho San Antonio County Park.

The original 430-acre Windmill Pasture was the generous gift of Frank and Josephine Duveneck to the Midpeninsula Regional Open Space District. The Duvenecks' Hidden Villa Ranch is well-known for its environmental education programs, its farm tours, its interracial summer camp, and its youth hostel, the first in the West, which celebrated its 50th anniversary in 1987. Since the death of the Duvenecks, the Hidden Villa programs and its ranch and wilderness lands are owned and operated by a private, nonprofit corporation, the Trust for Hidden Villa. MROSD has an easement over 1435 acres of Hidden Villa's wilderness lands.

Hidden Villa Ranch is open during the school year, but closed during the summer camp period. Since the ranch is nonprofit, there is an entrance fee to help maintain its facilities. Its private trails are open to hikers and equestrians; no bicycles are allowed, except on the ranch entrance road.

Eight miles of trails wind through the Duveneck Windmill Pasture Area's fragrant bay-tree and oak woodlands, across sloping, grassy meadows, up the steep shoulder of Black Mountain and down to the floor of the rancho.

How to Get There: From I-280 take El Monte Ave. exit west; just beyond Foothill College turn left on Moody Rd., then in 0.5 mile turn left on Rhus Ridge Rd. Continue for 0.2 mile, then turn right down to a small parking place at gated trail entrance. Do not park on Rhus Ridge Rd. or block the private home driveway.

A SHORT HIKE
TO A SECLUDED MEADOW

SEE MAP ON PAGE 201

A half-hour's hike takes you to a high, hidden pasture in the shadow of Black Mountain.

Distance: 2 miles round trip

Time: 1¼ hours

Elevation Change: 500' gain

From the preserve entrance in a forested glade, take the trail, which is a patrol road, up a wooded canyon. In spring, flowers bloom along the trail, and ferns—wood fern, gold back, and maidenhair—line the road banks. By summer the gold back and maidenhair have dried up, but the wood fern still clothes the hillsides with green.

As you round the last bend, pause on the threshold of the meadow, which the Duvenecks named the Windmill Pasture after an old windmill that stood until 1991. Behind you are the cities of the Santa Clara Valley. But take a few more steps along the trail and you'll find yourself in a secluded pasture removed from that urban scene. Handsome oaks border the pasture, and Black Mountain rises beyond.

This is a place to enjoy at your leisure. Short trails through the pasture invite you to explore it and to find hilltop spots to sit in the sun or watch the changing light on Black Mountain. Look along the lower border of the pasture for the sign that tells the story of the windmill.

In the mid-1800s the pasture was a part of the Rancho San Antonio, an early Mexican land grant. Before that time, these woodlands and meadows, so rich in fruits, berries, seeds, and game, were the territory of the Ohlone Indians, who had a village beside Adobe Creek in the valley below. A summer day might have found them gathering seeds here or beating the grass to round up grasshoppers, which they considered a delicacy when lightly roasted.

Nowadays, early-rising residents with a thermos of coffee, a roll, and an orange in a backpack find this a great site for a breakfast walk. And it is just right, too, for a leisurely picnic supper at the end of a warm summer day.

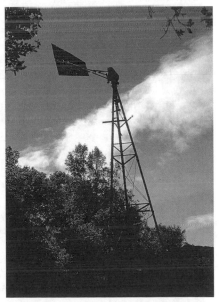

Long-gone namesake of Windmill Pasture

TREK TO BLACK MOUNTAIN

From the Windmill Pasture hike up a steep trail to the highest mountain in the Sierra Morena.

Distance: 9.6 miles round trip

Time: 5+ hours

Elevation Change: 2380' gain

This trail is closed to bicyclists and seasonally may be closed to equestrians. Plenty of water in your pack and an early start are requisites for this trip. From the Rhus Ridge parking area, take the 0.9-mile trail to the Windmill Pasture. After pausing there to survey the peak you will be climbing, veer right to dip into shady oak woodland. Traverse a chaparral ridge and then go back into a clump of trees, where you watch for a side trail on your right. Stay to the left here on the Black Mountain Trail, passing through a swale that drains into one of Permanente Creek's tributaries. Now begin your steady upward climb.

Shortly, out on the open ridge that divides the drainages of Adobe and Permanente creeks, your views on both sides are of wilderness lands, too steep to have been farmed. Across the deep canyons to the left lie the High Meadow trails of Rancho San Antonio, now accessible from the Duveneck Windmill Pasture Area via the Chamise Trail. To your right are the private wilderness lands of Hidden Villa.

Beautiful pink clusters of wild currant will delight you on an early spring trip, as well as graceful ferns on banks above the trail. Look for white limestone rocks of the kind mined in the Hanson (formerly Permanente) cement quarry on the southwest side of Monte Bello Ridge.

After about 2.75 miles of this unrelenting ascent with intermittent tree cover, you zigzag around switchbacks and wooded ravines dripping with winter rivulets. Here on a wide transverse ridge is a forest of tall madrones and oaks that invite you to pause.

Tall towers anchored on this ridge support the power lines spanning the upper reaches of Adobe and Permanente Creek canyons and running northward on the east side of the ridge through Wunderlich and Huddart parks and the town of Woodside. You cross under the power lines and emerge from the woods on a broad, bare, and steep service road cut through chaparral. Now, with communications towers in view and a second wind in your lungs, you head for the 2800-foot top of Black Mountain. From its summit there are marvelous views west into Stevens Creek Canyon and thousands of acres of open-space lands along the Skyline ridge. Turn around to behold the entire Bay Area spread out before you.

For a lunch break you could explore the MROSD backpack camp, downhill to the west near the site of the old Morrell farmhouse on gated Monte Bello Road (see Loop Trip on Indian Creek and Bella Vista Trails page 154. With an advance reservation, you could stay there overnight. For your return trip, you could arrange a shuttle to meet you at the west entrance of Monte Bello Open Space Preserve on Page Mill Road or you could return the way you came. Whatever your route, you have the satisfaction of having climbed the highest mountain in the northern Santa Cruz Mountains.

CHAMISE TRAIL TO ROGUE VALLEY

SEE MAP ON PAGE 201

Tread the high-line route from pasture to pond.

Distance: 6.6 miles round trip

Time: 4 hours

Elevation Change: 500' gain

Start from the Rhus Ridge parking area and climb the steep road through oak woodland and patches of chaparral, as in the first trip in this section (A Short Hike to a Secluded Meadow). If you take this trail in spring, note the small chinquapin trees beside the trail. Their slightly curled, yellow-backed leaves and prickly seed pods are easy to distinguish. Here too, are silk-tassel trees, another small tree that is easy to identify in spring by the long strand or tassel of gray-green flowers at the branch tips that become berries in fall. You may also be lucky enough to spot some beautiful orange wind poppies waving gracefully in sunny openings.

When you reach the Windmill Pasture, bear left (east) on the well-worn trail crossing the middle of the meadow. At the end of the meadow you rise through a little gap and follow the wide Chamise Trail, an old road that traverses the lands purchased from an adjoining landowner in 1993. From openings along the trail, there are glimpses of the midpeninsula and San Francisco Bay to the north. To the south lie the steep forested ridges enfolding Permanente Creek and its tributaries. You are often in dense chaparral, but occasionally you dip into oak woods. The trail takes its name from the tiny leaved, erect, brownish green chaparral shrub that covers the slopes on the south side of the trail. In the company of manzanita and mountain mahogany, chamise makes a dense, prickly, almost impenetrable cover, except for resident rabbits, quail, mice, and voles.

Soon you begin a long, gradual descent and your view is down into the Rogue Valley, which lies at the base of a lovely east-facing ridge. You wind around little knolls and past some very badly eroded ridges below the trail. When you reach a trail junction, turn right (south) to reach the little pond which sits at the Rogue Valley Trail junction. (When the authors reached this trail junction in the fall, we spent 10 minutes watching a covey of quail taking dust baths, completely unperturbed by us.) You can see the pond before you reach it. Here beside its reed-lined waters in spring, you could stop for a snack before starting back up the hill. This valley, formerly occupied by horse stables and corrals, is being restored with native plants. The return trip on the south-facing ridge should be taken in the early morning or late afternoon of a summer day, but it is delightful on a sunny winter day.

Or, you could continue on the Rogue Valley Trail, following it 1.1 miles to the Deer Hollow Farm to see the animals. From there it is 1 or 2 miles (depending on your route) to parking areas in Rancho San Antonio County Park, where you could have friends meet you for a picnic at tables in the meadow.

Stevens Creek County Park

The park encompasses a foothill canyon surrounding a reservoir fed by year-round streams. In an early description of this rugged area, Padre Pedro Font, a cartographer who accompanied Colonel Juan Bautista de Anza to California in 1776, wrote, "This place of San José de Cupertino has good water and much firewood, but nothing suitable for settlement because it is among the hills very near the range of the cedars . . . and lacks level land" (the "cedars" were what we know today as the redwoods).

Elisha Stephens settled on Cupertino Creek and set out vineyards there in the 1850s. Stephens was the leader of the Stephens, Murphy, Townsend Party that crossed the Sierra in 1844 (before the fateful journey of the Donner Party). Sometime after 1860, he left his lands and moved on to less "heavily populated" areas.

In 1893 the Jesuits of the University of Santa Clara purchased the Villa Maria, a 30-acre farm and winery here. It contained a chapel, villa house, winery, and barn, with grape vineyards and orchard of walnts, apples, and chestnuts. The buildings are gone, but remnants of the orchard and vineyards remain.

Later, the Arroyo de San José de Cupertino, which included Stevens Canyon and the Villa Maria, was named for Stephens (the spelling was changed) and today a busy thoroughfare is named for him and Cupertino Creek is known as Stevens Creek.

Hiking trails originate from (1) the north entrance to the park off Stevens Canyon Road in what is known as the Villa Maria Area, below the dam and its spillway, and (2) upstream above the reservoir near the intersection of Stevens Canyon and Mt. Eden roads. In the north and south ends of the park are connections with trails in the adjoining Fremont Older Open Space Preserve. The Zinfandel Trail (for hikers only) connects the park with the Picchetti Ranch Open Space Preserve.

Jurisdiction: Santa Clara County: 408-355-2200 (administration), 408-355-3751 (reservations)

Facilities: Visitor center; picnic areas for families and groups; trails chiefly for hikers

Rules: Open from 8 A.M. to ½ hour past sunset; multi-use allowed on the Rim Trail, the Canyon, and the Mt. Eden Trail; equestrian parking at Mt. Eden trailhead; pets on leash in picnic area; no pets on trails

Maps: Santa Clara County brochure *Stevens Creek County Park*; MROSD brochures *Fremont Older OSP, Picchetti Ranch OSP*; USGS topo *Cupertino*

How to Get There: From I-280 take Foothill Blvd. south, which becomes Stevens Canyon Rd., and reach north entrance of park in about 2 miles. For Villa Maria Area and visitor center, turn left at park entrance sign. For other trails, continue on Stevens Canyon Rd., which runs through the park and intersects Mt. Eden Rd. near the south end.

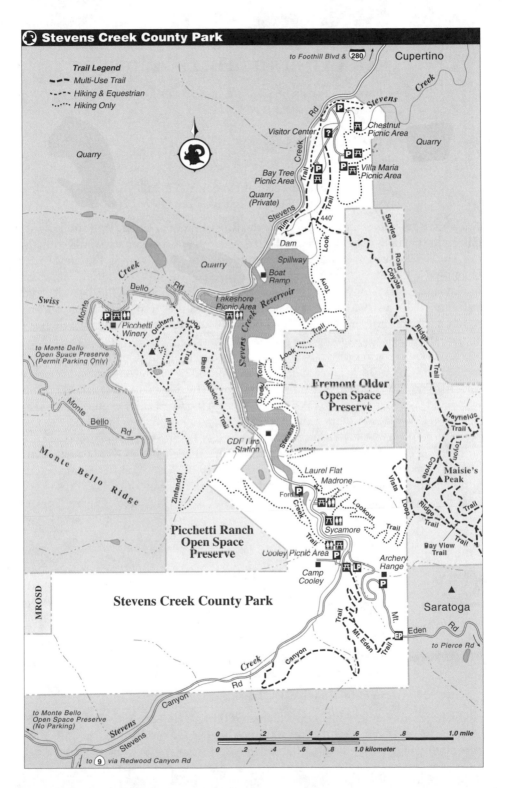

Stevens Creek County Park

Trail Legend
- Multi-Use Trail
- Hiking & Equestrian
- Hiking Only

to Foothill Blvd & 280
Cupertino

Stevens Creek

Quarry

Visitor Center

Chestnut Picnic Area

Quarry

Bay Tree Picnic Area

Villa Maria Picnic Area

Quarry (Private)

440'

Dam

Spillway

Boat Ramp

Lakeshore Picnic Area

Picchetti Winery

Swiss Creek

Bello

Monte Creek Rd

to Monte Bello Open Space Preserve (Permit Parking Only)

Monte Bello Rd

Monte Bello Ridge

Orchard Loop Trail

Bear Meadow Trail

Zinfandel Trail

CDF Fire Station

Stevens Creek Reservoir

Look Trail

Tony Look Trail

Coyote Ridge Trail

Service Road

Fremont Older Open Space Preserve

Hayfields Trail

Tony Creek

Laurel Flat

Madrone

Ford

Sycamore

Cooley Picnic Area

Camp Cooley

Picchetti Ranch Open Space Preserve

Vista Loop Trail

Lookout Trail

Coyote Ridge Trail

Toyon Trail

Maisie's Peak

Bay View Trail

Archery Range

Stevens Creek County Park

MROSD

to Monte Bello Open Space Preserve (No Parking)

Mt. Eden Trail

Canyon Trail

Saratoga

Mt. Eden Rd

to Pierce Rd

Stevens Creek Canyon Rd

Stevens

to 9 via Redwood Canyon Rd

0 .2 .4 .6 .8 1.0 mile
0 .2 .4 .6 .8 1.0 kilometer

HIKE TO THE RESERVOIR
AND CLIMB THE HILLS ABOVE

Hikers have two destinations for trips in this foothills park—a short trip to a shady picnic site or a longer hike.

Distance: 2.7 miles one way

Time: 1½ hours

Elevation Change: 200′ gain to oak-shaded flat; 600′ gain returning on Coyote Ridge Trail through Fremont Older OSP

From the visitor center all users take the Rim or Stevens Creek Trail south under tall spreading oaks, climbing gently for 0.6 mile toward the dam. Near the spillway the Rim Trail goes left to join the Coyote Ridge Trail in adjoining Fremont Older Open Space Preserve. At this junction near the spillway, hikers continue south on the Stevens Creek/Tony Look Trail and cross a small meadow on the 0.4 mile, level trail that circles partway around the reservoir to another trail junction. If you turn right on this trail for another 300 yards through oak groves by the water, you reach an oak-shaded flat—a good place for a picnic.

However, to continue over the hill above the reservoir, turn left onto a section of the Stevens Creek/Tony Look Trail, built in 1987–88 by volunteers under the sponsorship of the Trail Center. As this 2-mile trail winds in and out of ravines through oak woodlands, you glimpse the water below through the trees. After rounding an open, chaparral-covered ridge, you walk on a fenced ledge above the reed-rimmed lake and descend into oak forest again near the upper end of the reservoir at Laurel Flat.

The trail ends above Stevens Canyon Road near a cluster of picnic areas. Here you can pick up the 0.7-mile Lookout Trail to join the Vista Loop Trail and return to the visitor center by way of the Coyote Ridge Trail in Fremont Older Preserve, a total distance of 6 miles. (See Coyote Ridge Trail to Stevens Creek County Park in Fremont Older OSP section, page 220).

LOOKOUT TRAIL

Try this climb through the woods to a ridgetop Lookout Point for views of Stevens Creek Canyon and connecting trails on either side of the canyon.

Distance: 1.4 mile round trip

Time: 1½ hours

Elevation Change: 440′ gain

Take Stevens Canyon Road past the reservoir and turn left into parking for the Madrone Picnic Area. Find the trail entrance behind the restrooms. The trail crosses a small ridge that separates this picnic area from the Sycamore Picnic Area.

Another trail comes up from behind the Sycamore Picnic Area and joins this one about 200 yards up a small ravine.

The trail, for hikers only, ascends a steep hill on switchbacks under oaks and toyons, a shaded walk for warm weather. In spring the hill is lush and green when ferns and undergrowth are fresh from the rains, and irises, wild currants, and roses are in bloom. In fall and winter, toyons are bright with red berries.

In 15 minutes you are at the first ridge, from which you can look south to the park's Mt. Eden Trail. Then, at the 1000-foot-high Lookout Point, you can see west far up the canyon and east over the Fremont Older Preserve. At Lookout Point, go through the stile leading out of the park into the preserve. Before returning, walk along the ridge to a lunch spot overlooking the meadow, where you will often have the pleasure of watching horses cantering over the trails in this preserve.

For a loop trip, continue across the meadow and follow the last section of the previous trip (I like to the Reservoir and Climb the Hills Above), or return the way you came.

SEE MAP ON PAGE 211

CREEK TRAIL

Take the children for a short walk before a picnic lunch.

Distance: 1 mile round trip

Time: ½ hour

Elevation Change: Nearly level

At the intersection of Stevens Canyon and Mt. Eden roads, find the hikers-only trail going downstream from the Cooley Picnic Area. This trail makes for a leisurely stroll under alders and sycamores. From parts of the trail you can look down from the high banks of the creek into its pools and watch for fish in its depths. If you see perched in a tree a blue-grey bird, somewhat larger than a jay, with white stripes and a rumpled crest on his outsized head, it is a kingfisher, who also is watching for fish in the creek.

This trail ends at the creek, but in times of low water you can cross the creek to parking on Stevens Canyon Road, and you could extend your walk across the road and continue onto one of the previous two trips.

To a Southern Ridgetop on Multi-Use Trails

Find striking views of the Santa Cruz Mountains at the end of the trail.

Distance: 1.6 miles round trip

Time: 1 hour

Elevation Change: 300' gain

From the parking area off Mt. Eden Road at the south end of the park, the Mt. Eden Trail climbs south briefly, then levels off to a gentle grade heading northwest. It is an easy stroll under great bay trees and oaks. Blue wild lilacs bloom here in summer. In 0.2 mile you meet the Canyon Trail (a fire road), on which you turn left sharply (southwest) to climb a chaparral-covered slope. If you are picnicking at the Cooley or Canyon picnic area in the south end of the park, take the Canyon Trail to its junction with the Mt. Eden Trail and proceed as described here.

Along your way on the right is a great craggy limestone outcrop, a good place to pause for the views up the canyon and down the reservoir. In 0.25 mile from the junction you reach the high point of the trail and sweeping vistas of the Santa Cruz Mountains. You can continue down the fire road if you welcome the exercise of the climb back. But you may want to linger near the summit, where there are several fine spots for spreading out your picnic.

Beyond the ridgetop the slopes are covered with oaks, bays, and buckeyes. There are firs here and there on the way down to Stevens Canyon Road. However, there is no parking at the trail's lower end, so the trip should be taken as a round trip from Mt. Eden Road.

Picchetti Ranch Open Space Preserve

A visit to the Picchetti Ranch is an opportunity to enjoy the flavor of a foothill winery and ranch of the late 1800s, an experience now all but vanished. The ranch was in the Picchetti family from the 1870s until the Midpeninsula Regional Open Space District acquired it in 1978. Vincenzo Picchetti came to the Santa Clara Valley from Italy in 1872, and soon after bought the ranch and planted orchards and vine-yards on its hillsides. Early family quarters, the family home, the winery, and the orchards remain.

Today the buildings of the Picchetti Ranch form the centerpiece of the preserve. Listed in the National Register of Historic Places and in the Santa Clara County Resource Inventory, these buildings were restored with grant funds for historic preservation. The first to be completed was Homestead House, built by the Picchetti brothers in 1882, as a temporary home. Later it housed ranch hands, and was used as storage for gallon wine jugs and even an aviary.

A private party leases this restored building and offers wine made from grapes grown on the property. The building again carries the name Picchetti Winery and is open daily from 11 A.M. to 5 P.M. for wine tasting. The inviting picnic tables and grounds at the winery make a pleasant stop here after a hike or ramble through the preserve.

Restoration of the large barn across the courtyard from the winery preserved much of the original siding and foundation rock work. In conjunction with a previous lessee, MROSD completed the fermentation building for wine-making. MROSD finished restoring the original blacksmith shop and the little Picchetti family house. With grant funds for historic preservation MROSD is upgrading the winery to comply with new seismic requirements.

The ranch's 308 acres extend past an old orchard and up gentle hills. Four miles of trails take you to oak groves, meadows, and wooded slopes. A 10-minute spring stroll through a flowery orchard brings you to a small, tree-shaded, seasonal pond. Another five minutes along the trail and you are in a parklike meadow dotted with oaks.

Jurisdiction: Midpeninsula Regional Open Space District: 650-691-1200

Facilities: Trails for hikers and equestrians; historic winery; wine tasting; picnic tables; restroom

Rules: Except for winery and adjacent buildings, preserve open dawn to dusk; no dogs

Maps: Map on page 217 MROSD brochure *Picchetti Ranch Open Space Preserve* and USGS topo *Cupertino*

How to Get There: From I-280 go right (south) on Foothill Expwy, which becomes Foothill Blvd. and then Stevens Canyon Rd. Continue about 3 miles beyond entrance to Stevens Creek Reservoir in Stevens Creek County Park. Just beyond a quarry on your right, turn right, uphill, onto Monte Bello Rd. and go 0.6 mile to Picchetti Ranch on your left.

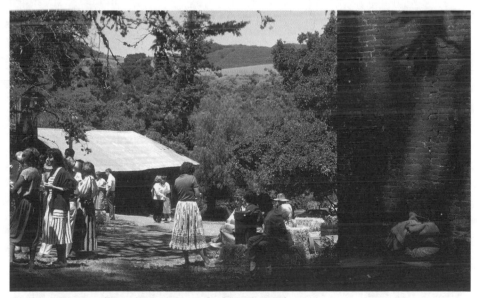

Picchetti Winery offers wine tasting at the historic ranch

A STROLL TO PICCHETTI POND
AND A HILLTOP VIEW

A short easy trail for a family outing takes you uphill through the old orchard.

Distance: 1 mile round trip

Time: 45 minutes

Elevation Change: 140' gain

Start from the parking lot to the right of the winery gate on the Zinfandel Trail that crosses a bubbling stream, Swiss Creek, on a small bridge. (You may be serenaded by the winery's resident peacocks.) Take the old ranch road, now called the Zinfandel Trail, by the abandoned orchard, ignoring the first side road leading down to your left. After less than a half mile you pass the north leg of the Orchard Loop Trail on your left, also an old road, and reach the Bear Meadow Trail that circles left around a small pond. This trail is for hikers only. This pond is home to a frog chorus in the rainy season, but usually dries up in summer.

Take this trail around to the east side of the pond to a fork, from which you follow the left-hand trail that winds gently northeast to the summit of a small hill (elevation 1080 feet). You will meet the right-hand trail, the Bear Meadow Trail, later on this trip. Shaded by live oaks, this hill offers superb views in three directions.

To the north is the quarry you passed on the road, where the machinery makes quite a noise on weekdays. Other noises you can hear on weekends are shots coming from the Sunnyvale Rod and Gun Club just east of the quarry. Beyond this quarry and through a gap in the northern ridge you can see buildings of the much larger Hanson Quarry in the hills behind Cupertino. Limestone from this quarry was used to make the cement for Shasta Dam in 1945. The East Bay is faintly visible through this gap on a clear day. Filling the foreground to the northeast are the Stevens Creek Dam and the reservoir behind it. Farther to the east are the slopes of Fremont Older Open Space Preserve. Think, as you survey all before you, that if some people hadn't the foresight to form the Midpeninsula Regional Open Space District in 1972, the nearby hills would not have been preserved for future generations to walk on.

As you descend east from the small hill, be careful of your footing on this very steep trail. You join the north leg of the Orchard Loop Trail, a patrol road, and turn right (east) through chaparral vegetation. This stretch can be very hot in summer, but in spring the ceanothus blossoms fill the air with scent. After only 0.25 mile you come to a junction where a patrol road leads left downhill to Monte Bello Road. However, this trip turns right on the Bear Meadow Trail (here a patrol road), and after about only 100 feet takes a trail going right uphill on which you can return to the pond and back the way you came.

To visit a lovely meadow and shady oak woodland from the Orchard Loop/Bear Meadow Trail junction described above, continue right on the Bear Meadow Trail and pass the foot trail that returns to the pond. On the right another trail bypasses the wide patrol road for a short distance, goes uphill, and then

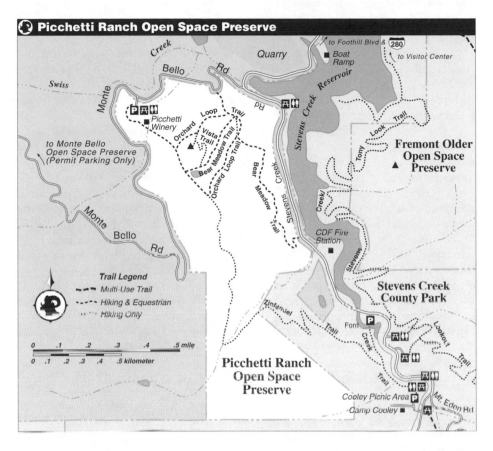

Picchetti Ranch Open Space Preserve

bends around to cross the patrol road to meander 0.7 mile southeast past an oak-bordered meadow and through the woods down to parking on Stevens Canyon Road opposite the reservoir.

SEE MAP ON PAGE 217

THE ZINFANDEL TRAIL TO STEVENS CREEK COUNTY PARK

Contour through forest and chaparral to the Cooley Picnic Area.

Distance: 3.8 miles round trip

Time: 2 hours

Elevation Change: 600′ loss

Begin this trip from the winery parking lot on the 1.9-mile Zinfandel Trail as in the previous trip (A Stroll to Picchetti Pond and a Hilltop View). If you do not wish to return the same way, you can leave another car at the Cooley Picnic Area in

Stevens Creek County Park. (The entrance to this picnic area is on Stevens Canyon Road just west of the Mt. Eden Road intersection).

Passing the Picchetti Pond and the two ends of the Orchard Loop Trail patrol road, continue south over a bridge and through a stile on the Zinfandel Trail. This gently sloping trail leaves the meadows behind and enters thick woods. Multiple-trunked bay trees shade you on hot days. In chaparral-covered openings in the bay-tree forest, occasional fir trees reach for the sky.

Pass several side creeks, rushing during winter rains, and keep a lookout past a small wooden bridge for a clump of California nutmeg trees on the downhill side of the trail. Note the very sharp needles shining in the canyon light. After 1.2 miles you enter Stevens Creek County Park, where there is a good view of the Stevens Creek Dam, the reservoir, and the Santa Clara Valley spreading to the east. A trail in Fremont Older Open Space Preserve is visible on the opposite hillside, tempting you to extend your hike to that preserve.

Soon you begin to switchback down through former ranchlands, seeing a huge barn roof on private property below you. Some buildings of the Santa Clara County Park maintenance yard lie ahead; your trail, becoming very narrow, jogs left on a patrol road, and then the trail, much narrower, resumes on the right (note these turns carefully for your return trip). You wind down through the forest to join the Creek Trail and turn right on it to reach the Cooley Picnic Area by Stevens Canyon Road.

Fremont Older Open Space Preserve

The preserve is part of the old William Pfeffer Ranch, later owned by Fremont Older, a noted San Francisco newspaper editor, and his wife Cora Bagley Older. In the 1920s Mrs. Older designed their ranch home, known as "Woodhills," with a flat roof and many pergolas, a departure from the prevailing style of the times. The house, in a state of disrepair when the Midpeninsula Regional Open Space District acquired the ranch in 1975, was restored by a leaseholder and is now listed in the National Registry of Historic Places. Woodhills is open for occasional house tours. (Call the district for information on the tour schedule.)

Meanwhile, 739 acres of the ranchlands are open to hikers, equestrians, and bicyclists, who can take the old ranch roads that wind across the rolling hayfields to old orchards and climb its long central ridge. The preserve is heavily used by equestrians from nearby stables and by bicyclists who enjoy the challenge of its many hill climbs. Trails leading to streets in neighboring subdivisions have no designated parking areas.

Jurisdiction: Midpeninsula Regional Open Space District: 650-691-1200

Facilities: Trails for hikers, equestrians, and bicyclists

Rules: Open dawn to dusk; approved helmets required for all bicyclists; dogs on leash allowed on all Fremont Older trails

Maps: MROSD brochure *Fremont Older OSP*, Santa Clara County *Stevens Creek County Park* and USGS topo *Cupertino*

How to Get There: From I-280 go south on Hwy 85, take DeAnza Blvd./Saratoga Sunnyvale Rd. exit and go south. Turn right on Prospect Rd. and go 1.3 miles to MROSD parking area.

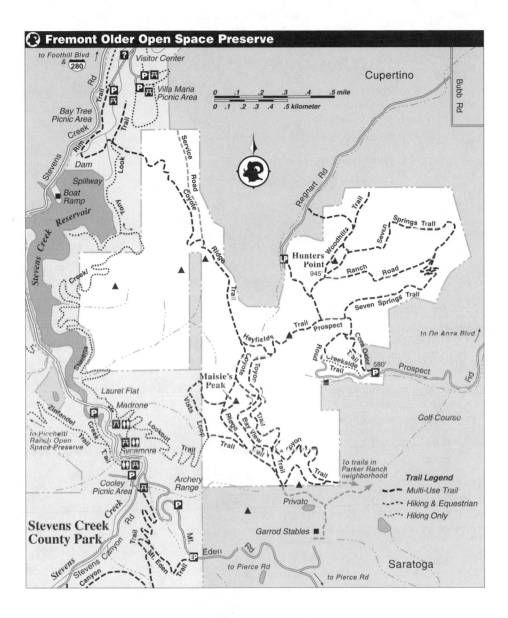

Fremont Older Open Space Preserve

to Foothill Blvd & 280

Visitor Center

Villa Maria Picnic Area

Bay Tree Picnic Area

Creek Rim Trail

Stevens Creek Reservoir

Dam

Spillway

Boat Ramp

Tony

Look

Creek

Cupertino

Bubb Rd

0   .1   .2   .3   .4   .5 mile
0 .1 .2 .3 .4 .5 kilometer

Service Road

Coyote

Ridge

Trail

Regnart Rd

Hunters Point
945'

Woodhills

Seven

Springs Trail

Ranch   Road

Seven Springs Trail

to De Anza Blvd

Stevens

Hayfields

Trail   Prospect

Cora Older

Trail

Creekside Trail

Road

580'

Prospect

Rd

Maisie's Peak

Coyote

Toyon

Trail

Canyon

Golf Course

Laurel Flat

Madrone

Zinfandel   Creek

to Picchetti Ranch Open Space Preserve

Sycamore

Lookout

Trail

Vista   Loop

Ridge

Bay View

Trail

Creek

Trail

To trails in Parker Ranch neighborhood

Trail Legend
— — Multi-Use Trail
- - - Hiking & Equestrian
······ Hiking Only

Cooley Picnic Area

Archery Range

Private

Garrod Stables

Stevens Creek County Park

Stevens

Stevens Canyon

Canyon

Mt. Eden Rd

Mt. Eden Trail

Eden

Rd

to Pierce Rd

to Pierce Rd

Saratoga

COYOTE RIDGE TRAIL TO STEVENS CREEK COUNTY PARK

Exhilarating views, steep climbs, and long descents make this trip a worthy work-out.

Distance: 4.8 miles round trip

Time: 3 hours

Elevation Change: 400' gain

Hikers and equestrians leave the parking lot on the road that goes along the creek under oak and bay trees. Beyond the first bend in the road, hikers can take the marked Creekside Trail to the right to rejoin the road beyond the gated entrance to the Fremont Older house. Bicyclists must use the 0.4-mile Cora Older Trail on the north side of the parking lot and join the road 0.1 mile uphill from the Bay View Trail. Equestrians continue on the road for 0.5 mile to join hikers and bicyclists. All users continue north beside rolling hayfields, pass the Seven Springs Trail on the right and turn left on the Hayfields Trail to a saddle on the ridge. In spring the green of the sprouting grass in the fields is brilliant against the trunks of old fruit trees. As the oat grass dries, these round hills are golden and billowing for a brief time.

Turn left (southwest) at the saddle and wind uphill for 0.5 mile on the ranch road lined with a few old walnut trees. On the way from the hayfields to the ridgetop you pass the Toyon Trail on the left, but you continue uphill on the ranch road. In a last steep climb from this junction you reach the Coyote Ridge Trail, running north and south along the spine of the preserve.

Bear right at the ridgetop to reach Stevens Creek Park. This trail goes through tall chaparral—wild cherry, wild lilac, mountain mahogany, and scrub oak. This brush gives cover to a number of wild creatures, most of which you will not see because they are nocturnal or shy. But when the path is dusty or muddy, you can see by the tracks that it is a busy thoroughfare—the pointed, wedge-shaped hoof prints of deer, the pads of coyotes, the engaging little handlike prints of raccoons, and bird tracks, particularly quail. You may even see these plump birds scurrying across the trail ahead of you. And remember, this is rattlesnake country.

Along with the tracks of small animals there will be horseshoe prints,

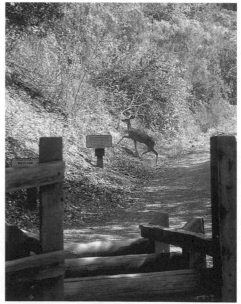

Deer like Fremont Older trails, too.

bicycle-tire treads, and marks of hiking boots. There are other signs of human impact on the ridge as well. The preserve borders a residential subdivision, so in some places the trail is close to houses built on these hills.

As the trail turns and starts around a ridge toward Stevens Creek Canyon, the views of the valley and the mountains are sweeping—golf clubs, subdivisions, and quarries below, straight ahead the hangars of Moffett Field, San Francisco Bay, and the East Bay hills. To the northwest, Monte Bello Ridge rises from the bend in Stevens Creek and extends to its summit at Black Mountain. Its quarry-scarred face seen from the trail belies the name given to the ridge at a time long before our needs for cement and gravel resulted in the massive excavations. However, the rest of the ridge is beautiful indeed, and someday even this quarry will be grown over with chaparral and trees.

After 0.5 mile along the Coyote Ridge you pass a trail on the right, round a few switchbacks, and then descend rapidly for 0.7 mile into Stevens Creek Park. A short service road leads to the Stevens Creek/Tony Look Trail by the reservoir. You could turn right toward the visitor center and perhaps have a creekside lunch in the shade at the nearby Villa Maria or Bay Tree picnic area. A car left at the Bay Tree parking lot could make this a shuttle trip and, of course, a much shorter hike.

For a longer trip you can take the Stevens Creek/Tony Look Trail south. At the first junction, one trail goes right partway around Stevens Creek Reservoir, but the hikers only trail veers left up the hillside and down, returning to Fremont Older Open Space Preserve by way of the Lookout Trail, which connects to the Vista Loop and Fern Trails and then the southern Coyote Ridge Trail. This makes a loop, adding almost 4 miles to your trip. See the Loop Trip South to Maisie's Peak below, and the first two trips in Stevens Creek Park, (Hike to the Reservoir and Climb the Hills Above, and the Lookout Trail; see page 212 for detailed directions and trip descriptions.)

LOOP TRIP SOUTH TO MAISIE'S PEAK

Skirt the east side of the southern ridge and return over the top of the preserve's highest point.

Distance: 4.8 miles round trip

Time: 2½ hours

Elevation Change: 580' gain

Start this trip as in the previous trip, turning left at the saddle. In 0.3 mile from the saddle, take the Toyon Trail, which veers left toward the stables and the southern ridges. Past tall eucalyptus and in and out of secluded canyons you contour along the east side of the ridge. In spring, pink-blooming wild currants and blue ceanothus brighten the trail. Here and there blossoming fruit trees remind you of earlier ranching days.

At the first junction you can veer right on the Bay View Trail, staying high on the ridge and following it up and down over high vista points. Crowned with spreading oaks, these hilltops make good picnic destinations. However, if you take the left-hand fork and continue south on the Toyon Trail, you traverse a hillside of chaparral interspersed with patches of oaks. Then out in open, rolling meadowlands the Bay View and Toyon trails meet.

The Toyon Trail circles east and then south, passes a gate into the preserve, and then turns west over Nob Hill to rejoin the Bay View Trail at another gate on the southern preserve boundary. This 1.3-mile loop is especially favored by riders from nearby stables.

If you eschew the Toyon Trail loop, continue south on the broad, well-used Bay View Trail to the south end of the preserve and turn north on the Coyote Ridge Trail. To reach the park's 1160-foot high point, stay on the Bay View Trail to a fork in the trail marked by a sign for Maisie's Peak, named for Maisie Garrod. She and her brother, R.V. Garrod, purchased this property in 1910, grew hay, pastured horses, and planted orchards here. Their heirs sold these southern ridgetop acres to the MROSD in 1980 but kept the property on which the present stables are located, just to the south.

A rocky trail goes straight up one side of the peak, but the 360° views from the fenced vista point are worth the steep climb. In the broad meadowlands west of and below the peak is the 1-mile Vista Loop Trail. Across the meadows to the southwest is Lookout Point, on the boundary between Stevens Creek Park and Fremont Older Preserve. A trail from the point joins the Vista Loop. (See Coyote Ridge Trail to Stevens Creek County Park for a description of a loop trip to and through Stevens Creek Park.)

Now, return to the trail from your summit climb and follow it north. At the third trail junction you turn right and descend on the Hayfields Trail past the old walnut trees, where deer often rest in the shade. At the saddle in the hayfields you turn right and return to the preserve entrance.

HUNTERS POINT

An easy walk to an old apricot orchard is delightful for an early supper hike.

Distance: 2 miles round trip

Time: 1 hour

Elevation Change: 365' gain

Start from the Prospect Road parking lot, as in Coyote Ridge Trail to Stevens Creek County Park. At the saddle in the hayfields turn right and take the trail to Hunters Point. You will pass two trails on the left that go down off the ridge, but you head straight for the hilltop, where the trees of an old apricot orchard still have a foothold. Here on the knoll called Hunters Point you can see the whole Santa Clara Valley spread out before you. To the west is the steep ridge that crosses the preserve; beyond are the heights of the Santa Cruz Mountains.

In summer, when the days are long, the short walk to Hunters Point is ideal for a picnic supper. With a festive spread in your pack you can walk to the top of the hill and have enough time left to enjoy a leisurely supper as you watch the sunset and its glow on the East Bay hills. When the lights begin to go on in the valley, it is time to pack up to get back to the parking lot by dusk, when the park closes.

SEE MAP ON PAGE 219

SEVEN SPRINGS TRAIL

Loop around Hunters Point before you climb it.

Distance: 3.5-mile loop

Time: 2 hours

Elevation Change: 365′ gain

Leave the parking lot and proceed toward the saddle on the Hayfields Trail as in Coyote Ridge Trail to Stevens Creek County Park. As the trail curves left before reaching the saddle, look for the Seven Springs Trail cutoff on your right. Take this trail and contour north on it, first around a grassy knoll, then gently down through a shady forest kept green by underground springs, which give the trail its name and once provided water for adjacent ranches. Today houses fill former orchard lands, but moisture from the springs still seeps down to the canyon floor. Look for a small grove of sycamores on your right—you may spot a red-tailed hawk nesting near its top.

Reaching the valley and a patrol road leading from the preserve boundary, you cross through an old walnut orchard and start uphill toward Hunters Point. The Seven Springs Trail veers north a little and then climbs west up the nose of Hunters Point. Immediately after passing a side trail on the right, you come to a fork and follow the right-hand trail to a hilltop encircled by large oak trees with a toyon understory. Beyond this tree-sheltered hilltop, a small flat supports remnants of a little apricot orchard. A short, steep climb from the orchard brings you to Hunters Point and the downhill return to the parking area.

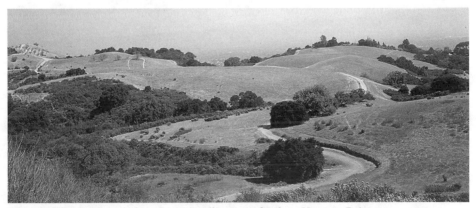

The Hayfields Trail meanders through rolling grasslands to Hunters Point

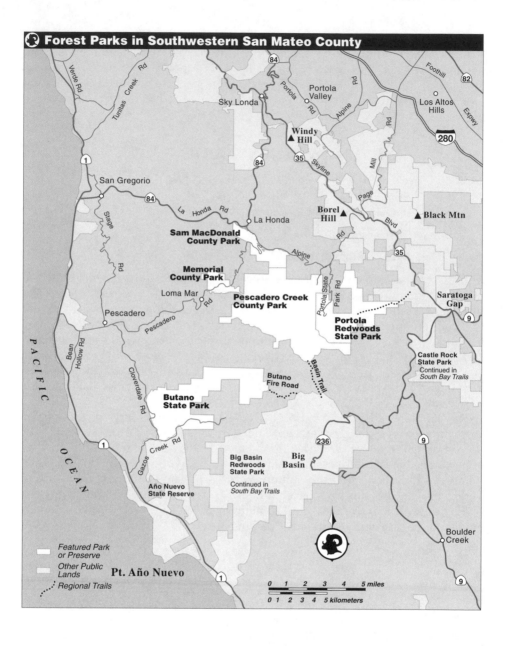

Forest Parks in Southwestern San Mateo County

Verde Rd
Tunitas Creek Rd
84
Portola
Portola Valley
Sky Londa
Foothill
82
Los Altos Hills
Windy Hill
35
Alpine
Rd
280
1
84
Skyline
Mill
San Gregorio
84
Page
Borel Hill
Black Mtn
La Honda Rd
Blvd
La Honda
Stage Rd
35
Sam MacDonald County Park
Alpine
Rd
Memorial County Park
Portola State Park Rd
Saratoga Gap
Loma Mar
Rd
Pescadero Creek County Park
9
Pescadero
Pescadero
Portola Redwoods State Park
Bean Hollow Rd
Castle Rock State Park
Continued in South Bay Trails
Cloverdale Rd
Basin Trail
PACIFIC
Butano Fire Road
Butano State Park
1
Gazos Creek Rd
236
9
Big Basin Redwoods State Park
Big Basin
OCEAN
Año Nuevo State Reserve
Continued in South Bay Trails
Boulder Creek

Featured Park or Preserve
Other Public Lands
Regional Trails

Pt. Año Nuevo
1

0 1 2 3 4   5 miles
0 1 2 3 4 5 kilometers
9

◆ Forest Parks in Southwestern ◆ San Mateo County

The large parks southwest of the Skyline lie in the heart of a remarkable aggregation of stately redwoods and mixed hardwood forests, midway between ridge and ocean. Creased by deep canyons where perennial streams flow west, these beautiful parks offer more than 14,000 acres of rugged mountainsides, superb second-growth and several virgin redwood groves, high ridges with ocean and mountain vistas, clear, deep pools in shady canyons, and a network of interconnecting trails. Each of these parks has a fine interior trail system; now trails connect these parks east to the Skyline ridge and southwest to state parks in Santa Cruz County and thence to the sea.

The magnificent redwoods preserved in these parks were first noted by Fray Juan Crespi when traveling with Don Gaspar de Portolá on his search for Monterey Bay in 1769. Crespi described them as "very high trees of a red color, not known to us" and named them *palo colorado*, red tree.

Over the intervening years many botanists studied the trees, eventually assigning their qualities of great height and long life to the genus *sequoia*. It is generally thought that the Hungarian botanist Stephen Endlicher gave it this generic name in honor of the Cherokee nation chief, Sequoyah.

The parks that make up this unique acreage include the three San Mateo County parks, Pescadero, Memorial, and Sam McDonald, and two state parks, Portola Redwoods and Butano.

The trips described in these forest parks lead visitors on short nature walks and long-distance trails to behold splendid specimens of this remarkable tree.

❖ Pescadero Creek County Park Complex ❖

San Mateo County's three parks in the La Honda area are Pescadero Creek, Memorial, and Sam McDonald parks. Together they comprise some 8027 contiguous acres in the drainage basin of Pescadero Creek. They were acquired at different times but have interconnecting trails and share many characteristics. Each is typical of the Santa Cruz Mountains habitat—redwood and Douglas fir forests, mixed evergreen forests, and dense riparian vegetation along the streams. Rainfall is heavy on this western side of the mountains, and most of the streams run year-round.

According to Frank Stanger's *Sawmills in the Redwoods*, logging began in this area when John Tuffley built a mill upstream from the town of Pescadero in 1856. Logging has occurred intermittently since then. However, due to its remote location, the area was never completely clear-cut. The difficulty of trips over the Santa Cruz Mountains on wagons hauled by oxen also prevented total clearing. But enterprising loggers, such as William Page, built a road over the Skyline to haul shingles to Mayfield and the Bayside. Other loggers hauled their shingles to Pigeon Point and sent them by boat to San Francisco.

Names of creeks and roads in the area remind us of the stalwart men and their families who built mills and established homes here. Blomquist and McCormick creeks were named for early mill owners. The steep hill between La Honda and Memorial Park known as Haskins Grade was once part of 500 acres owned by Aaron Haskins, who also had a mill on McCormick Creek. The road between Memorial and Pescadero parks was named for Henry Wurr, an immigrant from Germany who gave land for the Wurr School which remained in use until 1935.

Memorial Park, the first of the complex acquired by San Mateo County, owes its existence to Roy W. Cloud, the county superintendent of schools in the 1920s. When visiting schools in this outlying area, he was struck by the beauty of the forests and streams near the old Wurr School. In the Spring of 1923 he appealed to the County Board of Supervisors to buy land for a park here. After studying possible sites, a citizens committee recommended that the County buy 310 acres for $70,000, the beginnings of today's Memorial Park. It was named in honor of the San Mateo County men who lost their lives in World War I. During President Franklin Roosevelt's era veterans of World War I worked on WPA projects here building roads, picnic sites, and restrooms, some of which remain today.

Sam McDonald Park, the wooded retreat of a longtime employee of Stanford University, was bequeathed to the university in 1957 and one year later purchased by San Mateo County. McDonald began buying land in the La Honda area in 1917 and eventually owned more than 400 acres along Alpine Creek in the northwest corner of today's park. McDonald, a descendant of slaves, was born in 1884 in Louisiana, and came to Mayfield (part of today's Palo Alto) in 1903. His first employment was at Stanford University as a teamster, from which he rose in over fifty years to become Superintendent of Athletic Grounds and Buildings. Sam McDonald was particularly fond of children, and he wanted his land to become a park for the benefit of young people. In 1976 the County bought additional acres southwest of McDonald's holdings and the 37-acre Heritage Grove Preserve,

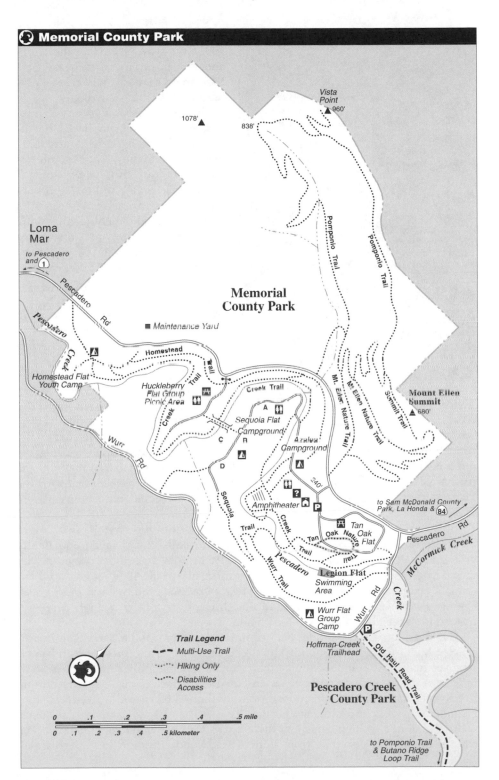

Memorial County Park

Vista
Point
▲ 960'

1078' ▲

838'

Loma
Mar

to Pescadero
and ①

Pescadero Creek

Pescadero Rd

Pomponio Trail

Pomponio Trail

**Memorial
County Park**

■ Maintenance Yard

Homestead Trail

Homestead Flat
Youth Camp

Huckleberry
Flat Group
Picnic Area

Creek Trail

Creek Trail

A

Mt. Ellen Nature Trail

Mt. Ellen Nature Trail

Summit Trail

**Mount Ellen
Summit**
▲ 680'

Wurr Rd

Sequoia Flat
Campground

C

B

D

Azalea
Campground

240'

?

P

to Sam McDonald County
Park, La Honda & ⑧④

Pescadero Rd

McCormick Creek

Amphitheater

Sequoia Trail

Tan Oak Nature Trail

Tan
Oak
Flat

Tan Oak
Trail

Pescadero Creek

Wurr Trail

Legion Flat
Swimming
Area

Wurr Rd

Creek

Wurr Flat
Group
Camp

P

Old Haul Road Trail

Trail Legend
– – – Multi-Use Trail
······· Hiking Only
········· Disabilities
　　　 Access

Hoffman Creek
Trailhead

**Pescadero Creek
County Park**

0　　.1　　.2　　.3　　.4　　.5 mile
0　.1　.2　.3　.4　　.5 kilometer

to Pomponio Trail
& Butano Ridge
Loop Trail

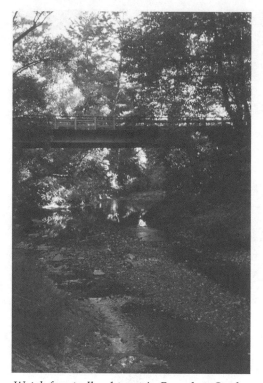

Watch for steelhead trout in Pescadero Creek

bringing the total acreage to today's 1002. It is most fitting that the camp-sites in this park that bears Sam McDonald's name can be reserved by organized youth groups only.

Pescadero Creek Park, the largest of the three, was purchased by the County following the controversy over plans to build a dam on the creek to supply water to the Pescadero area and to provide water-oriented recreation on a deep-water lake behind the dam. Proposed for the site of today's Worley Flat, this dam would have flooded the entire creek canyon, including some of today's Portola Redwoods State Park. In 1968 the county agreed to buy 4736 acres from the Santa Cruz Lumber Company in six yearly purchases through 1973. The company could take all the trees above 400 feet, the elevation of the proposed dam, in specified logging areas, beginning on the north side of the creek. San Mateo County had the option to purchase significant trees or outstanding groves of trees selected by the county forester before timber cutting by the company. Accordingly, during the three years following this agreement, San Mateo County purchased many of the park's monarch trees. Fortunately, many areas of the park were difficult for the loggers to reach and thus some trees that the county could not purchase were saved.

However, public opposition to the size and height of the dam, its flooding of many Portola State Park redwoods, and its enormous cost delayed and finally brought a halt to plans for a dam. In March 1971 a new agreement provided that the county would purchase all remaining timber above the 400-foot level and the lumber company would cease all logging operations. Today, Pescadero Creek County Park's 46 miles of trails pass through impressive re-grown redwood and fir forests, especially along Jones Gulch and Towne creeks.

The Pescadero Creek County Park complex does not stand alone in southwestern San Mateo County. Surrounded by a tapestry of parks and preserves and a network of trails, this is indeed one of the most remarkable public open space areas in California. Immediately upstream on Pescadero Creek is the 3000-acre Portola Redwoods State Park, making a total of more than 11,000 acres of redwood environment for public use and enjoyment.

In addition, two long trails join these parks to other public open spaces. The 6.8-mile Basin Trail extends from Portola Redwoods through Pescadero Creek

Park and on an easement through private lands reaches Big Basin Redwoods State Park in Santa Cruz County. Another long-distance trail links the Old Haul Road Trail in Pescadero Creek Park with the Slate Creek Trail in Portola Redwoods State Park, which connects to the Ward Road Trail in Long Ridge Open Space Preserve on the Skyline ridge. In the planning stage is a connection from Skyline Ridge Open Space Preserve down the Old Page Mill Road that could enter Portola Redwoods State Park at the Peters Creek Loop and continue to Pescadero Creek Park on the Pomponio or Old Haul Road Trail. These trail links will further enhance an already outstanding recreational experience and will provide back-packing routes that will challenge sturdy outdoor enthusiasts. Overnight stays in the trail camps in Portola Redwoods and Big Basin Redwoods state parks and in Pescadero Creek County Park can be reserved by calling each park's number listed in Appendix III.

Due to the parks' proximity to the Pacific Ocean, summer fogs and strong winter storms affect their weather. Trails near creeks and under the redwood trees can be damp late into summer. Visitors should carry sweaters and jackets. Spring and fall are delightful times to enjoy the trails, picnic sites, and camping at the parks.

Jurisdiction: San Mateo County: 650-363-4020; reservations: 650-363-4021; the main office for the complex is at Memorial Park: 650-879-0212

Facilities: Trails for hikers and some trails for equestrians; picnic tables; camp-sites; group facilities by reservation; two trail camps (each park in the complex has different facilities, described under that park's description)

Rules: Open 8 A.M. to sunset; horses on designated trails only; bicycles on designated roads only; no dogs; no ground fires allowed; reservations required for all organized youth groups, regardless of size or activity for group campsites, picnic areas, trail camps, and Jack Brook Horse Camp; reservations are not accepted for family camping and picnicking; fees

Maps: San Mateo County brochures *Pescadero Creek County Park, Memorial Park* and *Sam McDonald Park* and USGS topos *La Honda, Mindego Hill,* and *Big Basin*

How to Get There: Access to Pescadero Creek County Park complex is along some rather tortuous roads—La Honda, Pescadero and Alpine roads—to five park entrances: (1) Sam McDonald County Park (see below). (2) Pescadero Park (see below). (3) Memorial Park—On Pescadero Rd. pass the Wurr Rd. sign and go straight ahead (west) 0.25 mile to park entrance on left. (4) Pescadero Park, Tarwater Creek Trailhead—From Hwy 35 (Skyline Blvd) west of Palo Alto, take Alpine Rd. south for 3.1 miles and bear right past Portola State Park Rd. Continue 0.4 mile to Camp Pomponio Rd., turn left onto it, continuing 1 mile to a small unpaved parking area on left just uphill from gated entrance to County Jail. (5) Trails in eastern part of park complex are also accessible from Portola Redwoods State Park (see page 271). From Hwy 1 take Hwy 84 to La Honda and follow Pescadero Rd. as described above.

Sam McDonald County Park

This 1003-acre San Mateo County park lies on both sides of meandering Pescadero Road near La Honda. The 400 northeast-facing acres that drain into Alpine Creek are mostly redwood forest with understories of huckleberry, creambush, and hazelnut and a lush ground cover of redwood sorrel. On the southeast side of Pescadero Road are the sunnier grasslands and oak/madrone woods on south-facing Towne Ridge. On the north side of this ridge lies the 38-acre Heritage Grove on the banks of Alpine Creek. Here are specimen old-growth redwoods and a fine second-growth redwood/fir forest preserved following a citizens fund drive that culminated in the County's acquisition of the grove. Parklands stretch from the grove west to Pescadero and La Honda roads.

Trails for hikers loop through the redwood forest and pass the group campsites on the north side of Pescadero Road. On the south side trails wind through a stately redwood forest to the Heritage Grove and uphill to Towne Ridge and the Hikers Hut. Equestrians use the unpaved park service roads to reach both sides of the park and other trails in adjoining Pescadero Creek County Park.

A well-kept horse camp on Towne Ridge, named in honor of former parks and recreation director Jack Brook, is open by reservation for equestrians only.

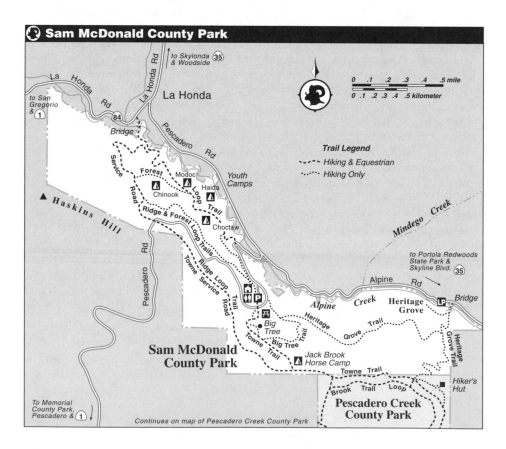

Facilities: Trails for hikers and equestrians; picnic sites; group campsites reserved especially for youth groups; Hikers Hut and Jack Brook Horse Camp; restrooms at park office and in campsites

Rules: All youth groups must make reservations; picnic sites available on first-come, first-served basis; no dogs or pets; no bicycles; fee for group camping

Maps: San Mateo County brochure *Sam McDonald Park* and *Pescadero Creek County Park*, USGS topos *La Honda* and *Mindego Hill*

How to Get There: There are two access points: (1) Park office on Pescadero Rd.—From Hwy 84 (La Honda Rd) in La Honda on west side of Skyline, turn left (southeast) on Pescadero Rd., go 1.1 miles to a triangular intersection with Alpine Rd., turn sharp right and continue 0.5 miles on Pescadero Rd. to park entrance on right. (2) Heritage Grove on Alpine Rd.—go 1.2 miles east of Pescadero/Alpine Rd. junction to parking on south side of road.

TWO LOOP TRAILS NORTH FROM PARK OFFICE

Find the Wolf Tree in a quiet redwood grove.

Distance: 2.6-mile—Forest Loop; add 1 mile for service road extension; 3.6-mile—Ridge Loop

Time: 1½ hours

Elevation Change: 300′ gain

Start this hikers-only trip on a trail to the right (east) of the park office and walk immediately uphill under beautiful redwood trees. At the first junction turn left on the foot trail (bear right to reach the campsites) winding up and down past many burned-out shells of giant redwoods and some splendid living trees. Some of these long-lived trees are fire-scarred; others are hollow and yet still living. As you meander along the steep-sided trail, note the beautiful, graceful ferns flourishing in this shady forest. Ferns can prosper without much sunlight because they reproduce by spores instead of by pollination, which is dependent on insects and flowers. Because redwoods groves create dense shade, plants that don't need direct sunlight or insects to pollinate them can flourish.

Here and there are seats cut out of redwood stumps or fallen logs, pleasant stopping places to contemplate the magnificent trees. After about a mile on this trail, look on your right for a fallen monarch, a branch of which resembles a wolf's head.

The forest floor is covered with redwood and tan oak duff, often carpeted with three-leaved redwood sorrel enlivened with small pink-petalled blossoms in spring. Look for occasional hazelnut bushes overhanging the trail, whose velvety, light green leaves emerge in spring and whose nuts become favorite food for squirrels in fall. You may see the shells underfoot, but seldom on the bush.

After 1.3 miles you reach a junction where the Forest Loop Trail goes right and the Ridge Trail left. Take the Forest Loop Trail (north), joining the unpaved service road for a very steep downhill stretch. Watch on the right for a small sign pointing right to continue on the 2.6-mile Forest Loop Trail, which goes east to the Chinook campsite. If you continue on the service road, you will have a longer loop hike north past the park's water-storage tank, then up, down, and around bends heading north, then east to the banks of Alpine Creek. Here you are at the park boundary, where private homes sit below the road. Stay on the road as it turns south and climbs out of the creek canyon. Five-finger ferns drape the trailside, and trillium bloom here in spring—both plants that thrive in this moist, shady environment.

About 0.25 mile after turning due south you enter the Modoc group site, where there are picnic tables, barbecues, restrooms, and a little circle of log seats for evening gatherings. You follow the unsurfaced park road here past other group campsites with Native American names, such as Haida and Choctaw, above a near-vertical canyon wall. When you round the head of this deep canyon beyond the Choctaw camp, find the Forest Loop Trail leading off the road on your right, follow this foot trail uphill to the junction where you started this loop and then descend to the park office.

BIG TREE TRAIL SOUTH FROM PARK OFFICE

Try this loop trail before a picnic at one of the tables in the redwoods.

Distance: 1-mile loop

Time: ¾ hour

Elevation Change: 200' gain

Begin by the Pescadero Creek signboard across the parking lot from the ranger station on a trail through the trees that quickly emerges at Pescadero Road. Carefully cross to the other side and step onto the Big Tree Loop Trail for hikers only. (Do not take the Towne Trail leading to Pescadero Park.) Begin your uphill trip under second-growth redwoods already reaching 175 feet skyward. Underfoot are branchlets and cones of the redwoods, making very pleasant footing. Pass a road to a few private inholdings in the park, and continue to a park sign on the right that points left to the Heritage Grove Trail and right to the Big Tree Trail. You take the latter one and climb steadily uphill on a shady north-facing slope. This is a lovely, cool hike on a hot day, with sunlight filtering through the trees and Steller's jays squawking in the canopy.

Continuing uphill, you bend south and then slowly descend west past a big green water tank. Paralleling the Towne Trail service road, you head downhill left (northeast), descend some steep steps, go around some switchbacks and finally reach the Big Tree, with its 15-foot diameter and hollow core. Fire-scarred and open on two sides, this venerable giant is alive and well. Apparently when redwoods are burned, they tend to sprout from the base, which may account for the multiple, fused trunks.

SEE MAP ON PAGE 230

You could stop for rest and a picnic lunch at a nearby table, or cross Pescadero Road to where other tables under the trees offer a pleasant place to reflect on the wonders of these magnificent trees.

SEE MAP ON PAGE 230

HERITAGE GROVE LOOP

Following a well-built hikers' trail to redwoods along the Creek, you rise gradually to Towne Ridge and return downhill.

Distance: 5-mile loop

Time: 2½ hours

Elevation Change: 550' gain

This route on the north side of Towne Ridge, a cooler, more gradual, but longer way to the ridge and Hikers Hut than the Towne Trail (service road), starts as described in the previous trip (Big Tree Trail South from Park Office). When you see the sign for the Heritage Grove pointing left, take that trail. Meandering through a forest of widely spaced redwoods and Douglas firs, you nip into little ravines, cross a stream with a little waterfall that is known as Gorge Creek, and cross another intermittent but unnamed creek.

Where the trail bends north, you can hear Alpine Creek coursing over rocks and fallen trees at the bottom of the slope. There are stumps of cut redwoods with slots for springboards on which the early loggers stood to use a two-handled saw. Then after 1.2 miles you will see a sign on a hefty redwood post pointing left to the Heritage Grove. Five minutes take you to the fenced flat where the largest and best trees remain, thanks to citizen fund-raising and the County Board of Supervisors who purchased the grove. Beyond, down a pretty trail are two bridges over Alpine Creek and a small parking area on the creekside of Alpine Road. This short trail from Alpine Road makes an excellent introductory redwood-ecology walk.

After savoring the sight and sound of the creek and its riparian trees and shrubs, retrace your steps to the grove, and then turn left (due south) at the redwood signpost to begin the climb to Towne Ridge and the Hikers Hut. From here to the ridge you traverse a mixed forest of oaks, bays, maples, and some Douglas firs. Around a wide turn you pass a knoll where the canopy is high above the ground and the

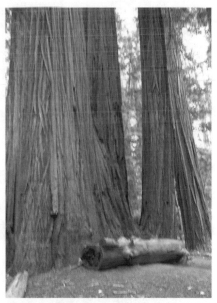

Heritage Grove's remarkable trees

understory is a tangle of creambush, berry and honeysuckle vines, and hazelnut trees. This different environment might indicate a clear-cut or fire occurred here in recent past.

When you reach the ridgetop grasslands, look to your left for the 0.25-mile trail through the woods to the Hikers Hut (see the Pescadero Park trip, Brook Trail Loop). After a short detour to experience the wonderful view across Pescadero Creek Canyon and up to Butano Ridge, you can return to the Towne Trail and go west 1.75 miles to visit the Jack Brook Horse Camp. Although this is reserved for equestrians only, you can walk up to see the corrals, campsites, and the little cottage that once belonged to the Towne family, who sold these 400 acres on the south side of the ridge to San Mateo County.

From the junction of the horse camp trail take the Towne Trail (service road) downhill along the west side of a redwood-filled canyon, pausing on the steep descent to savor the healthy trees whose tops tower high above the trail. At some point your eyes are almost at the level of the lower tree branches 100 feet above their trunks.

An alternate route to return to the park office follows the Ridge Trail out to Pescadero Road, crosses it, and mounts a few steps to reach the service road. Then you proceed downhill about 800 feet to the junction of the Forest Loop Trail. Turn right here and wind up and down along the 1.3-mile trail on the north-facing ridge to the park office (route described in reverse in the first trip, Two Loop Trails North from Park Office). This would add about 3 miles to your trip, but would make a fine overview of Sam McDonald Park.

Pescadero Creek County Park

This 6486-acre park, the keystone that ties Memorial and Sam McDonald parks together, encompasses seven miles of Pescadero Creek as it meanders through the canyon between Towne and Butano ridges. Joined by 19 intermittent streams that tumble down the steep sides of these ridges, Pescadero Creek forms the centerpiece of the park. More than 40 miles of trail reach its highest points, follow its creeks, and penetrate its great forests. When combined with the adjacent 3000 acres of Portola Redwoods State Park, this vast open space is premier country for long, strenuous hikes and horseback rides.

Trails leading to the banks of Pescadero Creek offer short jaunts for casual walks. The canyons are heavily forested, especially on north-facing, 2000-foot Butano Ridge, while the southwest-facing slopes of 1200-foot Towne Ridge offer pockets of grassland with inspiring views in all directions. Included here are trips that sample Pescadero Creek Park's splendid, remote, almost-wilderness acres, less than an hour from the urban Bayside.

Jurisdiction: San Mateo County

Facilities: Trails for hikers and equestrians; trail camps by permit from Memorial Park office

Rules: Bicycles on Old Haul Road only; no dogs; no fires

Maps: Map on pages 236-237 San Mateo County brochure *Pescadero Creek County Park*, USGS topos *La Honda*, *Mindego Hill* and *Big Basin*

How to Get There: (1) West entrance—From Hwy 84 (La Honda Rd.) in La Honda on west side of Skyline, turn left (southeast) on Pescadero Rd., go 1.1 miles to a triangular intersection with Alpine Rd., turn sharp right, pass Sam McDonald Park on right and go about 4 miles to sign on left pointing straight ahead (west) to Memorial Park and another small street sign marking Wurr Rd. Turn left on Wurr Rd. and continue 0.25 mile to Hoffman Creek Trailhead and a small parking area there. (2) Tarwater Creek Trailhead: From Hwy 35 (Skyline Boulevard) west of Palo Alto, take Alpine Rd. south for 3.1 miles and bear right past Portola State Park Rd. Continue 0.4 mile to Camp Pomponio Rd., turn left onto it, continuing 1 mile to a small unparved parking area on left just uphill from gated entrance to County Jail. (3) Trails in eastern part of park complex are also accessible from Portola Redwoods State Park (see page 243).

A SHORT WALK TO PESCADERO CREEK AND WORLEY FLAT

When the water level is low, take a backpack picnic to an easy destination for families with young children.

Distance: 2 miles round trip to creek; 3 miles round trip to Worley Flat

Time: 1 to 2 hours

Elevation Change: 50' gain to creek; 100' gain to Worley Flat

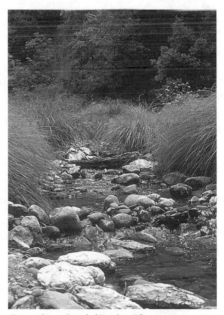

Choose a sunny day for this trip, pack a lunch, take dry socks and extra clothing and start from the Hoffman Creek Trailhead at the Wurr Road entrance to the park, access point (1), above. You set off across a sturdy bridge over Hoffman Creek and pass a few picnic tables by a kiosk on your left. After orienting yourself at the park map here and learning about its wildlife, follow the wide, unpaved Old Haul Road. Still used for occasional logging on nearby private property, this road/trail undulates up and down through a clearing and a former orchard, then dips into redwoods on an easement through adjoining private lands, where second-growth trees are intermittently

Pescadero Creek lined with grasses

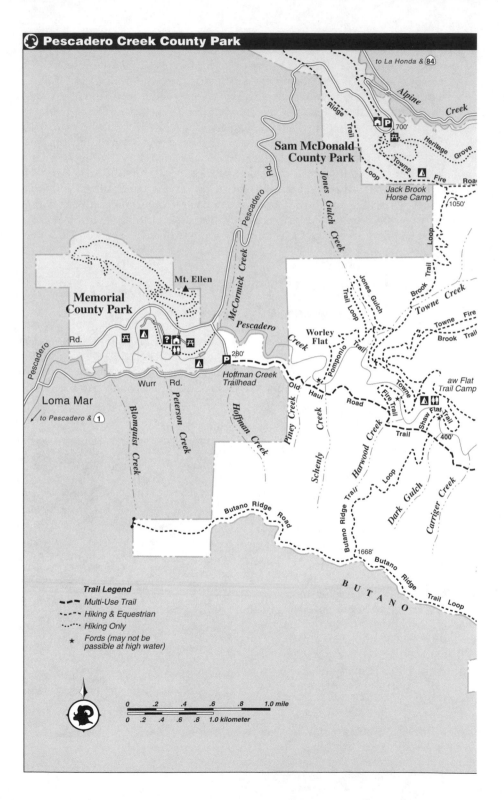

Pescadero Creek County Park

to La Honda & ⑧④

Alpine Creek

Ridge Trail

700'

Heritage Grove

Sam McDonald County Park

Towne Loop

Fire Road

Jack Brook Horse Camp

1050'

Jones Gulch Creek

Brook Trail

Towne Creek

Memorial County Park

Mt. Ellen

McCormick Creek

Pescadero Rd.

Jones Gulch Trail Loop

Towne Fire

Brook Trail

Worley Flat

Pomponio Trail

Pescadero Creek

Pescadero Rd.

280'

Hoffman Creek Trailhead

Wurr Rd.

Loma Mar

to Pescadero & ①

Blomquist Creek

Peterson Creek

Hoffman Creek

Piney Creek

Old Haul Road

Schenly Creek

Harwood Creek

Towne Fire Trail

aw Flat Trail Camp

Shaw Flat Trail

400'

Trail

Dark Gulch

Loop

Carriger Creek

Butano Ridge Road

Butano Ridge Trail

1668'

Butano Ridge Trail Loop

B U T A N O

Trail Legend

- – – *Multi-Use Trail*
- - - - *Hiking & Equestrian*
- ⋯⋯ *Hiking Only*
- ★ *Fords (may not be passible at high water)*

0   .2   .4   .6   .8   1.0 mile

0   .2   .4   .6   .8   1.0 kilometer

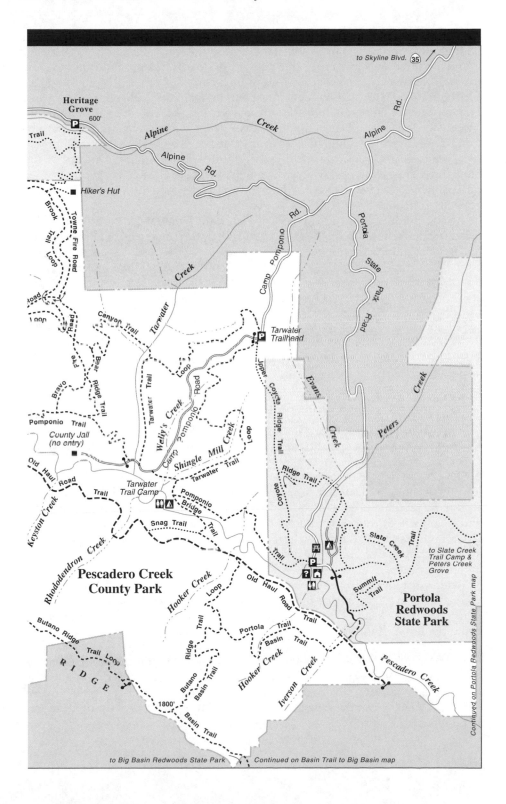

Heritage Grove
600'

Alpine Creek

Alpine Rd.

Alpine Rd.

Alpine

to Skyline Blvd. 35

Trail

Hiker's Hut

Brook Trail Loop

Towne Fire Road

Camp Pomponio Rd.

Portola State Park Road

Creek

Canyon Trail

Tarwater Creek

Road

Loop

Tarwater Trailhead

Evans Creek

Peters Creek

Bravo

Bear Ridge Trail

Tarwater Trail

Welly's Creek

Camp Pomponio Road

Loop

Shingle Mill Creek

Coyote Ridge Trail

Loop

Pomponio Trail

County Jail (no entry)

Old Haul Road

Tarwater Trail Camp

Tarwater Trail

Ridge Trail

Coyote Trail

Keyston Creek Trail

Pomponio Bridge

Snag Trail

Trail

Slate Creek Trail

to Slate Creek Trail Camp & Peters Creek Grove

Rhododendron Creek

Pescadero Creek County Park

Hooker Creek

Loop

Old Haul Road Trail

Summit Trail

Portola Redwoods State Park

Butane Ridge

Ridge Trail

Portola Trail

Basin Trail

Trail Loop

Butano Basin Trail

Hooker Creek

Iverson Creek

Pescadero Creek

R I D G E

1800'

Basin Trail

to Big Basin Redwoods State Park   Continued on Basin Trail to Big Basin map

Continued on Portola Redwoods State Park map

harvested. Although the ancient redwood forest was logged many years ago, remnant stumps of old monarchs still stand beside the trail attesting to the size and grandeur of the ancient forest. Some trees are hollow and tempt little ones to crawl through. Others are blackened by fires of long ago.

About 0.5 mile through the cool forest you pass Piney Creek, after which watch for the signed Pomponio Trail turnoff on your left. As you drop down under a canopy of deciduous alder and willow trees to the creekside, you find a portable foot bridge (removed at high water) over Pescadero Creek. Here the creek tumbles over scattered rocks, tugs at clumps of graceful grasses, laps at mossy stream banks, and brushes against willows that arch overhead. Here children can float leaf boats downstream, watch skeeter bugs on the water, and see dragonflies flitting above the stream.

After a picnic in the shade at creekside or in the sunny meadow at Worley Flat, just another ten minutes up the Pomponio Trail, return on the Old Haul Road from a delightful children's outing.

BROOK TRAIL LOOP

SEE MAP ON PAGE 236

Climb out of the creek canyon to sunny meadows and wide views.

Distance: 8-mile loop

Time: 5 hours

Elevation Change: 650′ gain

Begin at the Hoffman Creek Trailhead on Wurr Road [access point (1)] and follow the directions to Worley Flat as in the previous trip, A Short Walk to Pescadero Creek and Worley Flat. Then continue on the Pomponio Trail past the wide meadow and curve right (east) across its north end. On the far side of the meadow follow the Pomponio Trail left onto a graveled tread and go uphill through oak woodland. Soon you cross a wide, closed-off trail, the former Jones Gulch Trail, and take the foot trail down a long traverse. In sunny patches look for blue iris blooming in spring and red rose hips and orange-red poison oak leaves in fall. On switchbacks you descend to the creek, which you can hear gurgling in the canyon after heavy rains.

After 1.6 miles from your starting point you reach another trail junction, where the sign tells you that the Pomponio Trail goes right and the Jones Gulch Trail goes left. Ahead of you is the Jones Gulch Bridge, which you will take to begin the Brook Trail Loop. Turn sharply left (north) at the junction, go right onto the bridge and you have reached a magical part of Pescadero Park. If you pause here under the towering redwood trees, look into the depths of the creek canyon carved out of Butano sandstone to see five-finger ferns and moss draping its high banks and little waterfalls dropping over fallen logs. Carpets of pink-flowered redwood sorrel adorn the forest floor in this idyllic spot—a cool destination for a hot day's hike.

In 500 feet you bear right on an unpaved patrol road, the Jones Gulch Trail, cross Towne Creek in a culvert, go 300 feet farther on the patrol road, and turn sharply left. On a rare, hot morning, it would be cooler to ascend the other side of the loop, which is shaded in the morning, and then descend on this side. A sign farther along the patrol road points right to the other leg of the loop.

Slowly climbing through a forest of ancient and second-growth trees on the west side of the Brook Trail Loop, you find new trees sprouting from fallen ones, tan-bark oaks growing out of sawn-off redwoods and slanting light filtering through the forest canopy. You may be puzzled by the presence of an occasional monarch tree remaining near a clump of redwood stumps. A possible explanation is that some trees were too inaccessible, too scarred by fire or just too difficult to haul out of the forest.

About midway up the mountain the trail narrows and skirts a deep ravine, then makes 10 or 11 switchbacks through mixed forest to a chaparral clearing. From here you can look down into the deep, heavily wooded canyon of Towne Creek and east across it to the route of your return trip. To the south lies Butano Ridge rising above the Pescadero Creek Canyon. Then after more switchbacks through a forest of fir, oak, and madrone, you emerge on a gentle grassy slope with a view of the Skyline ridge. (Occasionally, you can hear sounds of target practice from a gun club off Skyline Boulevard east of here.) Trail signs point south to destinations in Pescadero and Memorial parks and east to the Hikers Hut and the continuation of the Brook Trail Loop. In a few steps you are on a wide, unpaved road, which you can take, but you may prefer to stay on the foot trail which parallels this road around the head of the Towne Creek canyon. You are now in Sam McDonald County Park.

In about 0.5 mile look for the left turnoff sign (north) to the Hikers Hut. To reach this attractive Sierra Club hut, follow the trail 0.25 mile uphill into the woods. Shortly you come to a sturdy cabin with a million-dollar view. Thanks to Ollie Mayer and a dedicated team of Sierra Club volunteers, this hut was imported from Denmark and assembled on this park site in 1977. You can reserve the hut for an overnight or a weekend by calling the Loma Prieta Chapter of the Sierra Club (see Appendix III). However, if you are just visiting for the day, you can sit on a log seat in front of the hut and enjoy the vista of forested Butano Ridge and Pescadero Creek canyon. After a rest and snack here, begin the next leg of your trip.

Return to the Brook Trail Loop and proceed downhill about 0.5 mile through a fir forest. When the trail crosses the patrol road, you can climb up to a ledge where two picnic tables and another fine view of southwestern San Mateo County's beautiful evergreen forests await you. Following this short digression, take the narrow foot trail through beautiful, quiet redwood groves on the west-facing side of the canyon. When you come to the Towne Fire Road, cross it, and at the next junction angle sharply right to stay on the Brook Trail Loop. If you go left and uphill from here, you will be on the Bear Ridge Trail, which is discussed in the next trip, A Loop around the Tarwater Creek Basin.

For approximately 0.5 mile the Brook Trail Loop levels off, paralleling the fire road. Then it joins the road for about 500 feet, after which you leave the road, go right, uphill, and zigzag through deep redwood forest to another trail junction, where the Brook Trail Loop goes right onto the Pomponio Trail heading north.

Shortly you cross another fire road, the Jones Gulch Trail, and continue to Grangers Bridge across Towne Creek, signed ELEVATION 270 FEET. From this bridge you can look upstream to the confluence of Towne and Jones Gulch creeks. Little waterfalls drop into a pebbly pool shaded by huge redwoods, its banks festooned with graceful ferns. Just a bit farther is the Pomponio/Brook Trail junction where you began the Brook Trail Loop. Take a last look at the lively creek as it tumbles over a sandstone shelf, bounces off a fallen tree, and continues on its way to join Pescadero Creek.

Now you bear left on the Pomponio Trail, retrace your steps on a few switchbacks uphill, cross Worley Flat, and head southwest to the ford of Pescadero Creek. Shortly you reach the graveled Old Haul Road, where you turn right (west) to return to the Hoffman Creek Trailhead.

A LOOP AROUND
THE TARWATER CREEK BASIN

Explore up and down the east-facing slopes of the Tarwater Creek canyon.

Distance: 5 miles

Time: 3 hours

Elevation Change: 650' loss to trip's lowest point

Start from the northeast corner of the park at the Tarwater Trailhead on Camp Pomponio Road, access point (2).

Take the west leg of the Tarwater Trail Loop just across the road from the parking area and go northwest about 0.25 mile through open grassland to a sharp turn left, then meander along a narrower trail into a pretty oak/bay woodland. Emerging from the woods you follow the east edge of a long meadow, then cut across it to skirt the forest above a branch of Tarwater Creek. As you walk under the trees, continue around a huge, lone redwood and look for a side trail cutting over to a small building with corrugated tin roof under a cluster of tall eucalyptus trees, known as Tie Camp. Just a few steps lead you to it and a peek at the thick redwood sides and floors of this long-deserted dwelling, later used as a barn. The fence across the lower end of this meadow and bailing wire scattered about recall the days when a dairy farmer rented the site, kept goats and cows in the meadow and transported milk and cheese out of the canyon to local customers.

This barn is all that remains of an extensive layout for the Moore, Fisher, and Troupe mill operation that cut redwood trees into railroad ties here in 1915-16. Some present-day residents of this area remember that descendants of the mill operators later came here for holidays in the new-growth redwoods. After exploring the exterior of this deserted site (not safe to enter it), get back on the main trail and contour around the barn's south side into a little swale where an early settler planted a double row of pear trees, now quite aged, and then switchback downhill into the shade of big redwoods.

When you reach the junction of the Tarwater and Canyon trails, bear right onto the Canyon Trail, an old logging road, and pause to admire the huge redwood tree on the left side of the trail. It must have been left by the loggers because of some defect or because the county purchased it during the negotiations for the park. A little farther along in the hushed silence of the ancient forest, descend to the Tarwater Creek crossing. You are now on the north side of a tributary of Tarwater Creek. In this canyon where horsetails, ferns, and huckleberry thrive, begin a climb of several hundred feet on a narrow trail, closed to horses in wet weather. Switchbacks carry you up and up past a few pools in the creek, a huge logjam, and a marshy spot where wild boars have been at work. From an elevation of about 900 feet you make a long climb south and then round a sharp switchback to look north through the trees to Towne Ridge and the houses along Alpine and Camp Pomponio roads.

About two hours from the trailhead you reach the Bear Ridge Trail and turn left (south) on it through a forest with a high canopy. Swing along on this trail up a little hump and then downhill to intersect the Bravo Fire Road, on which you descend briefly before angling left on the Bear Ridge Trail again. With the steep canyon of Tarwater Creek on your left, you contour along this hillside through big Douglas firs, then cross to the west side of the ridge.

After meeting a fence across an old trail, you pass the white plastic pipes where treated wastewater from the jail is sprayed on the hillside. This is not a good place to pause for lunch. Shortly you meet a trail junction and turn left (southeast) on the Pomponio Trail. If you go west on this trail, you reach the eight Shaw Flat Trail Camps, which are reservable by calling the Memorial Park office. You must carry your own water, food, and sleeping bag; there are restrooms. However, if you are not going to Shaw Flat, follow the Pomponio Trail downhill into a huckleberry hollow and then out to the paved Camp Pomponio Road. Here a big sign tells you that the jail (a men's correctional center) is just west of here and only official visitors may enter. Therefore, go left, following the road across a steel trussed bridge over Tarwater Creek, climb up a short hill, and turn left (north) around a split-rail fence onto the wide, west leg of the Tarwater Trail Loop.

Now you hike up a little rise, then drop down, but gradually ascend along the east bank of Tarwater Creek under tall redwoods and Douglas firs, with cut logs bordering much of the trail. In fall, there is often a beautiful display of shelf fungus in shades of salmon pink and cream on these logs. When you reach the Canyon Trail junction, bear right between redwood posts and retrace your steps to the Tarwater Trailhead where your trip began.

BUTANO RIDGE TRAIL LOOP

Innumerable switchbacks take you up and down on a day-long workout.

Distance: 13.3 miles

Time: 8 hours

Elevation Change: 1750′ gain

Note: If you do this trip in reverse, you take the long leg on the wide, graveled Old Haul Road at the beginning of the trip and enjoy a gentle downhill leg along the Butano Ridge Trail Loop from east to west at the end of the trip.

Even if you don't take the entire loop, a climb partway up the western leg of this loop trail offers the experience of a second-growth forest relatively untouched since the logging of the late 1960s. With an early start from the Hoffman Creek Trailhead, access point (1) on page 235 you can do the uphill stretch in the cool of the morning. Carry extra sweaters, a windbreaker and plenty of water and food for this trek to the top of the ridge. In fall, days can be delightfully warm and sunny; summer can bring drippy fogs and chilly, damp days.

On the Old Haul Road you follow the same route as in the first two trips, A Short Walk to Pescadero Creek and Worley Flat and the Brook Trail Loop, but after reaching the Pomponio Trail turnoff, you continue another 1.5 miles, passing the marked crossings of Schenly and Harwood creeks. Occasional dense groves of alders fill hollows along the wide, unpaved road and ferns clothe its shady banks. But the stately redwoods are the main attraction along this road in the bottom of Pescadero Creek canyon.

Two trails cross to the north side of the creek—Towne Fire Road and the Shaw Flat Trail—and lead to the Shaw Flat Trail Camp on the Pomponio Trail. Just opposite the Shaw Flat Trail, look for the entrance to the western leg of the Butano Ridge Trail Loop on your right (south). Now you step onto this well-designed, comfortably graded trail that goes up and around ridges, between giant redwoods, past burned-out shells of monarch redwoods and continues zigzagging upward for nearly 2 miles. Underfoot your way is carpeted with duff and small branchlets; occasionally a tree root protrudes across the trail. About two thirds of the way up the mountain, you hit a southeast-trending ridge where there should be views of the coast, but thick, second-growth forest intervenes. However, you traverse this minor ridge until you finally reach the road on the ridgetop, the Butano Ridge Trail Loop.

This road follows the park boundary except for one Pescadero Creek County Park piece that extends downhill to the south. There may be a sunny spot along the ridge where a fallen log provides a resting place, although no picnic sites appear. The wide road continues in rollercoaster fashion for more than 2 miles until a gate bars further travel. Look on the left here for the Butano Ridge Trail Loop, which angles sharply uphill. When this trail levels off, you trend left (northeast) and contour under tall redwoods and Douglas firs until you reach a massive sandstone wall, at least 30 feet high and 150 feet long.

Shortly beyond this exposed sandstone is the Basin Trail sign on your right. From here it is 5.5 miles to Big Basin Redwoods State Park and 21 miles to Waddell Creek. (See The Basin Trail to Big Basin Redwoods State Park, Portola Redwoods State Park, page 256). Another sign points you sharply left on the Butano Ridge Trail Loop. Now you begin a series of innumerable switchbacks that carry you rapidly downhill in a lovely evergreen forest.

At the next trail junction take the left fork, the Butano Ridge Trail Loop. The right fork, the Portola Trail (also called the Basin Trail) will reach the Old Haul Road about a mile farther east and across from the trail into Portola Redwoods State Park (see The Basin Trail to Big Basin Redwoods State Park in that park). Continuing on the Butano Ridge Trail Loop, you drop down into a damp little glade, then descend to a flatter area near the Old Haul Road. At the junction with this road are several wax myrtle trees that bear closely spaced, long, glossy, narrow leaves. At first glance these small trees could be mistaken for California bay trees, a much larger tree whose leaves have a distinctive, aromatic scent.

Now you turn left on the wide, graveled Old Haul Road and follow it uphill past Hooker Creek, the Snag Trail to the Tarwater Trail Camp on the right, and Rhododendron Creek on the left. When you see the sign for Keyston Creek, look for a small waterfall upstream in a shady ravine. Then just past Dark Gulch, you will see the other leg of the Butano Ridge Trail Loop on which you started your climb to the ridgetop. From here you retrace your steps to the Hoffman Creek Trailhead, winding up and down some small hills, past exposed, fractured shale road cuts and under the redwood canopy to the broad clearing before crossing the Hoffman Creek bridge at the Wurr Road parking area.

Portola Redwoods State Park

Portola Redwoods State Park's 3000 acres nestled at the base of Butano Ridge lie along the northeast side of Pescadero Creek on ridges bisected by Peters, Evans, Evergreen, and Slate creeks. Some of the largest redwoods in San Mateo County can be found in its shady canyons. The park adjoins San Mateo County's 8027-acre complex of Pescadero Creek, Memorial, and Sam McDonald county parks. On its northeast corner it abuts Long Ridge Open Space Preserve, which lies along the crest of the Santa Cruz Mountains amid thousands of acres of contiguous open space. The park offers miles of hiking trails through stately redwoods and mixed evergreen forests that tie in with these adjoining parks. Across the Old Haul Road the Portola and Basin trails in Pescadero Creek County Park wend their way south for 6.8 miles to Big Basin Redwoods Park

The first known European settler in this area, Christian Iverson, a former Pony Express rider, came here in the 1860s and built a small redwood cabin on a high bank above a meander of Pescadero Creek. Only a few timbers of this cabin—hard hit by the 1989 earthquake—remain, but you can view an excellent scale-model of the cabin, produced by one of the park's volunteers, in the park's visitor center.

After the Gold Rush, lumbermen came to this area seeking wood first to build and then rebuild San Francisco. They cut the giant redwoods along the streams and hillsides and made them into shingles and shakes, then hauled them by oxen teams over the Skyline ridge to the Embarcadero in present-day Palo Alto.

William Page, who lived in Searsville in present-day Woodside, developed a mill on Peters Creek which was later moved to Slate Creek, the latter within today's park boundaries. The road he built from old Mayfield in today's Palo Alto, Page Mill Road, is still in use on the east side of Skyline Boulevard. Beginning on the west side of the Skyline, the Old Page Mill Road Trail descends 2 miles through Skyline Ridge Open Space Preserve and may continue as a public trail to the Peters Creek Loop Trail in Portola Redwoods at a future date. This loop is about a mile upstream from the site of the original Page's Mill, now on private property.

In the early 20th century, San Francisco residents seeking quiet and relaxation in these magnificent forests established summer retreats here. John A. Hooper, a San

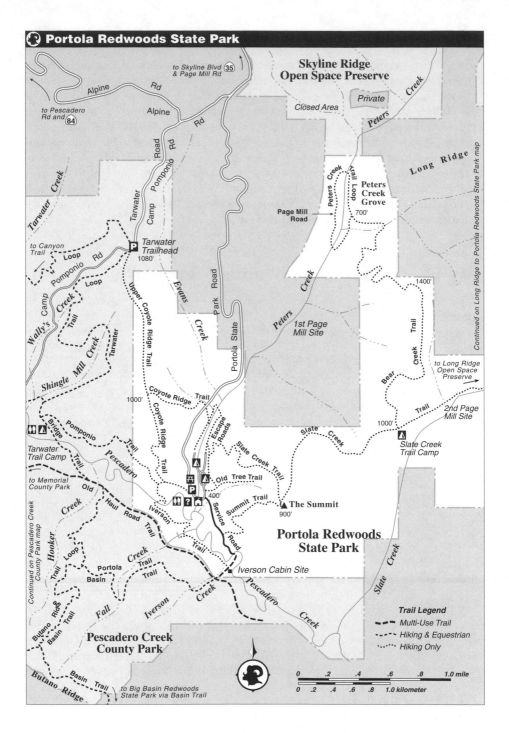

Portola Redwoods State Park

Skyline Ridge
Open Space Preserve

to Skyline Blvd
& Page Mill Rd (35)

Alpine   Rd

to Pescadero
Rd and (84)

Alpine   Rd

Closed Area   Private

Peters   Creek

Long   Ridge

Tarwater   Creek

Pomponio   Rd

Tarwater
Camp   Road

P Tarwater
Trailhead
1080'

Peters   Creek

Trail Loop

Peters
Creek
Grove

Page Mill
Road   700'

to Canyon
Trail

Pomponio   Rd
Loop
Loop

Wally's
Camp

Creek

Tarwater   Trail

Shingle Mill Creek

Upper Coyote Ridge Trail

Evans   Creek

Park Road

Portola State

1st Page
Mill Site

1400'

Bear   Creek   Trail

to Long Ridge
Open Space
Preserve

1000'

Coyote Ridge

Coyote Ridge   Trail

Trail

Escape
Roads

Slate Creek Trail

Slate   Creek

1000'

2nd Page
Mill Site

Slate Creek
Trail Camp

Pomponio
Ridge

Tarwater
Trail Camp

to Memorial
County Park

Old   Haul   Road

Iverson   Trail

Old

Pescadero   Creek

Trail

P
?

400'

Old
Tree Trail

Summit Trail

Service   Road

The Summit
900'

Portola Redwoods
State Park

Continued on Pescadero Creek
County Park map

Hooker   Trail

Portola
Basin

Loop   Trail

Creek

Iverson   Creek

Trail

Pescadero   Creek

Iverson Cabin Site

Fall   Creek   Trail

Butano Ridge   Basin   Trail

Basin   Trail

Trail Legend
— — Multi-Use Trail
- - - Hiking & Equestrian
······ Hiking Only

Slate   Creek

Pescadero Creek
County Park

Butano   Ridge

to Big Basin Redwoods
State Park via Basin Trail

0   .2   .4   .6   .8   1.0 mile
0   .2   .4   .6   .8   1.0 kilometer

Continued on Long Ridge to Portola Redwoods State Park map

Francisco banker who had moved to the former Mountain Home Ranch in present-day Woodside, built a large summer residence on Pescadero Creek. In 1924 a San Francisco Shrine group purchased 1600 acres in this area which were bought by the State of California in 1945. The Save-the-Redwoods League donated many acres in the last 50 years, swelling the present-day acreage to over 3000 acres. Today, hikers and campers drive the winding road to enjoy a dayhike or a picnic or to take a longer camping trip.

At the park office/visitor center are exhibits of the outstanding natural features of the park. Preserved specimens of many animals and samples of trees, flowers, and shrubs are displayed in life-like settings.

Trails starting from the park office offer trips of one to 13 miles, some on short nature trails around Pescadero Creek, several on longer loop trips, and still other trails that connect to adjoining Pescadero Creek County Park, Long Ridge Open Space Preserve, and Big Basin Redwoods State Park. With the opening of the Basin Trail in 1995 and the Butano Fire Trail Extension, there is the opportunity for extensive backpacking trips between Portola Redwoods State Park and other state and regional parks in the area.

Spring, summer, and fall are the best times for hiking, picnicking, and camping. The many campsites for families, groups, and backpackers willing to walk to trail camps are very popular during summer, especially on weekends. The campsites fill by reservations on all weekends between Memorial and Labor Day.

Dayhikers will find parking at pleasant picnic areas near the park office convenient to all the trailheads. Those who stay in the campsites can get an early start on long hikes to the outer edges of the park and on to neighboring parks. All trips in this park are described from the park office/visitor center at the creek level (400') and most go uphill from there. Following are seven trips of different length and difficulty to suit varying interests and abilities.

Jurisdiction: State of California, Department of Parks and Recreation: 650-948-9098; reservations: 800-444-7275; reservations for Slate Creek Trail Camp: 831-338-8861.

Facilities: Trails for hikers; visitor center; amphitheater; camping for families, groups, and backpackers; picnic areas with barbecues, restrooms; fee for parking and camping

Rules: Hikers only on trails; bicycles allowed on Old Haul Road Trail in adjacent Pescadero Creek County Park; no dogs on trails; dogs on leash in camp and picnic areas; fishing prohibited in order to protect native steelhead trout population

Maps: Portola Redwoods State Park brochure, USGS topos *Mindego Hill* and *Big Basin*

How to Get There: From Hwy 35 (Skyline Blvd) west of Palo Alto, take Alpine Rd. south for 3.1 miles to left turnoff onto Portola State Park Rd. Continue 3.4 miles to park office in visitor center, then proceed to parking areas nearby.

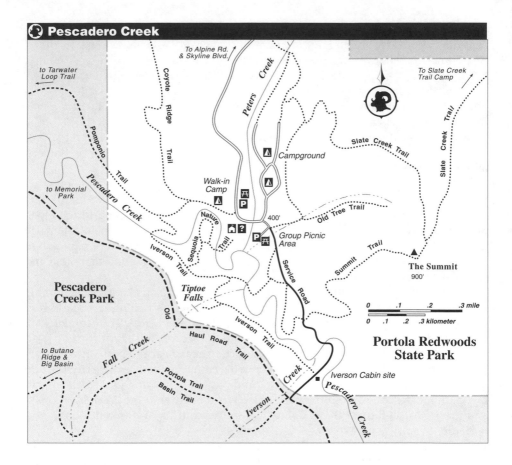

Pescadero Creek

To Alpine Rd. & Skyline Blvd.

to Tarwater Loop Trail

Coyote Ridge Trail

Peters Creek

To Slate Creek Trail Camp

Pomponio Trail

Slate Creek Trail

Slate Creek Trail

Campground

Pescadero Creek

to Memorial Park

Walk-in Camp

Old Tree Trail

400'

Nature Trail

Group Picnic Area

Summit Trail

The Summit 900'

Pescadero Creek Park

Sequoia Trail

Iverson Trail

Tiptoe Falls

Service Road

0   .1   .2   .3 mile
0 .1 .2 .3 kilometer

Portola Redwoods State Park

Old Haul Road Trail

Fall Creek

to Butano Ridge & Big Basin

Iverson Trail

Iverson Creek

Iverson Cabin site

Pescadero Creek

Portola Trail

Basin Trail

Iverson Creek

SEE MAP ABOVE

EXPLORING ALONG PESCADERO CREEK

Meander down to the creek through tunnels of huckleberry bushes on Sequoia and Iverson trails.

Distance: Sequoia Trail, 0.75-mile loop; Iverson Trail, 3-mile loop

Time: Sequoia Trail: ¾ hour; Iverson Trail: 1½ hours

Elevation Change: 90' loss

The Sequoia Trail, a must for understanding redwood-forest ecology, is well-described in the park brochure and is available at the park office for a small price. After you have wandered along this fascinating route and learned about the soil, root system, and effects of fire on these magnificent trees, try your newfound knowledge on the Iverson Trail. It begins just a few yards north of the park office opposite the Madrone picnic area. Turn left (northwest) onto the trail and walk between tall huckleberry shrubs under red-barked madrone, mossy-trunked Douglas fir, and good-sized redwoods to a fenced overlook of Pescadero Creek. At least 75 feet below the steep canyon wall the creek flows along its bed carved over the centuries into sandstone uplifted from under the Pacific Ocean. You follow the Iverson Trail left at two junctions, the first where the Coyote Ridge Trail goes right and the next where the Pomponio Trail also goes right.

Continuing downhill, sometimes descending steps braced by redwood planks, you go beside moss-covered logs edging the trail and arrive at creek level. In summer a fine, portable aluminum bridge makes its crossing easy. In winter all these bridges are removed, and the creek can be treacherously swift and full.

On the other side of the creek you bear left and rise through the forest, past a swampy area of serrated edged grasses, to a junction with the Sequoia Trail in a high huckleberry hollow. Proceeding straight ahead on the Iverson Trail, you climb switchbacks through redwoods of all ages, some burned but still living, others with hollow cavities in their trunks, to two lookouts over Pescadero Creek. Through openings framed by alders, firs, and tanbark oaks, you see and hear the creek far below.

At the next junction you can go left on an unnamed trail to cross Pescadero Creek and return to the park office. However, if you go 0.15 mile straight ahead, you cross Fall Creek on a little bridge and then go right on the well-marked trail to reach Tiptoe Falls.

Here this lively creek drops over a corrugated shelf of shale or sandstone into a lovely little pool in a basin flanked on two sides by high rock walls clothed with overhanging ferns, shrubs, and trees. Upstream in a narrow canyon the creek splashes over a jumble of fallen logs, visible but inaccessible.

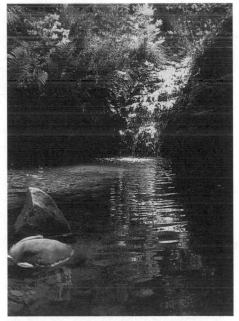

Leaving this cool canyon, return to the main trail by going to your right up a bank and through a grove of widely spaced, second growth redwoods. Heavy winter storms took out a section of this trail; watch for signs that direct you up to the Old Haul Road and follow it to your left (east). In less than 100 yards, you find the Iverson Trail on your left, take it and continue past a group of ancient stumps with notches cut for inserting the springboards on which early loggers balanced to fell these huge trees.

Shortly the Iverson Trail crosses a bridge over Iverson Creek and goes uphill to the park service road. Step out onto this road and turn left (north) to

Tiptoe Falls, Portola Redwoods State Park

see, beside the trail, a few timbers remaining upright from Christian Iverson's 1860s cabin.

To return to the park office, bear left on the trail just beside a road barricade, descend along the east bank of Pescadero Creek, and then cross it on the service road bridge. From here you can follow the paved road back to the park office, stopping at a fenced overlook to gaze again at the creek flowing below its high northeast canyon wall.

Alternatively, you can follow the foot trail described in reverse in the following trip, the Summit and Slate Creek Trails Loop. The trail junctions are marked along the service road.

SUMMIT AND SLATE CREEK TRAILS LOOP

SEE MAP ON PAGE 244

Climb out of the canyon through mixed evergreen and oak/madrone forests to experience fine views of Butano Ridge to the southwest.

Distance: 2.5-mile loop; add 1.2 miles for side trip to the Old Tree

Time: 1½ hours; add 30 minutes for side trip

Elevation Change: 550′ gain

From the park office turn right on the entrance road, cross the bridge over Peters Creek, and turn right again. Just past the amphitheater the road becomes a service road for park vehicles only. Look on your right here for a trail that leads to Tiptoe Falls. On it you immediately step into an understory of shiny-leaved huckleberry bushes with long, pliant branches that grow under tall, second-growth redwoods. After 0.3 mile go left on a short trail back to the park service road and continue on it to an opening overlooking Pescadero Creek flowing 200 feet below in a sheer-sided canyon. Just beyond the overlook, reenter the forest on a trail where more huckleberries are interspersed with graceful fern fronds, long-leaved iris, and climbing honeysuckle. On a series of small ups and downs you pass several double-trunked redwoods and one huge virgin redwood. When the trail again hits the service road, cross it and take the Summit Trail.

Shortly you come upon two water tanks, then switchback uphill past several redwoods scarred by fire, yet still living. As you gain elevation, there are tan oak, live oak, and madrone, some Douglas fir, and fewer redwood trees. Heading steadily upward you contour below a ridge and then hike atop a narrow, knife-edge ridge where cream-colored clusters of Fremont lilies blossom in spring, and pink wild roses bloom on small-leaved, thorny bushes in summer. Then, as the trail curves east, you see south over a patch of chaparral—toyon, manzanita, chamise, and honeysuckle—to densely-forested Butano Ridge. Here is a good rest stop, just a few feet from the summit at 950 feet.

From here you descend through redwoods to the junction of the Summit and Slate Creek trails. You could go northeast 1.3 miles on the Slate Creek Trail to the backpackers camp, the "Slate Creek Trail Camp," continue another 0.5 mile to

Page's Mill Site, and forge uphill 2.5 miles more to the boundary of Long Ridge Open Space Preserve. However, to take the return leg of this loop trip, turn due north on the Slate Creek Trail.

Now traversing a west-facing ridge, you nip back into the heads of ravines, round bends, and get deeper into redwood forest. The Save-the-Redwoods League and the Sempervirens Fund long ago initiated a program through which donors can honor friends and family by dedicating a tree or a grove of trees. Here in Portola Redwoods State Park, you will pass several of these groves, preserved for all of us to enjoy. Money from these dedications goes to purchase more redwood acreage for the state park system.

When you reach a trail junction sign that points right, 0.3 mile to the campground, stay left (heading due south), contouring along a narrow trail with mossy banks. Stay on this ridge through the redwoods for 0.5 mile. Here some recently fallen trees remain as seats beside the trail. At the next junction you can take the Old Tree Trail left (east) for a 0.5-mile round trip into a quiet canyon to see a grand old redwood giant, at least 12 feet in diameter, surrounded by a split-rail fence to preserve its fragile root system.

If you choose the Old Tree side trip, return to the Slate Creek Trail junction, continue straight ahead to the service road and go to your right on it to the park office. If you don't take the trip to the Old Tree, bear right (west) at the Old Tree Trail junction and go less than 0.2 mile to the park service road and then right to the park office.

COYOTE RIDGE LOOP TRAIL AND UPPER COYOTE RIDGE TRAIL

You may not see coyotes, but these high grasslands are favorite hunting sites.

Distance: 2.2 miles—Loop Trail, plus 4 miles round trip—Upper Coyote Ridge Trail

Time: 3 hours

Elevation Change: 630′ gain

Starting from the park office, go left on the entrance road for about 30 feet, turn left on the Iverson Trail, and in 0.1 mile turn right onto the Coyote Ridge Loop Trail. Shortly you cross a paved road leading to the walk-in campsites and switchback uphill through oak- and bay-tree forest. As you climb, note the burnt trunks of still-living trees, and several redwoods that have developed double trunks, probably due to repeated stress from fires. Researchers now know that forests benefit from fire, since burning the undergrowth reduces competition so seedlings can flourish. It is also known that fire helps some seeds to sprout.

Shortly you reach a low ridge where a large fallen tree in a small clearing makes a pleasant place for a rest or early lunch. This would be a good short destination for a children's hike. In spring there are violets and trillium blooming, wind whispering in the trees, and the scent of blossoming madrones.

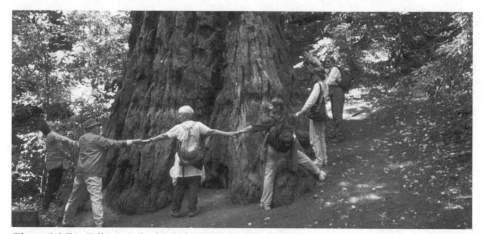

Eleven Walkie Talkies circle the Old Tree in Portola Redwoods State Park

Climbing steadily, you reach the junction of the two Coyote Ridge trails (elevation 960 feet), where you turn left onto the Upper Coyote Ridge Trail. This trip description will follow the Upper Coyote Ridge Trail, return to this junction and then descend on the other leg of the Coyote Ridge Loop Trail. If you eschew this 4-mile round trip, bear right and begin your descent to the park office following directions found later in this trip.

Bear left on the Upper Coyote Ridge Trail under large madrone trees, whose big, shiny-green leaves, orange-red berries, and rich, red-brown trunks add color to hillside trails. In a series of gentle ups and downs you traverse a long north-trending ridge, first on its west side, then on the east. From openings in the forest there are views of Butano Ridge southwest and of Towne Ridge north in Pescadero County Park. In summer, fog hangs over the beach beyond coastal ridges, sometimes enveloping not only this park but the entire western half of San Mateo County.

When the trail shifts to the east side of the ridgetop, you are in the hushed shade of great redwood, Douglas fir, and bay trees. Near the boundary with Pescadero Creek County Park, look for a row of mossy green posts and a wire fence going east past two large bearing trees. "Bearing tree" is a surveyor's term meaning a point that could be seen when determining property lines. On one tree with a sign showing land-survey numbers, the tree's bark has grown around the fence wire, embedding it at least ten inches.

Now you walk along an open hillside above grasslands that drop into the Evans Creek Canyon. East across this canyon the Portola Park Road meanders along the ridge between Evans and Peters creeks. Beyond lie the high ridges forming the crest of the Santa Cruz Mountains. Continuing on this trail, you soon dip into oak woods and shortly arrive at a clearing where there is a small dirt parking lot on Camp Pomponio Road (gated downhill from here to the San Mateo County Jail), and the end of this trail.

You can rest in sun or shade here and then retrace your steps on the Upper Coyote Ridge Trail. As you step onto this trail, note on a nearby signpost that the Tarwater Trail Loop (see the following trip) also reaches this parking area.

Returning to the Coyote Ridge Trail junction, look for the shade-loving maroon trillium in spring or the magenta masses of sun-loving clarkia in late spring and summer. At any season you can see graceful woodland grasses swaying in the breeze. When you reach the junction, angle sharply left and start your steep descent via numerous switchbacks. Along the way there is a charming little meadow ablaze with yellow, cream, pink, and blue wildflowers, still blooming when the authors visited here one August. Beyond, climb three steps cut into a tree fallen across the trail and then, in a deep ravine, cross a plank bridge over a little creek that splashes into a pool about 20 feet left of the trail. Abruptly you drop down to the main park road, cross it, descend wooden steps to a bridge over Evans Creek and shortly cross the longer Peters Creek bridge with chain-link fenced sides. With the sounds of rushing water filling the air, you reach the junction with the Slate Creek Trail (east) and the Upper Escape Road. Turn right (south) on the Upper Escape Road through a fine redwood grove and follow the fairly level road back to the campground and on to the park office.

SEE MAP
ON PAGE
244

TARWATER TRAIL LOOP

Through forests and meadows a two-park sampler reaches a deserted barn and the source of the trail's name.

Distance: 5 miles

Time: 3 hours

Elevation Change: 630' gain

Although most of this trip is in Pescadero Creek County Park, beginning in Portola Redwoods State Park makes it possible to start uphill and end going down. Therefore, go a few steps north beyond the park office and take the Iverson Trail, which is just across the park entrance road from the Madrone picnic area. Follow the Iverson Trail past the first junction, where the Coyote Ridge Trail turns right. You continue on the Iverson Trail for 0.12 mile to the next junction, where you go straight onto the Pomponio Trail and the Iverson Trail goes left. Signs here read PESCADERO COUNTY PARK 0.5 MILES, MCDONALD COUNTY PARK 4.0 MILES and MEMORIAL PARK 7.0 MILES. Signs also warn that the trail, which is narrow and has some steps, is unsafe for and closed to horses.

Shortly the Pomponio Trail widens and becomes an unpaved road as you enter Pescadero Creek County Park. Climbing gradually through Douglas firs, oaks, madrones, and redwoods, you reach a big crossroads and another sign: left, on the Bridge Trail to the Old Haul Road Trail, among others, and right, continuing on the Pomponio Trail 0.1 mile to the Tarwater Trail Loop, which you take.

As you follow the wide Pomponio Trail, watch on your right for a small sign that marks the beginning of the narrow Tarwater Trail Loop. Step onto this hikers-only trail and into a dark grove of second-growth redwood trees. Ferns and moss-covered rocks line the trail and Shingle Mill Creek courses through and around the grove. This area, easily accessible to logging through the 1960s and early '70s, has regrown tall and dense since then. Huge stumps encircled by new growth attest to the size and tenacity of the ancient trees.

Now on an unpaved road, you swing west, cross Shingle Mill Creek enclosed in a culvert, and ascend past scattered woods and meadows. As you turn north, the banks on the right side of the road are chalky limestone, characteristic of many soils on the west side of Skyline. Still gaining elevation on this road, you come upon a tremendous old redwood perched at the top of the steep hillside on the left. At least 12 feet in diameter with a burned-out heart and two huge elbow-shaped limbs high above the ground, this ancient monarch is worth watching for.

After crossing the deep ravine of Wally's Creek, you might pause at a high, grassy meadow on the left which is bordered on the north by a fence and woods of oak and Douglas fir. Probably used as pastureland before the park acquisition, this meadow is now a good place for a picnic and offers views across the deep canyon of Pescadero Creek and its many tributaries to the wooded heights of Butano Ridge in the southwest. In meadows and clearings such as this, listen for birds singing and bees buzzing, and watch for dragonflies and colorful butterflies. Here too, you will find lovely spring wildflowers, and if you are very quiet, you may see deer browsing or rabbits scurrying into the brush.

Continuing along the trail, you soon reach a gate at the parking area on Camp Pomponio Road where this leg of the Tarwater Trail Loop and the Upper Coyote Ridge Trail converge. Looking north from here, about 3 miles as the crow flies, you can see the rounded south side of 2143-foot Mindego Hill, creased by a big canyon and fringed with trees on its lower slopes.

To continue the loop, cross the road and take the signed Tarwater Trail Loop northwest about 1.25 mile through open grassland to a sharp turn left, then meander along a narrower trail into a pretty oak/bay woodland. Emerging from the woods you follow the east edge of a long meadow, then cut across it to skirt the forest above a branch of Tarwater Creek. As you walk under the trees, continue around a huge, lone redwood and look for a side trail cutting over to a small building with corrugated tin roof under a cluster of tall eucalyptus trees, known as Tie Camp. Just a few steps lead you to it and a peek at the thick redwood sides and floors of this long-deserted dwelling, later used as a barn. The fence across the lower end of this meadow and bailing wire scattered about recall the days when a dairy farmer rented the site, kept goats and cows in the meadow, and transported milk and cheese out of the canyon to local customers.

This barn is all that remains of an extensive layout for the Moore, Fisher, and Troupe mill operation that cut redwood trees into railroad ties here in 1915–16. Some present-day residents of this area remember that descendants of the mill operators later came here for holidays in the new-growth redwoods. After exploring the exterior of this deserted site (not safe to enter it), get back on the main trail and contour around the barn's south side into a little swale where an early settler planted a double row of pear trees, now quite aged, and then switchback downhill into the shade of big redwoods.

The trail zigzags downhill through the redwoods past a horsetail-fringed wallow dug up and rooted in by wild pigs. Although these big creatures, descended from European pigs brought here for sport hunting, may not be in sight, respect them for their long teeth and unpredictable nature. At its junction with the Canyon Trail the narrow Tarwater Trail Loop widens, and you bear left (south) to continue this trip. However, if you go right (north) a short distance on the Canyon Trail, you will cross the main trunk of Tarwater Creek and discover the meaning of its name. Observe its surface for globs of thick, shiny, iridescent material. Clue: San Mateo County once had an exploratory lease with a petroleum company just southwest of here.

Now following the wide Tarwater Trail Loop, make a gentle rise and continue south about one mile through sizable redwoods above the east side of Tarwater Creek. Huckleberries, iris, and ferns line the trail's edge in these quiet woods. At the next junction, go through a gate in a split-log rail fence onto Camp Pomponio Road and turn left following the road (also the Pomponio Trail here) for about 200 feet. Then veer off right onto the narrow Pomponio/Tarwater Trail Loop. With another gate on your left, go right onto an unpaved road, still the Pomponio/Tarwater Trail Loop, in a small clearing bordered by high ceanothus. Just watch the signs and remember to go generally east.

Soon you cross Wally's Creek, then Shingle Mill Creek, and note on your left the other leg of the Tarwater Trail Loop, on which you started several hours before. You now retrace your steps on the Pomponio Trail by going left on it at the Bridge Trail junction. As you wind through the forest of bay trees and redwoods, your path is littered with fallen leaves and branchlets. Soon the sign for Portola Redwoods park office assures you that it is 0.5 mile to the end of a very beautiful hike.

PETERS CREEK LOOP

A full day's trip to Old Page Mill Road and spectacular redwoods spared in old logging days.

Distance: 13+ miles round trip

Time: 8 or 9 hours

Elevation Change: 1000' gain

Start this trip early in the day, take plenty of water and food, and allow ample time to negotiate the steep climb out of Peters Creek on the return leg. You could spend the night at Slate Creek Trail Camp, 3 miles from the park office and do the 7-mile loop up and down to Peters Creek on the second day. Reserve the campsites by calling 831-338-8861.

To begin this trip, take the Summit Trail, as in the Summit and Slate Creeks Trails Loop, to its junction with the Slate Creek Trail. From this junction at 940 feet, go right (northeast) along an east-facing ridge under a high forest canopy of redwoods, Douglas firs, and occasional oaks growing in more open zones. In many places the huckleberries form high walls on either side of the trail, making it seem

as if you were going through a leafy, green canyon. Gently gaining a little elevation, you swing around to the north-facing slope and in 1.3 miles you reach Slate
Creek Trail Camp. Here six separate campsites with picnic tables screened by low
native shrubs sit under high madrones and tan oaks. If there is a free campsite, this
is a good place for an early lunch or snack before beginning the next uphill leg of
your trip.

When you've explored a bit and are ready to start off, return to the junction
where the Bear Creek Trail takes off north, and begin the 7-mile round trip to Peters
Creek. The trail is an old jeep road that climbs around a west-facing knoll, swings
east, and then north up a steep canyon above an intermittent creek, a tributary of
Slate Creek. In a few places you must climb over fallen trees or go around big boulders, not serious obstacles on your steadily upward trek. Under redwoods at first,
you eventually rise to more open country where firs, oaks, and bays thrive and the
old road ends at about the 1380-foot level.

From this point a narrow trail leaves the damp canyon and enters a high wooded bowl. You meander close to private property—stay on the trail through this
area. Under tall Douglas firs and a dense tangle of berry vines, veer a bit west, and
emerge in chaparral made up of hardy manzanita, chinquapin, and some knobcone
pines. These pines, which need fire to germinate their seeds, corroborate the
authors' impression that fire must have cleared the old forest here. You are now at
the highest point of your trip, about 1440 feet. From this chaparral area you can
briefly look northwest to the ridge that Alpine Road traverses, the route you took
to get to Portola Redwoods State Park.

Soon you traverse a forest of spindly Douglas firs, possibly the site of an old
lumber camp (as evidenced by an old, tilted wooden privy) and proceed up and

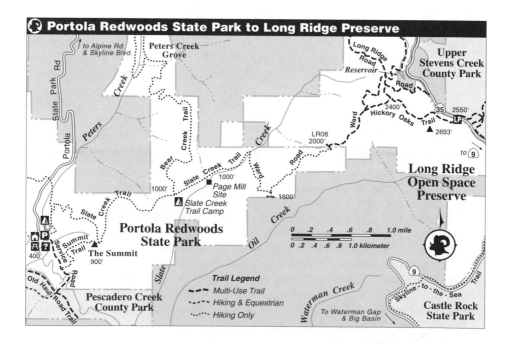

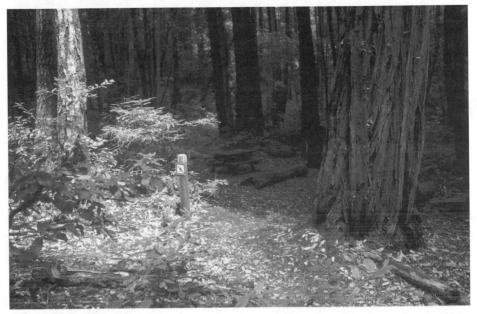

Slate Creek Trail Camp

down a southwest-facing ridge to an opening high on its north side. Here are a few brief views of the Peters Creek Canyon, upstream from your intended destination.

Now you begin the downhill leg of your trip on a foot trail that can be slippery if the litterfall is damp or the soil muddy. On foggy days the air is fragrant with bay leaves crushed underfoot, and moisture drips from trees overhead. Steadily downward you go, zigzagging into and around ravines on a west-facing slope. Small cones of Douglas firs and acorns from tan oaks and live oaks litter the trail. After you cross a little plank bridge over Bear Creek, you make a sharp turn left (west), traversing a side slope above the creek thickly covered with fern fronds, redwood sorrel and trailing yerba buena.

Soon you are in the depths of a magnificent redwood grove at the confluence of Bear and Peters creeks. Here is a magical place of monarch redwoods, pervaded by a hushed silence broken only by the sounds of the creek slapping against rocks and tree roots, and tumbling over fallen logs and boulders. You can rock-hop the creek and make a loop around the grove to see more trees and the signs that honor families and organizations from whom donated funds purchased this land and preserved the trees. Then choose a fallen log on which to sit and contemplate why these trees, many at least 12 feet in diameter, are still standing. Perhaps it was too steep to haul the cut lumber or shingles out of here. Maybe the woodcutters saw flaws unperceived by today's hikers. Perhaps they were just tired of sawing these giant trunks by hand. Regardless, they are worth the trip to behold.

On your return you will be climbing the steepest part first—an elevation gain of 760 feet in about a mile. After you reach the trip's high point, it is almost all downhill. Allow plenty of time to enjoy the trees, flowers, ridges, and canyons.

UPHILL TO LONG RIDGE
OPEN SPACE PRESERVE

This trip is described in the Long Ridge section as a 7-mile, downhill-all-the-way excursion with car shuttle (Downhill to Portola Redwoods State Park). When the Old Page Mill Road is opened as a trail all the way to the Peters Creek Loop in Portola Redwoods State Park, this trip could be combined with the previous trip, Peters Creek Loop, for an approximately 16-mile loop trip with an overnight at Slate Creek Trail Camp. As of this writing, about 2 miles of Old Page Mill Road are open.

THE BASIN TRAIL TO BIG BASIN
REDWOODS STATE PARK

A surfeit of switchbacks up Butano Ridge leads to an easement trail through private land and thence to Big Basin Redwoods State Park.

Distance: 6.8 miles

Time: 5 hours

Elevation Change: 1917' gain

Although this trip for hikers and equestrians begins in Portola Redwoods State Park, the first half is mostly in Pescadero Creek County Park. However, starting from one of the Pescadero Park trailheads would add 3 to 6 miles to your trip. So, this trip description starts from the Portola Redwoods park office. Follow the service road to the right (east) and either take the foot trails described in Summit and Slate Creek Trails Loop or the service road past the Summit Trail turnoff. Continue past the park maintenance area, cross Pescadero Creek and proceed on an elevated bank above a tight meander of the creek beyond the old Iverson Cabin site. Just 50 feet farther you enter Pescadero Creek County Park at the Old Haul Road. On the other side of this road/trail, pick up the Basin Trail (also called the Portola Trail) heading uphill under alders, toyons, and oaks. At first paralleling Iverson Creek, you then cross it and contour through a pretty dell under some second-growth redwoods enlivened in late summer by orange redwood lilies and yellow mimulus.

Following the east side of Fall Creek you climb steadily and then cross it in an opening in the forest. Just before the creek crossing is a lively little waterfall and farther upstream a cascade rippling over mossy rocks. Look here for blue-flowered iris and white-blossomed, fragrant azalea in spring. Around more zigzags and out on a few knolls you continue upward through redwood and Douglas fir forest.

At a fork in the trail, go left on the Butano Ridge Loop Trail; the other fork heads north to Old Haul Road. Now seriously climbing, you gain altitude at every switchback as you round shoulders of the ridge, go between great redwoods, and pass burned shells of monarch trees. You will find small caves in great sandstone

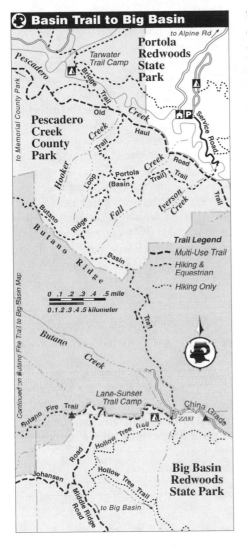

boulders worn away by wind, rain, and chemical action. Look for trees growing out of the rock and other rocks that have broken loose and tumbled down the hillside.

Occasional madrone or tan oak trees have sprung up in gaps where old or diseased trees have fallen. But in general, this is a very shady redwood/fir forest, cool in summer, and exposed to ocean winds and fogs that condense on tree branches and fall on the ground (and on hapless hikers). This environment is just right for white milkmaids, creamy-white and maroon trillium in spring, pretty little bluebells in summer, and the predominant, evergreen huckleberry shrub.

At one of the numerous switchbacks look for a deep ditch that loggers once used to haul logs up the mountain on a cable attached to trees at top and bottom of the ridge. Near this ditch are cut ends of two large trees that were buried when the ditch was dug some 60 or 70 years ago.

At the Basin Trail/Butano Ridge Loop Trail junction, the Basin Trail goes left 5.5 miles to Big Basin Redwoods State Park, while the Butano Ridge Loop Trail veers right, trending northwest to the ridgetop. This trail follows the unpaved Butano Ridge Road, and eventually descends to the Old Haul Road on a west segment of this trail. (See the Butano Ridge Trail Loop in Pescadero Creek County Park).

However, following the Basin Trail you turn left (southeast), round the nose of a ridge, and contour 0.8 mile through scattered redwoods and Douglas firs to a small clearing, the Scenic Overlook, a good place for lunch with a view. If the day is fair, many high points along the Skyline ridge are visible—Mt. Melville in Russian Ridge Open Space Preserve, Lambert and Peters creek canyons, which feed into Pescadero Creek, and the high grasslands in Long Ridge Open Space Preserve. Bring binoculars to identify other features of the southern Peninsula.

The next leg, about 2 miles, ambles along the ridgetop, gaining about 300 feet in elevation before reaching China Grade Road in Big Basin Redwoods State Park. After reaching the boundary of Pescadero Creek County Park, just 0.2 mile from the overlook, this segment of the Basin Trail goes through the private Redtree

Properties L.P., formerly the Santa Cruz Lumber Company, which granted an easement to Sempervirens for a 15-foot-wide hiking and equestrian trail. No bicycles
are allowed. Logging roads intersecting the trail are blocked off, but are used to
haul logs during the regular harvesting season, which follows a 16- to 20-year sus-
tained-yield cycle. Sempervirens Fund, the oldest land-conservancy organization
in California, negotiated the arrangements for this important connector.

Volunteers from the Santa Cruz Mountains Trail Association under the direction
of Tony Look, first executive director of Sempervirens Fund, and Robert Kirsch
built this section of trail; volunteers patrol and maintain the trail. It undulates up
and down along a ridgetop under Douglas firs and redwoods on a carpet of leaves.
At a few points you can look east to other lands of the State Park system on
Highway 9, which descends from the Skyline ridge—Big Basin and Castle Rock.

As you approach Big Basin Redwoods, watch the signs for the China Grade
Road trailhead and the boundary of the park. You can have a shuttle car waiting
for you here, or if you carry gear in your backpack, you can stay in nearby
Lane-Sunset Trail Camp by making advance reservations with Big Basin
Redwoods State Park trail camp office, 831-338-8861. For a mostly downhill trip,
you can take this trail in reverse by starting at the Basin Trail/China Grade Road
junction.

Butano State Park

Not the smallest or the largest of state parks, nor the most isolated, 3500-acre
Butano State Park nevertheless has a special quality of solitude, and after short
acquaintance one can get a feel for the whole park as a unit, despite its diverse
habitats. Centered around the valley of Little Butano Creek, with riparian habitat
along its banks, the slopes of the park rise gently on three sides, enclosing the park
between ridges that form the watershed of this pretty stream.

Butano (the preferred pronunciation is "Boo-" with the accent on the first sylla-
ble) was first visited by Native Americans, who fished the stream, burned the
underbrush to create open hunting and gathering grounds, and were supplanted
by more aggressive people of European descent. By the 1860s the Jackson family
had settled on the northern or Jackson Flats side of the canyon, and the Taylor and
Mullen families had settled on the southern, or Goat Hill, side. Together with
Purdy Pharis, who also logged the El Corte de Madera and Purisima areas, the settlers logged the redwood forest in the canyon bottom until about 1900, taking all
but a few of the forest giants. In the 1940s logging of giant Douglas firs took place,
as testified to by some remaining stumps. Count the rings on younger fallen firs—
you will find they are about 50 years old.

By the early part of the 20th century Timothy Hopkins, son of Mark Hopkins of
"Big Four" fame, owned most of the Butano and Little Butano Creek watersheds.
He left this property to Stanford University, and in the 1950s much of the area was
sold to private parties. An active preservation effort resulted in the State of
California purchase of the Little Butano Creek valley for a state park. In 1961 Butano
State Park became part of the state park system.

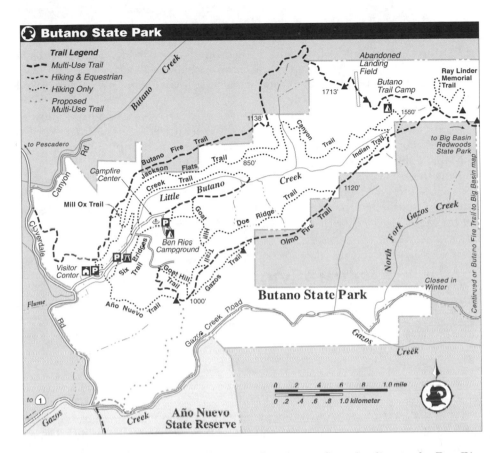

A paved road runs about a mile along the canyon floor, leading to the Ben Ries Campground (named after the park's first ranger, killed in an accident), and this road continues unpaved for service vehicles and hikers only, for another mile into the canyon. All the other trails in the park are narrow, for hikers only. Surrounding the park on the tops of the ridges are two fire roads: Butano Fire Road on the north, leads past an abandoned airstrip and turns east through the most recently acquired part of the park, Butano Crossing. The other fire road is Olmo Fire Road, running along the south ridge between Little Butano Creek and Gazos Creek drainages. Both these roads go through sections of private property.

A proposed trail connection, for hikers and equestrians only, would run between Butano and Big Basin Redwoods state parks beyond Butano Crossing on an easement through private lands along the existing Butano Fire Trail. Another proposed trail may be in the making at this writing—the ever-industrious Trail Center volunteers have it on their list for summer work parties.

Sempervirens Fund, a private land-conservancy that has acquired much of the land for Big Basin and Castle Rock state parks, recently bought a one-half interest in 1800 acres in the upper Gazos Creek drainage south of Butano State Park. State parks purchased a sizeable piece of this in 2004.

Jurisdiction: State of California Department of Parks and Recreation: 650-879-2040

Facilities: Thirty miles of trails for hikers; campground with 39 campsites—21 drive-in and 18 walk-in; picnic area; trail camp with 8 sites (backpackers must register at the park entrance or the visitor center and may camp only at designated sites); no drinking water available

Rules: Trails open dawn to dusk; no bicycles or horses; dogs on leash allowed in campground but not on trails; camping reservations advised from April 1 through Labor Day by calling 1-800-444-7275; day use and camping fees

Maps: California State Parks *Butano State Park*, USGS topo *Franklin Point*

How to Get There: Take Hwy 92 or Hwy 84 from I-280 to Hwy 1 on Coastside and turn south. At 4.6 miles south of Hwy 84 take Pescadero Rd. east for 2.6 miles, turn right (south) on Cloverdale Rd. and then go south 5 miles to park entrance on left (east).

SEE MAP ON PAGE 259

CIRCUMNAVIGATE THE PARK

Take the "high road" around the park, visiting all its habitats, on the Jackson Flats and Doe Ridge trails.

Distance: 10.3 miles

Time: 5 to 6 hours

Elevation Change: 1000' gain

From the entrance station parking lot take the Jackson Flats Trail heading north through second-growth Douglas fir and live oak trees following a gradual grade on the north side of the valley. After 10 minutes you enter second-growth redwood forest, and the trail widens to an old road paralleling the paved road below. In the open forest there are burned stumps, and the trail narrows to a single track.

Soon you pass a series of flat, swampy areas, probably the heads of large landslides. These wet areas are important winter breeding grounds for newts, where interesting marsh plants such as skunk cabbage and cattails flourish. Cross the Mill Ox Trail, which comes up from the valley floor on the right and joins the Butano Fire Road above.

After about 3 miles, at the junction where the Jackson Flats Trail veers left to join the Butano Fire Road, take the Canyon Trail to the right to circle around the head of the valley. Here at about 850 feet elevation, the vegetation changes significantly from the fir- and redwood-forest. You are now on the Santa Margarita Formation of shale and sandstone, which forms great banks of gravelly material on which grow knobcone pines, oaks, manzanita, and chinquapin. Notice also some California nutmegs, with sharp-tipped, shiny needles, a handsome small tree.

The Canyon Trail heads generally east, circling in and out of numerous small drainages. Some small redwood and fir trees are in the protected canyons, but the vegetation is mainly chaparral, with more nutmeg, manzanita, and possibly a canyon or a maul oak. Views are to the east and south, looking across Little Butano

Creek. This south-facing slope is sunny and hot. Working up and down this slope, you have gone just under 6 miles to reach an elevation of 1250 feet when you meet the junction with the Indian Trail. The Canyon Trail goes left to the trail camp, which is charmingly situated in a grove of second-growth redwoods and Douglas firs. It has 8 primitive campsites with rustic tables and stools, lovingly hand-crafted and maintained by volunteers from the Sierra Club Singleaires. There are pit toilets but no water, and campfires are not allowed. From this trail camp you can stroll on the nearby Ray Linder Nature Trail, which is 0.75 miles long.

Near the Canyon/Indian Trail junction is a footbridge across Little Butano Creek and a mossy sandstone seat, a convenient spot for lunch. The trickling stream is cooling on a hot day. This area, seldom visited by humans, has frequent animal visitors—look for bobcat or gray fox tracks in the dust. Here you are at the edge of chaparral, with plentiful tan oak and huckleberry.

After only half a mile the Indian Trail ends at the Olmo Fire Road, on which you also can reach the trail camp by a roundabout route. The fire road is wide on the ridge, with splendid views to the south, west, and north. Many bicycle tracks are on the road. After about a third mile you reach the Doe Ridge Trail on the right; no bikes are allowed. Here is an instant change of habitat. You are on the north-facing slope, in redwood- and fir-forest. This trail winds gently down and west to a junction with the Goat Hill Trail at 8.3 miles from the start of your trip.

Take the Goat Hill Trail right downhill to its junction with an unnamed trail leading to the Ben Ries Campground, and go left to the campground. There are 39 campsites in a nice open forest amid redwood trees and ferns. A nearby campfire center has benches facing a stage for interpretive programs. From the campground this trip continues west on a trail down an excessively steep grade to a side creek and a road leading to the ranger residences and the maintenance yard. Beyond this paved road the trail climbs up again just as steeply. Take heart, for you are nearing a different habitat at the end of your hike!

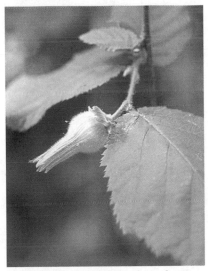

Passing the park office, you join the Six Bridges Trail. This last stretch is through riparian vegetation along Little Butano Creek and its north-flowing tributaries, and there actually are six bridges amid the willows, maples, alders, and herbaceous plants. This is sensitive habitat, so please stay on the trail. Note one huge fir tree that managed to survive the ax during earlier logging. This Six Bridges Trail would make a nice, easy stroll for a hot day.

At 10.3 miles from your start, you reach a junction with the Año Nuevo Trail going uphill to the left, and shortly thereafter, you are at the entrance station. Pause to look into the little visitor center here; it is maintained by a volunteer group, part of the San Mateo Coast Natural History Association.

Hazelnut blossom and velvety leaves

TO AN OVERLOOK
AND SOME UNUSUAL HABITATS

*Climb the south rim of the park for great views and
diverse vegetation.*

Distance: 3 miles

Time: 2½ hours

Elevation Change: 750′ gain

Park at the entrance station and take the Año Nuevo Trail on the south side, left
of the small nature center. Start out through riparian vegetation and cross Little
Butano Creek on a bridge, passing the Six Bridges Trail on your left. Climb uphill
through cow parsnip, thimbleberry, and wild cucumber spiraling around any nearby stem, and over tree roots through willows to reach a Douglas fir forest. In March
forget-me-nots are in bloom along the trail (not native plants but brought here by
European settlers) and red elderberry bushes are covered with white panicles of
bloom. Large horsetails, an ancient plant from the Cretaceous period, are evidence
that this trail has a number of springs to keep them moist year-round.

As you climb you can see through the trees all the way to the ocean, and long
clusters of lichen on tree branches indicate how often ocean fogs invade this
canyon. Rest on a handy bench to contemplate the view to the west. Here you see
some landforms that are rather puzzling at first glance. Little Butano Creek
emerges from its canyon and then turns sharply north before joining the main
Butano Creek; together they flow a bit farther north before going west to the ocean.
Parallel to Little Butano Creek is the intermittent stream, Arroyo de los Frijoles,
dammed into two little lakes for irrigation. A 400-foot-high ridge called the Mesa,
which apparently was formed by action of the San Gregorio Fault, blocks the direct
entrance of these streams into the ocean. Though low, this mesa tends to block
some of the summer fogs and strong ocean winds from reaching Butano State Park.
This ridge forms the centerpiece of a 5600-acre property under the management of
POST, some of which may become public open space linking Butano Park to the
Coast.

Continue on excellent, short switchbacks and then a last steady pull to reach the
Año Nuevo Overlook bench. This viewpoint is at 980 feet, and at one time commanded a bird's eye view of Año Nuevo Island to the south. The view now is somewhat obscured by growing forest, but there are many interesting things to look at
from this spot. You will have taken about 40 to 50 minutes to climb to this point.

As you rest, see how many of these plants you can identify from your seat on
the bench: live oak, Douglas fir, madrone, and tan oak trees; coffeeberry, huckleberry, and ceanothus bushes; poison oak, blackberry, and honeysuckle vines;
strawberry, sword fern, and Douglas iris plants.

Continue on the Año Nuevo Trail east along the ridge through a fir forest, with
hazelnut shrubs just leafing out in March. Stroke their leaves—they feel like velvet.
When you reach the Olmo Fire Road, you continue southeast along it to where the
road edges a shaley bank. In the spring elderberry bushes bloom in the valley and

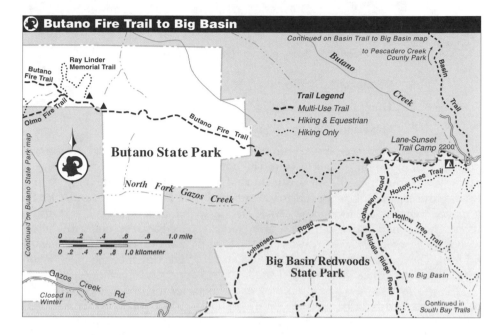

cream-colored zygadine lilies grow in the shade. Passing a trail to the right (not marked, and do not take it), you reach an intersection of the Goat Hill Trail Extension to the left and the Gazos Trail to the right. Go right (northeast) although the trail entrance is a little obscure, and travel on the Gazos Trail, paralleling the Olmo Fire Road but much above it. This is a sort of rollercoaster trail along the ridge, and has interesting views of the Coastside to the west and of the canyon of Gazos Creek to the south.

On the south slope of the ridge which the Gazos Trail follows is the same vegetation you saw in the previous trip (Circumnavigate the Park)—Santa Margarita shale formation broken into small chips growing knobcone pines, chamise, and bracken ferns, all adapted to hot, dry hillsides. Views east are of the forested Gazos Creek canyon.

When you reach the Olmo Fire Road and at the end of the Gazos Trail, take this road left (west) and downhill steeply through fir forest. Note one giant fir with an 8-foot-thick trunk and four large trunks diverging from it. In 0.5 mile take the Goat Hill Trail connection downhill to the right, and descend on its right-hand branch 0.9 mile to reach the maintenance road next to Little Butano Creek. From here you can either return along the trail discussed in the previous trip, a little over a mile, or take the Little Butano Creek Loop described in the next trip (Little Butano Creek Trail).

LITTLE BUTANO CREEK TRAIL

SEE MAP
ON PAGE
259

Stroll along the valley bottom through redwood forest.

Distance: 2.25 miles

Time: 1½ hours

Elevation Change: 30′ gain

As you go northeast from the entrance kiosk, watch across the park road for an old wooden flume on the north side. This was built early in the 20th century to carry water from a small dam upstream to irrigate fields in private lands farther west. From the end of the paved road leading to Ben Ries Campground take the unpaved maintenance road, now named the Little Butano Creek Trail, east up the creek. The original redwood forest was logged in the 1800s, but second-growth redwoods and even a few giants missed by the loggers make this a shady and beautiful trail. The road is surfaced with needles and it winds down to the creek where redwood sorrel grows in the deep shade.

On the way you pass a new building used for water treatment. At a small dam on the creek is a building used to pump water from the creek to this treatment building for campground and residence use. After crossing Little Butano Creek on a footbridge, the trail goes downstream on the north bank past large redwood stumps and small redwood trees. *Trillium ovatum* blooms in spring, a three-petaled white flower atop three spade-shaped leaves. You can also find *Clintonia andrewsiana* in spring, with its lovely rose-purple flowers brightening the shade. The trail crosses on small bridges back and forth over the creek several times. See if you can spot a strange, huge redwood burl near the junction of an unused trail just south of one of these crossings.

Soon on the north side of the creek, you reach a bench on which to rest while admiring the level area in this generally steep-sided canyon. Passing numerous side creeks bridged by boardwalks you reach a very boggy area where numerous yellow-flowered plants with huge leaves bloom in spring. This is yellow skunk cabbage, quite rare in California and known from only a few localities in the Santa Cruz Mountains growing in wet ground near perennial springs.

The trail crosses here to the south side of the creek, and 100 feet farther on reaches a paved road where there is a pullout for a few cars to park. Just ahead and downstream is the junction with the Mill Ox Trail, noted in the first trip (Circumnavigate the Park); you can avoid returning on the pavement by going up this very steep trail to the Jackson Flats Trail, then returning to the entrance station. The Mill Ox Trail has a tunnel tree in this segment which could easily accommodate child adventurers.

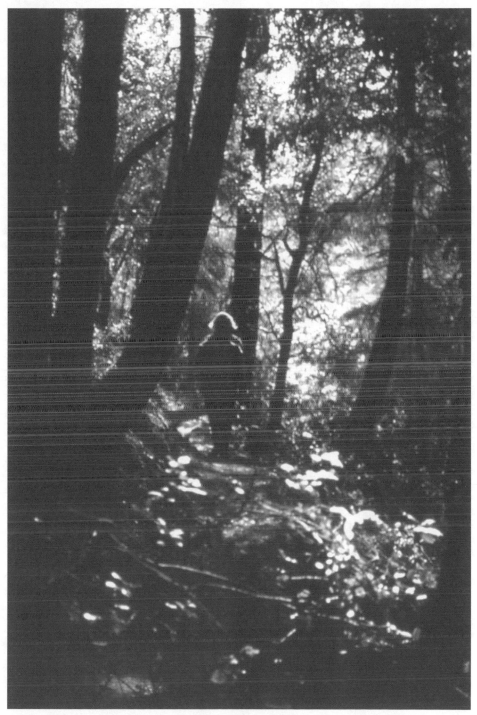

Author Betsy Crowder hiking in shady Butano State Park

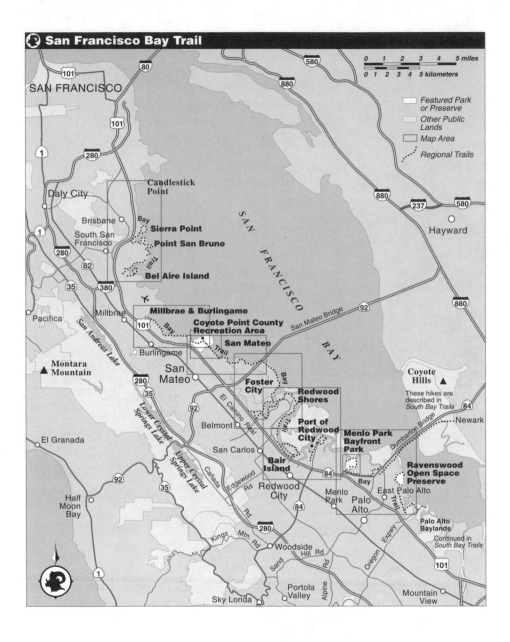

San Francisco Bay Trail

0 1 2 3 4   5 miles
0 1 2 3 4 5 kilometers

Featured Park
or Preserve
Other Public
Lands
Map Area
Regional Trails

80
101
SAN FRANCISCO
580
880

101

1
280

237
880
580
580

Candlestick
Point
Daly City
Hayward

Brisbane
Bay
Sierra Point
South San
Francisco
1
Point San Bruno

280
82
Trail
Bel Aire Island

35
380

S
A
N

F
R
A
N
C
I
S
C
O

880

Pacifica
Millbrae
Millbrae & Burlingame

San Andreas Lake
101
Bay
Coyote Point County
Recreation Area
San Mateo Bridge
92

Montara
Mountain
280
Burlingame
San Mateo
B
A
Y

Coyote
Hills
These hikes are
described in
South Bay Trails

35
San
Mateo
Foster
City

Redwood
Shores
84

Lower Crystal
Springs Lake
92

El Camino Real
Trail
Port of
Redwood
City
Menlo Park
Bayfront
Park
Dumbarton Bridge
Newark

El Granada
Belmont
Bay

Upper Crystal
Springs Lake
San Carlos
Bair
Island
84
Ravenswood
Open Space
Preserve

35
Cañada
Edgewood
Rd
Redwood
City
Menlo
Park
East Palo Alto
Trail

92
Half
Moon
Bay
84
Palo
Alto
Palo Alto
Baylands
Continued in
South Bay Trails

Kings
Mtn.
Rd
280
Woodside
Hill Rd
Oregon Expwy
101

Sand
Rd

1
Portola
Valley
Alpine
Mountain
View

Sky Londa

◆ San Francisco Bay Trail ◆

San Mateo County's trails by the Bay are as varied as its convoluted 100-mile shoreline. More than 43 miles of trail are in place and more are planned. Although there are a number of gaps between these trails, a Bay Area–wide plan for bicycle and hiking trails circling the Bay envisions a continuous trail down San Mateo County's Bay shoreline.

Today, landscaped paths overlook blue Bay waters that reflect massive airline buildings and tall storage tanks. Promenades edge lawns by restaurants and hotels. Paths through neighborhood Bayside parks are busy with bicyclists and strollers. Trails over a reclaimed trash mountain give walkers a perspective on the geometry of salt ponds below. Boardwalks beside sloughs take birdwatchers through wide expanses of marshes to find avocets, willets, and long-billed egrets probing for food in the mud.

The original Bay margin from the rocky promontory of Candlestick Point to Coyote Point was a series of low points of land and protected coves. South of Coyote Point to Palo Alto were broad marshes crossed by sloughs extending as much as 3 miles into the Bay.

More than two hundred years ago when Spanish explorers came up the Peninsula, they found the marshes an impassable barrier and followed inland paths worn by Indians on the solid ground near the alignment of present-day El Camino Real. From their villages on creeks, Indians traveled in reed boats, finding abundant fish, shellfish, and birds along sloughs.

During Spanish and Mexican times the boat trip to San Francisco from landings along navigable sloughs was easier than travel on the rough, muddy roads. Then Anglos built more landings and channeled sloughs to improve shipping, and by 1863 a railroad extended to San Jose. Here and there the newcomers drained the marshes for pastures and crops, and around the turn of this century built dikes around marshes to impound Bay waters for salt ponds.

As Peninsula communities grew, marshes gave way to subdivisions, industrial parks, and freeways. The Bay's edges became sites of city dumps, sewage-treatment plants and an international airport. The Bay became smaller and more polluted. Concern for the Bay and recognition of the values of marshlands gave rise to a Save-The-Bay campaign that resulted in passage of the Bay Conservation and Development legislation in 1968. This law not only limited filling of the Bay but also required public access to the Bay.

A trend toward trails by the Bay gained added momentum from the 1987 state legislation that mandated a plan for a continuous recreational corridor with a bicycle and hiking trail around San Francisco and San Pablo bays by 1989.

From Candlestick State Recreation Area just north of the county boundary down to the international airport several segments of trail take bicyclists and walkers beside the Bay waters. As construction continues in Brisbane and in South San Francisco, gaps in the trail will be filled. South of the airport through Burlingame are only a few breaks in the landscaped paths. From Coyote Point Recreation Area down San Mateo's shore and around Foster City, a bicyclist can ride an unbroken paved shoreline path for 12 miles. Now a bridge over Belmont Slough connects these paths to the long levee path around Redwood Shores. From Redwood Shores to Menlo Park there are some gaps in the Bay Trail, but pleasant paths front the Port of Redwood City and the new Pacific Shores Center. From Menlo Park to the Dumbarton Bridge some trail segments are in place and others are planned. These trails would complete an unbroken bicycle path to Palo Alto in Santa Clara County. From there continuous paths extend to Moffett Field.

By late 2005 we can look forward to more trails from San Francisco down the Peninsula to the South Bay at Alviso. Traversing these trails we can appreciate the magnificent setting of San Francisco Bay, enclosed and delineated by the Coast Range mountains. Bicyclist, runner, walker, and neighborhood stroller can enjoy the outlook across broad marshes or open water.

Look for the blue Bay Trail signs at entrance points along the route.

◆ Brisbane ◆

At the Sierra Point industrial park, sidewalks along the main roads and a paved path on the riprap seawall take the bicyclist and the walker out to a marina and a fishing pier. Although no trail exists from the Candlestick Point State Recreation Area, at the San Francisco boundary south along the Bay east of the Bayshore Freeway causeway, bicyclists can ride in the bike lanes along Marina Boulevard west of the freeway to reach Sierra Point.

CIRCLING SIERRA POINT

A walk, inline skating jaunt, or bicycle trip around the landscaped perimeter of an industrial park takes you to the edge of the Bay past a fishing pier and colorful marina.

Facilities: Landscaped picnic areas; restrooms; paved paths for pedestrians, skaters, and bicyclists

Map: San Francisco Bay Trail *San Francisco Peninsula SF to Foster City*; USGS topo *San Francisco South*

How to Get There: From Bayshore Hwy 101: Southbound—Take Sierra Point Pkwy exit, go south and then go under freeway onto Marina Blvd. Follow it east to any of several parking bays at the marina and north and south corners of Sierra Point. Northbound—Take Sierra Point Pkwy exit, go north to right turn on Marina Blvd. and continue to parking bays on northwest and southwest corners and east side of Sierra Point.

Distance: 1.5-mile loop

Time: 1 hour

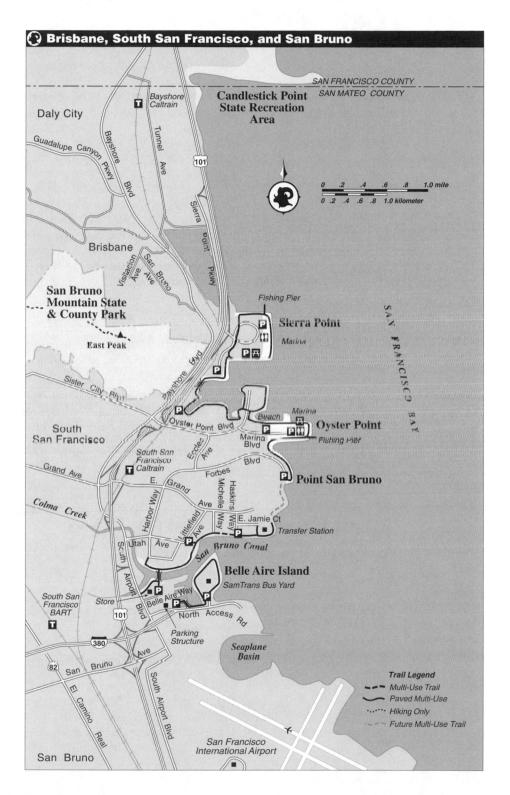

Brisbane, South San Francisco, and San Bruno

Daly City

Bayshore Caltrain

SAN FRANCISCO COUNTY
SAN MATEO COUNTY

Candlestick Point State Recreation Area

Guadalupe Canyon Pkwy

Bayshore Blvd

Tunnel Ave

101

Sierra Point Pkwy

0 .2 .4 .6 .8 1.0 mile
0 .2 .4 .6 .8 1.0 kilometer

Brisbane

Visitacion Ave

San Bruno Ave

San Bruno Mountain State & County Park

▲ **East Peak**

Fishing Pier

P
Sierra Point
Marina
P

SAN FRANCISCO BAY

Sister City Blvd

Bayshore Blvd

P

P

Oyster Point Blvd

Beach   Marina
P P **Oyster Point**
Marina Blvd   Fishing Pier

South San Francisco

South San Francisco Caltrain

Eccles Ave

Blvd

Grand Ave

E. Grand Ave

Forbes Blvd

P **Point San Bruno**

Colma Creek

Harbor Way

Littlefield Ave

Haskins Way

Michelle Way

E. Jamie Ct

P ■ Transfer Station

Utah Ave

San Bruno Canal

Belle Aire Island
SamTrans Bus Yard

South San Francisco BART

South Airport Blvd

Store
101

P
P
Belle Aire Way
North Access Rd

380

82 San Bruno Ave

Parking Structure

Seaplane Basin

El Camino Real

San Bruno

San Francisco International Airport

Trail Legend
– – – Multi-Use Trail
――― Paved Multi-Use
·········· Hiking Only
–·–·– Future Multi-Use Trail

Walk down to the quayside promenade from your parking area to enjoy the boating scene—sailors working on their boats, others lunching on deck or motoring out to set sail on the open Bay. Over the masts you see Mt. Diablo rising above its foothills.

From the marina take the paved path north to the fishing pier and continue west around the shoreline of Sierra Point. One gets a sense of spaciousness here beside the expanse of Bay water.

Past high-rise office buildings, the path turns to complete the circle around Sierra Point on the paved sidewalks toward the south shoreline. You will cross palm-lined, sidewalk-bordered Sierra Point Parkway, which offers a shorter route back to the marina parking. However, if you continue to the south shore, you will find an unpaved route along the riprap seawall easily passable on foot and favored by fishermen. This shore is more protected from strong Bay winds than the north shore. A recently laid paved path set on higher ground parallels the unpaved path.

For a longer trip, continue south along the Bay, cross a pedestrian/bicycle bridge to more paths in front of new condominiums and a small anchorage to join the attractively landscaped paths in South San Francisco.

◆ South San Francisco ◆

From the trail around Sierra Point in Brisbane through South San Francisco to the San Francisco International Airport, there are altogether more than 5.5 miles of Bayside paths. They take you on a number of short trips beside yacht harbors, through Point San Bruno Park, along Colma Creek and around Belle Air Island. Because of the present gaps between completed trails, these trails are more interesting for walkers than bicyclists. However, as new building construction fronting the Bay gains approval, trails will be required and gaps will be filled.

A STROLL AROUND OYSTER POINT AND ITS YACHT HARBORS

Enjoy quayside boating activity and savor long views over the open water.

Jurisdiction: Oyster Point Marina, San Mateo County Harbor District: 650-952-0808; Oyster Cove Marina, part of private industrial park

Facilities: Fishing pier; parks; two marinas; picnic areas; restrooms; paved pedestrian and bicycle paths

Maps: San Francisco Bay Trail map *SF to Foster City*, USGS topo *San Francisco South*

How to Get There: From Bayshore Hwy 101: Southbound—Take Airport Blvd. south and turn east on Oyster Point Blvd. After 0.9 mile turn right on Marina Blvd. and go through marina to public parking area near fishing pier. Northbound— Take Airport Blvd. exit, immediately turn left (north), go 0.2 mile, turn right (north-

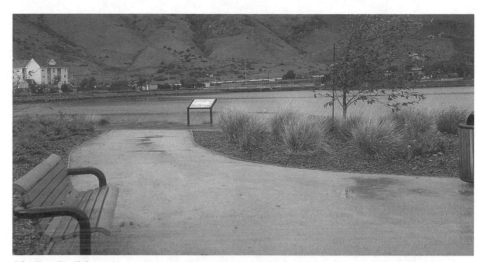

The Bay Trail from Sierra Point to Oyster Point at the base of San Bruno Mountain

east) on Gateway Blvd. and continue 1 mile to Oyster Point Blvd. Turn right (east), continue to Marina Blvd. and follow directions above. Day use fee at marina.

Other parking bays along the trail at the end of Shoreline Court in Oyster Point Park, near Oyster Cove Marina and on weekends at many industrial park lots.

Distance: 4 miles round trip

Time: 2 hours

From the parking area, walk out onto the fishing pier, installed by the San Mateo County Harbor District and the California Department of Fish and Game. At your approach, flotillas of white-faced black coots swimming near the pier take off with noisy flapping of wings and splashing, yet they barely leave the water. Soon they settle again, resuming their search for food beneath the surface.

From the pier walk around to the south side of the point on a path at the top of the sloping bank for a spectacular vista of Bay and distant mountains. The 80-foot tree-topped knoll of Coyote Point juts out into the Bay and the 182-foot hill above Point San Bruno stands just across the cove from you. The ridges of the Santa Cruz Mountains that you see above you on the west extend from San Bruno Mountain in the near foreground to Black Mountain in the south.

Your path curves right, crosses the road to the Harbormaster's office and returns beside the marina to the pier. On the path beside the marina you pass a fleet of boats berthed in the East Basin behind the breakwaters. Near the fishing pier you will find picnic tables tucked behind protective plantings.

A trail continues west from the Harbormaster's office for 0.5 mile to the West Basin, and then north past the swimming beach to the wide, paved paths around the office and industrial parks of Oyster Point. Now you walk on an attractively landscaped, paved path marked PUBLIC TRAIL at the edge of the Bay. Flanked by acres of parking lots, the high-rise buildings in this industrial park are deserted on weekends. From the benches along the trail you can see downtown San Francisco and, across the Bay, the wooded ridgetops behind Oakland and Berkeley. Just a few feet beyond the seawall white-winged terns wheel and dive for fish.

Continue around to the Oyster Cove Marina west of the point, where the blue of canvas sail covers repeats the blue roofs of the adjoining buildings. The trail goes around the marina past a strip of marsh and mudflat where avocets and egrets stand on long, thin legs. Two 8-foot slabs of marble placed beside the trail serve as benches from which to observe the marsh life. Shortly beyond the marsh the paved path continues north past new condominiums, crosses the bridge, and continues to the Sierra Point paths.

Marina parking is permitted only on weekends and holidays, but there are a few parking bays available for trail use during the week. If you park at this end of the trail, you can do this trip in reverse.

On the way back to your car you see different views of harbor and Bay. You may also see sunbathers and swimmers enjoying the beach just south of the high-rise buildings. This little beach, one of only two Bayside bathing sites in San Mateo County, is protected from the harshest northwest winds.

POINT SAN BRUNO PATHS

The views are splendid from this short stretch of trail.

Facilities: Picnic tables, parcourse

How to Get There: Follow directions in the previous trip (A Stroll around Oyster Point) to Oyster Point Blvd., turn right (south) on Eccles Ave. and go to Forbes Blvd. Go east on Forbes Blvd. to its intersection with Pt. San Bruno Blvd. Here is a little park Bayward from a large industrial plant complex. Ten parking spaces at this plant are reserved for midweek trail users. On weekends there are many parking places available close to the trail.

Distance: 2 miles round trip

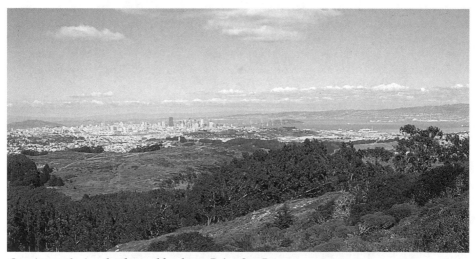

Curving paths in a landscaped border at Point San Bruno

Time: 1 hour

At Point San Bruno is a small park of manicured lawns, cypress trees, picnic tables, and paths. In an ideal location for workers in the nearby commercial and industrial buildings and for weekend visitors, the park's paved trails wind among lava boulders and seabreeze-tolerant plantings close to the Bay.

From the park, where a parcourse begins, paths lead north to the other exercise stops and to Bayside picnic tables and benches. You can walk north at low tide along a little pebbled beach or on the trail above it to the park at the Oyster Point Marina. Here at the water's edge the resting shorebirds—egrets, gulls, and willets—will fly off before you get close enough for a picture, no matter how quietly you advance.

SOME SHORT WALKS
ON THE TRAILS BESIDE COLMA CREEK

Views of marshes and the open Bay reward you for seeking out the paths along the creek banks.

Facilities: Landscaped, paved path for pedestrians and bicyclists; benches, interpretive plaques

How to Get There: From Bayshore Hwy 101: (1) **North bank Colma Creek;** Southbound—Take Airport Blvd. south to South Airport Blvd. and continue east of Hwy 101 to Utah Ave., where you turn east. Shortly after crossing Colma Creek, turn south on Harbor Way. At the curve where street name changes to Littlefield Ave., turn right onto 20-foot-wide access road to parking behind commercial buildings beside trail. Northbound—Take San Bruno Ave. Ext. exit, turn left (northwest) on South Airport Blvd., turn east on Utah Ave. and follow directions above. (2) **South bank Colma Creek**: Follow directions for north bank Colma Creek to reach South Airport Blvd. east of Hwy 101, then turn east on Belle Air Rd., and then turn left into parking area behind large discount store.

Distance: Two paths, round trips of 2 miles and 1 mile

Time: 1 hour and ½ hour

For the first stroll, on the north bank of the wide channel of Colma Creek and its fringes of marsh, park at Bay Trail parking behind buildings at Harbor Way and step out onto the trail. Surfaced and removed from the buildings, the trail runs through a broad band of fill for about 1 mile. At high tide the creek is full to its pickleweed-and-cordgrass borders. Ducks, mudhens, and seagulls near the banks dive for food in the water. At low tide, flocks of sandpipers and willets scamper at water's edge ready to pluck worms or clams from the mud.

As you walk east beyond the mouth of the creek, a few low islets of marsh dot the water, havens for the waterfowl. Across the channel lies the SamTrans maintenance facility on Belle Air Island and beyond is the San Francisco International Airport.

The trail is interrupted for a short stretch, but it can be reached again from the end of Haskins Way, which runs south from East Grand Avenue. Occasional landscaped seating areas with explanatory plaques along the trail make convenient sites for Bayside viewing. The paved trail ends at the parking area on the south end of Michelle Way. Under the shade of trailside trees are picnic table and benches. Beyond here an informal path continues to Haskins Way. There is off-street parking at the corner of Haskins and E. Jamie Court and a wide path leads to the Bay Trail.

Here the path resumes in a wide, landscaped corridor that reaches the tip of this craggy point, you look south over the broad mouth of Colma Creek to the San Francisco International Airport. Wind-surfers skim the choppy waters, airplanes roar on take-off, and nearby, behind a very tall, metal fence, the area's waste is processed and recycled.

The broad path continues around the point to a circular, landscaped area and picnic site. Across the mouth of a small creek, more construction signals new buildings atop San Bruno Point and the eventual tie-in with trails north of it.

As the creek widens you look out to the open waters of the Bay, across to Hayward and south to the airport. The expanse of water is a tranquil scene, attracting workers from nearby plants.

Another stroll, particularly suited to those who stay in the airport inns of South San Francisco or who shop at the discount store, is a 0.5 mile paved path along the landscaped south bank of Colma Creek. It begins east of a small bridge over Colma Creek on South Airport Boulevard, edges the parking areas and skirts the back of the store. Then it goes through a narrow, fenced aisle adjacent to the Water Quality Control Plant. Notable are the salt-tolerant plantings of native shrubs, yellow lupine, gray salt bush, and daisy-like grindelia, or yellow gum plant. These mature plants make a pleasant path for noon-hour exercise or an after-shopping stretch.

From the end of this trail is a fine pedestrian/bicycle bridge that takes you across Colma Creek to the creek's north side. If you follow the north-side trails it will extend your round trip by more than 2 miles.

SEE MAP ON PAGE 269

A Parcourse and Hike
on Belle Air Island

This well-surfaced loop path offers views of creek, Bay, and airport activity as well as a fitness course.

Facilities: Paved path for pedestrians and bicyclists; picnic tables; parcourse; benches

How to Get There: From Bayshore Hwy 101: Southbound—Follow directions for the previous trip Some Short Walks on the Trails beside Colma Creek) to South Airport Blvd., continue south to North Access Rd. and go east. Turn left (north) on causeway to SamTrans facility on Belle Air Island. Park on left side of entrance. Northbound—Take San Bruno Ave. Ext. east, turn left (north) on South Airport Blvd. and go right (east) on North Access Rd. Turn left (north) on causeway to parking.

Distance: 1-mile loop

Time: ½ hour to walk, longer if you use the parcourse

This little island, connected to North Access Road by a causeway, is circled by a paved path and parcourse built for the employees of the SamTrans maintenance station but also open to the public. The island lies off the mouth of Colma Creek between Point San Bruno's industrial-park development and the airport. The large-scaled white buildings with their blue and red trim lend a lively air to the island.

To the left of the entrance is parking for the public. By the water's edge, trees frame picnic tables for lunching in the sun. The 1-mile landscaped path has enough parcourse equipment along the way to keep the SamTrans staff in top condition. Benches at intervals accommodate those not so exercise-minded who want to enjoy the views of water and bird life. A run around the path is enlivened by the sight of planes from the airport taking off just beyond the tanks and hangars, by the view of ducks and coots feeding in the creek channel and, on still days, by the reflections of the strong patterns of the industrial plants in the water.

✦ Millbrae and Burlingame ✦

A continuous path follows the Bayside from Millbrae Avenue south to the west end of Coyote Point Recreation Area with one small interruption. Where the waterside path is interrupted, pedestrians can use the sidewalks along Airport Boulevard and bicyclists can ride in the bike lanes. Millbrae's Bayfront Park sits just south of the airport. Burlingame, one of the first cities in San Mateo County to meet BCDC's public shoreline access requirements, has waterfront walkways along almost all of its 3 miles of Bay frontage. These paths cross bridges over sloughs, pass an array of hotels and restaurants and reach parks with lawns, trees, and playgrounds. Described here are two walks along the Millbrae and Burlingame shoreline.

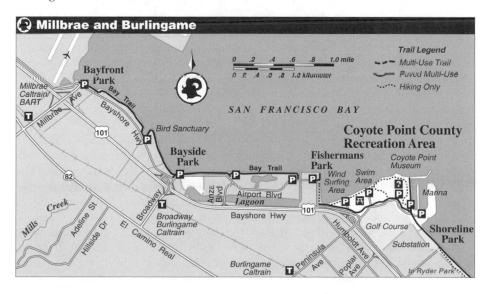

Facilities: Paved paths for bicyclists and pedestrians; fishing pier; benches; restrooms; some paths lighted in the evening

Maps: San Francisco Bay Trail map *San Francisco Peninsula SF to Foster City*, USGS topo *San Mateo*.

How to Get There: There are several public parking areas: (1) North Shoreline: (a) From Bayshore Hwy 101 take Millbrae Ave. exit, go east and turn right (south) on Bayshore Hwy (frontage road). Follow signs to Millbrae's Bayfront Park. (b) continue south on Bayshore Hwy turn left on Burlway Rd. to Shoreline Park; (2) South Shoreline: Southbound—From Bayshore Hwy 101 take Broadway exit, go under freeway overcrossing, turn right (north) on Rollins Rd. and immediately turn right (east) onto overcrossing. After crossing freeway, turn right onto Bayshore Hwy (frontage road) and go 0.1 mile. Turn left (east) on Airport Blvd., which curves south around Burlingame's Bayside Park. At Anza Blvd. turn left toward Bay and continue to signed shore parking areas near hotels beside Bay. Northbound—From Bayshore Hwy 101 take Anza Blvd. exit, go east on it across Airport Blvd. to designated parking areas as described in directions above.

NORTH SHORELINE—
MILLBRAE AVENUE TO BROADWAY

This walk takes you across two marshy inlets and in front of Bayfront establishments before continuing on sidewalks to the south-shoreline paths.

Distance: 2 miles round trip

Time: 1 hour

When you step out of your car at the north end of the trail at Bayfront Park parking area [(1) in the directions above], you look across a cove to the San Francisco Airport runways and their extensions. Start your walk by going north along the cove for a few hundred yards toward Millbrae Avenue to the handsome redwood pedestrian/bicycle bridge spanning an inlet. The marsh-bordered inlet attracts shorebirds, particularly the snowy white egret. Beyond the bridge a walkway continues through Millbrae's Bayfront Park to Millbrae Avenue. From benches here a visitor sees almost constant feathered- and metal-winged aerial activity accompanied by a cacophony of bird cries and engine roars.

If you turn southward from Bayfront Park, take the paved landscaped path beside the Bay that winds along past hotels and in front of car-rental establishments and motor inns. The restaurants beyond here, set back from the zigzag seawall, will install a path when the seawall is replaced.

For now, leave the Bayfront, go back out to the Bayshore Highway sidewalk and cross the pedestrian/bicycle bridge over the mouth of Mills Creek at Burlingame's Shoreline Bird Sanctuary. From this bridge you have an outstanding vista of tidal marsh and open Bay. The paved path continues on the south side of the creek in front of restaurants, hotels and businesses as far as One Bay Plaza, almost 1 mile from your starting point. You can retrace your steps from here or take the sidewalk along Bayshore Highway to continue south.

SEE MAP
ON PAGE
275

STROLL ALONG THE SOUTH SHORELINE: BROADWAY TO COYOTE POINT RECREATION AREA

Take this delightful Bayfront walk following a paved path fringed by lawns, shrubs, and trees and furnished with benches facing the Bay.

Distance: 4 miles round trip

Time: 2 hours

At the parking area at Anza Blvd. [(2) in directions above], BCDC signs note that the landscaped area and path curving along the Bay's edge in both directions is public shore. To the west the path goes in front of high-rise hotels and commercial buildings. It continues along the Bay's edge for 0.25 mile Bayward of Burlingame's Bayside Park. The path ends just beyond the park, near the Broadway exit from Highway 101.

If you go in the other direction from the Anza Blvd. parking area and east of the first high-rise hotel, you will find pleasant, landscaped paths along the Bay and around the Anza Lagoon linking hotels and restaurants. These paths, well-lighted

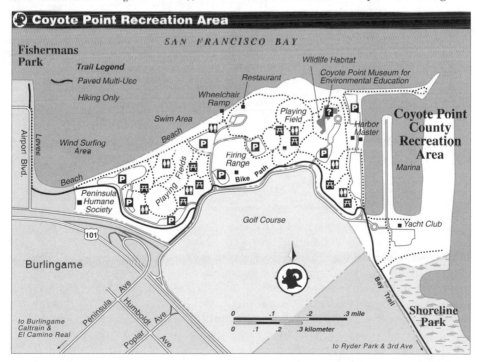

in the evening, make for delightful strolls. The Bay waters reflect lights from the airport and shorefront hotels. Around the lagoon pathside lights shimmer on the water.

For a daytime walk from the Anza Blvd. parking area you will find a fishing-access pier arcing out over the water. Even if you don't care about fishing, you can sit on the nearby benches and watch the fishermen's attempts to hook a big one. There are fish-cleaning sinks here and a restroom.

Where the Bayfront path meets the mouth of the lagoon, a striking pedestrian bridge vaults across the inlet, taking you to a shoreside restaurant on the other side. Here is 2-hour public parking at Bay View Place, from which you could start a walk.

Continuing farther east along the water, you can make your way along a strip of land in front of undeveloped property and soon come to the inlet for the Burlingame Recreation Lagoon. The lagoon, a slough resculptured by fill, is edged with cordgrass and pickleweed and inhabited by snowy white egrets stalking fish and frogs. Moored at the mouth of this lagoon is an old Oakland ferry, the Frank M. Coxe, once refurbished as a restaurant, and presently undergoing repairs. Plantings edge the Bay, and a parking area provides another access to the Bay Trail. The paved path resumes here, extending to the vehicle bridge across the inlet. On the far side and south along the waterfront a broad band of fill behind the seawall serves as an unpaved path.

Along the seawall at the point where it angles south is yet another access point, a paved parking area edged with plantings and picnic tables provided by San Mateo County and the Anza Corporation, known as Fisherman's Park. And indeed, many fishermen do cast their lines from the seawall, and on breezy days windsurfers skim the waters of the cove between here and Coyote Point. You can make your way along a rough path by the riprap seawall for 0.3 mile, paralleling Airport Blvd. Then turn east to follow the paved Coyote Point Park paths.

You have come 2 miles from your starting point at Anza Blvd., but if you want to walk or ride your bicycle farther, many miles of continuous, paved trails extend farther down the Bay, all the way to the San Carlos Airport.

◆ Coyote Point County Recreation Area ◆ and City of San Mateo Parks

Six miles of continuous paved paths edge San Mateo and Foster City's Bayfront from Coyote Point Recreation Area to Little Coyote Point at the San Mateo/Hayward Bridge. These paved paths for runners, walkers, and bicyclists connect four parks, passing a bathing beach, marshes, and a yacht harbor.

Jurisdiction: County of San Mateo: 650-363-4020; City of San Mateo: 650-522-7400

Facilities: Coyote Point Recreation Area: bathing beach with showers; restrooms; picnic areas with barbecues; playgrounds; Coyote Point Museum; yacht harbor; access for physically limited. City of San Mateo: two city parks with picnic areas and play equipment; dog walking park

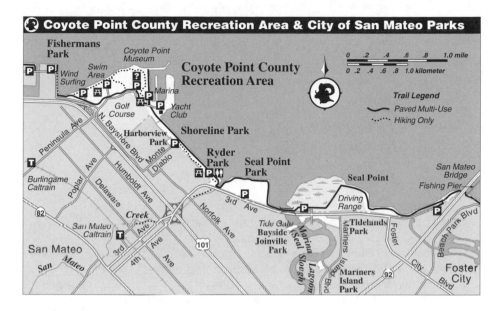

Rules: Coyote Point Recreation Area: fee; open sunrise to sunset; no pets allowed. City parks: open until 9 P.M.

Maps: Map on page 277 San Francisco Bay Trail map *San Francisco Peninsula SF to Foster City*, San Mateo County *Coyote Point County Recreation Area* and USGS topo *San Mateo*

How to Get There: Access points from north to south from Bayshore Highway 101: (1) Coyote Point Recreation Area—(a) Southbound—Take Poplar Ave. exit, turn right on Humboldt, right on Peninsula Ave. and go across freeway to park entrance, (b) Northbound—Take Dore Ave. exit, turn left on North Bayshore Blvd. and proceed to Coyote Point Dr. and park entrance. (2) Harborview Park—From North Bayshore Blvd., south of Coyote Point Dr., turn east on Monte Diablo Ave. to its end. Limited on-street parking, access to trail on levee. (3) Ryder Park—Take East Third Ave. exit from Bayshore Freeway for 0.5 mile to limited parking on left. (4) Tidelands Park—Take East Third Ave. exit from Bayshore Freeway to parking on north side of J. Hart Clinton Dr. near bridge over Marina Lagoon.

AN OUTING ON TRAILS THROUGH COYOTE POINT RECREATION AREA SOUTH TO SAN MATEO CREEK

Choose a leisurely stroll on part of the trail or a vigorous round trip through the park and along the high dike path to Ryder Park by the creek. For bicyclists it can be part of a 12-mile round trip ride to the San Mateo/Hayward Bridge.

Distance: 6 miles round trip

Time: 3 hours

Coyote Point Recreation Area, the County of San Mateo's 670-acre park, has a 2-mile shorefront trail, as well as a network of interior trails. The shorefront trail is for pedestrians only, but bicyclists can use a paved path that skirts the south edge of the park and emerges at its easternmost tip near a restored marsh.

For this trip, drive to Coyote Point Recreation Area's west parking area near the beach promenade. Pick up the broad, paved path and follow it eastward along the swimming beach. The beach at Coyote Point Recreation Area and the point itself are almost the only remaining fragments of the county's original shoreline. Here by the beach are a bathhouse, picnic areas, and playing fields.

After this promenade reaches the tree-topped knoll in the center of the park, it follows the bluff to two observation platforms overlooking the Bay. From the first you look northwest through the trees to the San Francisco Airport; from the second platform you see sailboats cutting through the water, and below you are more boats at their berths in the yacht harbor.

Atop the eucalyptus-covered knoll you'll find the Coyote Point Museum, the only Bay interpretive facility in San Mateo County. Don't miss the permanent exhibits about Bay ecology, featuring dioramas of birds in the marshes and aquariums of marine life. Changing exhibits treat fascinating subjects related to ecology of the Bay and regional sites.

Continuing through the park you descend past the yacht harbor to an elegant little marsh, restored and now attracting resident shorebirds and migratory waterfowl. At the marsh you are 2 miles from the parking area. You could turn around and retrace your steps or continue down the 1-mile dike trail of Shoreline Park.

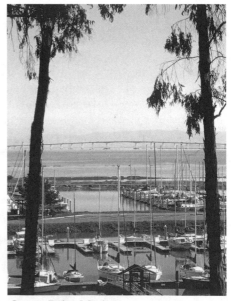

Coyote Point Marina

The city of San Mateo's Shoreline Park extends east from the Coyote Point marsh on a straight dike under the power lines. On top of the dike the paved path is popular with walkers, runners, bicyclists, and children in strollers. Close to neighboring homes and adjacent to Harborview and Ryder parks, Shoreline Park provides occasional benches from which to enjoy the Bay and the bird life in the band of marsh beside the dike. When you reach Ryder Park, you may want to explore the trail that continues 0.5 mile upstream beside San Mateo Creek.

A WALK OR BICYCLE RIDE FROM RYDER PARK TO THE SAN MATEO/HAYWARD BRIDGE

Past a converted mountain of trash, beside a healthy marsh, and atop a seawall this trip takes you on San Mateo and Foster City's paths to the bridge.

Jurisdiction: San Mateo and Foster City

Distance: 6 miles round trip

Time: 3 hours on foot; 1½ hours by bicycle

You can begin this trip at either Ryder or Tidelands park, or start on the far side of the San Mateo Bridge in Foster City. It is described here from Ryder Park.

On the southeast side of Ryder Park, San Mateo Creek flows into the Bay 7 miles from its source behind Crystal Springs Dam in the foothills. Spanning the creek is a handsome bridge which leads to a mile-long path around Seal Point Park, a mound created over the years from the city's refuse. Now the landscaped path around this landfill offers unobstructed views of the open Bay.

A new park project to be completed in 2005 will offer a road to the top of this mound, parking and viewing areas, and art panels decorating the trailside bayward of the summit. Ryder Park will have new picnic and children's play areas.

As the path returns to J. Hart Clinton Drive another pedestrian/bicycle bridge crosses the wide inlet to Seal Lagoon, now called Mariners Island Park. It's worth a stop here to see the flocks of shorebirds wheel and dive over the mouth of the lagoon. Then continue past the broad marsh, its colors subtly changing from green in spring to red-brown in fall.

As you continue east on the trail beside J. Hart Clinton Drive, you see across the street the green lawns and curving paths of San Mateo's Tidelands Park. Past the park you enter Foster City, where the Bay Trail stays on a levee next to East Third Avenue (Foster City's name for this section of the road) for about a mile. The path stays inland past an area of new construction, along the Bay beside a golf course and then near Foster City Boulevard it follows the Bay's edge on top of a seawall for the last 0.75 mile before the San Mateo Bridge. On this exposed section of the trail, waves splash against the rocks and invigorating breezes blow off the water. Several access ramps offer windsurfers starting points for Bay sails.

After passing under the bridge you come to the former San Mateo County Fishing Pier, a windswept section of the old low-level bridge, presently closed. Also fishing are the black-winged cormorants and the slender-winged terns you may see flying overhead.

You've come 3 miles from Ryder Park beside San Mateo Creek. You can retrace your steps from here or follow 6 more miles of trail circling Foster City. There is ample parking south of the bridge and a few picnic tables.

◆ Foster City ◆

From the San Mateo/Hayward Bridge the Bay Trail continues around the perimeter of Foster City. You can walk or ride a bicycle for more than 6 miles circling the city. Marshland, where resident shorebirds congregate and migratory waterfowl rest and nest, lies between the path and the Bay.

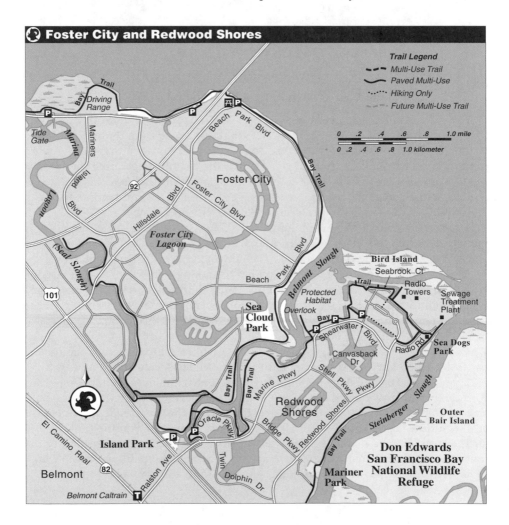

Foster City, once a marsh and tidelands threaded by a system of sloughs, is now a city of homes and apartments, shopping centers, and office complexes. In mitigation for the taking of these wetlands, BCDC required public access and marsh restoration at the Bay's edge.

Jurisdiction: Foster City

Facilities: Paved paths on levees for pedestrians and bicyclists; city parks nearby with restrooms, picnic tables, and play areas

Rules: Open during daylight hours

Maps: Map on page 282 San Francisco Bay Trail map *SF to Foster City*, USGS topos *San Mateo* and *Redwood Point*

How to Get There: From Bayshore Hwy 101 take Hwy 92 east. Turn right (southeast) on Foster City Blvd. and then left (north) on East Hillsdale Blvd. This street becomes Beach Park Blvd., which you follow to a parking area near the San Mateo Bridge at the Werder Fishing Pier, which may be under repair at this writing.

CIRCLING THE CITY ON FOOT OR BICYCLE

In the company of runners, bicyclists, joggers, and people pushing baby carriages, you will find a fascinating and diverse marine setting beside the Bay.

Distance: 6+ miles one way

Time: As long as you can spend

Starting from the San Mateo/Hayward Bridge, the Bay Trail is on a levee above the adjacent city street. Bayward, the tall transmission towers provide perches for birds. Especially noticeable are the large black birds sitting with outstretched wings—diving cormorants, whose feathers need occasional drying, unlike other waterfowl. An offshore lagoon is often filled with birds resting on the mudflats or probing the shallow waters with their long beaks. Avocets, distinguished by their black-and-white striped wings, sweep the water with upturned bills. The plain gray willet also has black and white stripes on its wings, seen only when it flies.

As the trail curves around the city, it leaves the water's edge, then returns to border Belmont Slough for 2 miles. This slough is a rich birding area, where great blue herons and white egrets stand tall in the marsh grasses. The tidal changes from ebb to flood attract a range of birds—those that dive in the water for their food and those that probe the mudflats.

After the path leaves Belmont Slough, it takes two courses—one follows a levee and continues north along Marina Lagoon, the former Seal Slough, until it reaches East Hillsdale Boulevard. The city of San Mateo's intermittent paths on the north side of Highway 92 follow Marina Lagoon back to Tidelands Park on East Third Avenue.

The other course continues along the Bay's circuitous shoreline, following the path southwest to Island Park. Here it crosses a handsome bridge over the slough to a paved trail adjacent to the parkway that circles the high-rise Oracle buildings in Redwood Shores.

◆ Redwood City ◆

Paths circle the island between Belmont and Steinberger sloughs in the community known as Redwood Shores. This large-scale development filled the former marshlands, but a rim of protected marsh lies outboard of the levee. Now the Bay Trail follows the sloughs on raised levees around the entire island. Small parking bays, benches, and landscaping make a walking or bicycling trip along this segment of the Bay Trail a very enjoyable experience.

Jurisdiction: Redwood City

Facilities: Pathways for pedestrians and bicyclists; restrooms at parks and Port of Redwood City Marina; wheelchair access at Marina, on some paths at Redwood Shores, and at Pacific Shores Center paths

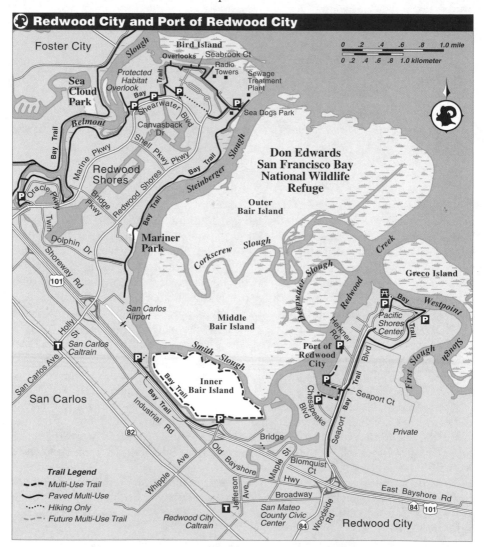

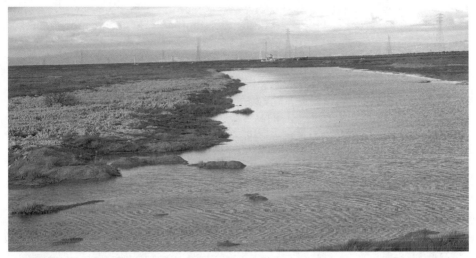

Steinberger Slough from the Bay Trail in Redwood City

Rules: Open 8 A.M. to dusk; all marshes by path protected by California Fish and Game Department; no dogs on path; port open 8 A.M. to 5 P.M.

Maps: USGS topo *Redwood Point*, San Francisco Bay Trail *Redwood Shores to Newark*

How to Get There: From Bayshore Hwy 101: (1) Redwood Shores—Take Marine Pkwy or Redwood Shores Pkwy (Holly Street) exit and park either at one of small parks along Oracle Pkwy which circles Oracle buildings, along Marine Pkwy or at Mariner Park at southeast end of Bridge Pkwy, one block southeast of Redwood Shores Pkwy. There you will find parking bays from which you can reach entrances to the Bay Trail. (2) Port of Redwood City: Southbound—Take Woodside Rd. exit, then go east under freeway to Seaport Blvd. and continue east to parking on Chesapeake Dr. or Seaport Ct; Northbound—Take Seaport Blvd. exit and go to parking.

Redwood Shores

Follow a nearly 10-mile levee path around the perimeter of Redwood Shores between Belmont and Steinberger sloughs. Bayward, Bird Island, a band of protected marsh washed by the tides, provides habitat for waterfowl.

Distance: 10 miles one way

Time: 5 hours

Start at one of the public parks edging the pathway. Along this levee top, fringed with a band of protected marsh, you find a variety of seabirds and shorebirds, both resident and migrant. In winter months the sloughs are a resting place for ducks on their way down the Pacific Flyway. Watch the waters for the great flat-bodied skates that inhabit the sloughs. Along the path is low-growing saltbush, which is host to the fingernail-sized pygmy blue butterfly.

The bicyclist or the energetic walker who gets to the outer rim of the path will see Bird Island across a slough. From the viewing platforms you can see over the green cordgrass of Bird Island to the blue Bay beyond. The island is a protected avian habitat, a nesting ground for snowy egrets and herons.

Among many species of shorebirds, the least tern nests here, an endangered species on the California coast. This tern looks like a small, slender gull with a slightly forked tail. Also nesting here is the cosmopolitan Caspian tern, gull-sized with a red beak. These terns are fishers, so you may see them plunging headlong into the water for their prey.

The nearly 10 miles of paths circling much of this island provide bicyclists a good ride, runners a satisfying workout, and walkers and birdwatchers trips of any length to suit their inclination.

The outer rim of the island adjacent to Bay Slough is closed to the public in order to protect the endangered species—salt marsh harvest house and clapper rail. But two viewing platforms on Seabrook Court provide opportunities to look across the slough and out to Bird Island and the open Bay. Near the short road at the east end of Radio Road is Shore Dogs Park and the private road to the Sewage Treatment Plant.

If you circumnavigate the island along Belmont and Steinberger sloughs, you will come to a dead end just southwest of Twin Dolphin Drive. The San Carlos Airport represents an obstacle that has yet to be solved. So, to return to your parking place, take the path along Twin Dolphin Drive to reach the parking areas on Belmont Slough

BAIR ISLAND

The connection between the southwest end of the Redwood Shores Trail and Inner Bair Island Road is proposed to follow levees bayward of Highway 101 on Inner Bair Island. There are unpaved trails that circle the interior of this island which are very popular with dog owners. Runners and walkers also frequent these paths at the noon hour and after work. To reach the island, drive across the Whipple Road bridge over Highway 101 and park at the point where the frontage road curves right.

◆ Port of Redwood City ◆

Short paved paths along the south bank of Redwood Slough take walkers to the Port of Redwood City and its marinas. From the historic embarcadero on this slough in the mid-1800s, lumbermen sent logs from the Pulgas Redwoods by raft or sailing schooner to build Gold Rush San Francisco. Today the Port of Redwood City accommodates seagoing vessels and its marinas berth hundreds of yachts.

In granting a 1984 permit for an additional wharf at the port, BCDC required public access to the slough. Now small parks and wharf-side paths invite visitors to watch port activities. A pleasant park by a new boat ramp was included in 1986 improvements at the port's marina.

EXPLORE THE PORT AND ITS COMMERCIAL CENTER

Strolls to urban seascapes await you at the municipal marina and the Port of Redwood City.

Several short strolls around the port are described here. Each takes off from Seaport Boulevard. On your way to the Port you will note beside Seaport Boulevard a paved and landscaped path on your right, a good walk on the edge of a salt pond.

For the first stroll turn left at Chesapeake Boulevard, a new, tree-lined street leading to an industrial park. Look for the small park to your right as you reach the yacht basin. Turn into the parking space by the small, two-story building that houses the offices of the Port of Redwood City's Harbormaster. At the park are tables by the water for lunch or checkers and a long bench for sheltered sunning or boat watching. Beyond are piers and a launching ramp. Across a narrow channel are berthed large yachts in surprising variety.

From the paved court of the little park and up a short flight of steps, a three-block-long boardwalk leads back out to Seaport Boulevard. This raised walk covers a slurry pipe from the salt pond to the salt company (no longer used since salt production ceased). From the walk you have more views of yachts across the channel. On a strip of marsh below, you may see great blue herons stalking fish.

After lunch in the sun and a walk down the boardwalk and back, you can move on to the next marine stroll. Turning left from Seaport Boulevard onto Seaport Court, you will find parking, two restaurants, trees, an exercise course, and an 800-foot strip of flower-bordered lawn beside Redwood Creek. Across Redwood Creek once rose a monsterous pile of salt at the former salt works.

The next stroll is along the wharves of the Port of Redwood City. Go two long blocks farther down Seaport Boulevard and turn left at Herkner Road. The entrance is more controlled than in the past, but check in with the attendant at the port gate and go on to the parking lot as directed. The port is open from 8 A.M. to 5 P.M. You will see by the ship channel the little Bay Access Park, with flower beds and benches from which to watch the action in the channel. Immediately downstream you may find a seagoing freighter or two tied up at the wharf, lending deep-sea flavor to this outing. Unless the vessel is loading or unloading, you can walk along the wharf beside it. The cargo might be redwood logs or scrap iron from a 25-foot-high pile by the wharf.

In the other direction a short path leads up the channel (left) to more wharves—for the Geodetic Survey ship and often for large yachts from other ports. It is the Bay Conservation and Development Commission requirements for public access that result in waterside parks and paths such as these all around the Bay.

Pacific Shores Center

A new business center has sprung up at the end of Seaport Boulevard in Redwood City. Situated at the edge of San Francisco Bay, it is inboard from Greco Island and separated from it by Westpoint Slough. On the west is Redwood Creek. From the Port of Redwood City, the Bay Trail follows the sidewalk along Seaport Boulevard due east to this new center. It circles the center and passes through it on a wide alignment past about six or eight tall office buildings. Between the buildings and along the illuminated paths are landscaped gardens, grassy mounds, and numerous benches for Bay viewing and bird watching. At this writing the buildings are not fully occupied, the parking areas have plentiful space, and the paths are uncrowded. As a condition for the building permit, BCDC required the installation of the Bay Trail. It offers another opportunity to appreciate the expansive waters of the South Bay.

◆ Menlo Park and East Palo Alto ◆

The city of Menlo Park's Bayfront Park and the Bay Trail to Highway 84 are close to populous neighborhoods and to many offices and plants. Noontime runners and families on weekend excursions find interest in the ever-changing marsh and Bay life. Although there are two short gaps in the Bay Trail south of Highway 84, most of the route is complete.

Jurisdiction: Caltrans, San Mateo County, Midpeninsula Regional Open Space District, cities of Menlo Park (Menlo Park's Bayfront Park: 650-322-1181), and East Palo Alto

Facilities: Pedestrian and bicycle paths; benches; parking

Rules: Bayfront Park open dawn to 5 P.M.; dogs allowed on leash; Bayfront Expressway path and Ravenswood Open Space Preserve open dawn to dusk

Maps: Map on page 289 San Francisco Bay Trail *South Bay-Redwoods Shores to Newark*, MROSD map *Ravenswood Open Space Preserve,* and USGS topos *Palo Alto* and *Mountain View*

How to Get There: From Bayshore Hwy 101: (1) Bayfront Park—Turn north on Marsh Rd., cross Bayfront Expwy to parking. The Bay Trail beside Bayfront Expwy and the Ravenswood Trail can also be reached from Hwy 84 at its junction with University Ave. Park at shore access area adjacent to Sun Microsystems on north side of Hwy 84 or at generous parking area at Ravenswood Pier (now closed) at east end of frontage road on south side of Hwy 84; (2) Southern Ravenswood Open Space Preserve and Bay Trail—Take Hwy 84 east, turn south on University Ave., then go east on Bay Rd. to its end at Cooley Landing and a parking area; (3) In Palo Alto, go east on Embarcadero Rd. to Geng Rd., then north to parking at Baylands Athletic Center.

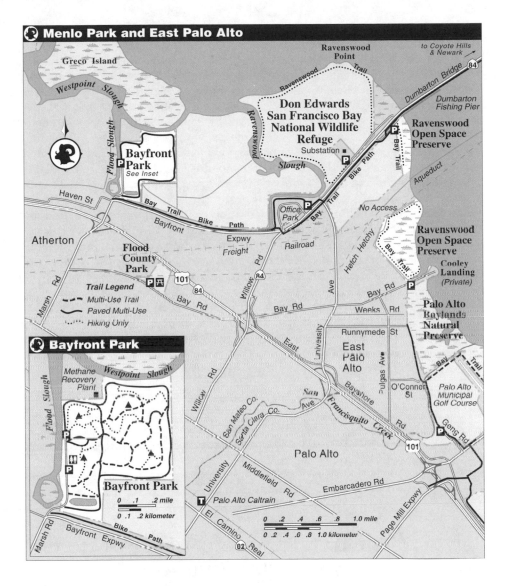

Menlo Park and East Palo Alto

Greco Island

Westpoint Slough

Flood Slough

Bayfront Park
See Inset

Haven St

Bay Trail Bike Path

Bayfront

Atherton

Flood County Park

Trail Legend
- Multi-Use Trail
- Paved Multi-Use
- Hiking Only

Ravenswood Point

Ravenswood Trail

Don Edwards San Francisco Bay National Wildlife Refuge
Substation

Slough

Office Park

Bay Trail Bike Path

Bayfront Expwy

Freight

Railroad

Willow Rd

101

84

Bay Rd

Willow Rd

Bay Rd

East

University Ave

San Mateo Co.
Santa Clara Co.

San Ave

Palo Alto

University Ave

Middlefield Rd

El Camino Real

El Camino Real

82

to Coyote Hills & Newark

Dumbarton Bridge 84

Dumbarton Fishing Pier

Ravenswood Open Space Preserve

Bay Trail

Aqueduct

No Access

Ravenswood Open Space Preserve

Cooley Landing (Private)

Palo Alto Baylands Natural Preserve

Hetch Hetchy Ave

Bay Rd

Weeks Rd

Runnymede St

East Palo Alto

Pulgas Ave

Bayshore

O'Connor St

Palo Alto Municipal Golf Course

Bay Trail

Geng Rd

101

San Francisquito Creek

Palo Alto

Embarcadero Rd

Page Mill Expwy

Bayfront Park

Methane Recovery Plant

Westpoint Slough

Flood Slough

Bayfront Park

0   .1   .2 mile
0 .1 .2 kilometer

Marsh Rd

Bayfront Expwy

Bike Path

Palo Alto Caltrain

0 .2 .4 .6 .8 1.0 mile
0 .2 .4 .6 .8 1.0 kilometer

SEE MAP
ABOVE

Bayfront Park—A Hike on the Hills or a Run by the Slough

Easy paths over gentle hills lead you to new views over marsh and Bay.

Distance: 2-mile loop

Time: 1 hour

Elevation Change: Relatively level

The 130-acre Bayfront Park at the end of Marsh Road, created on top of many years' accumulation of municipal refuse, brings you fresh views of the Bay from trails on its landscaped heights. From experimental plantings of salt-tolerant trees, small forests are springing up on the hills. Several miles of paths wind over the slopes and a 2-mile trail circles the park just above the marsh.

The park is surrounded by marshes and sloughs. Along Flood Slough to the left of the entrance road, ebb tide leaves mudflats by its banks, attracting white egrets. You cannot miss the lovely great white egret, standing nearly 3 feet tall, and the smaller snowy egret, which nests in reeds and cordgrass in the marsh and searches for fish in the shallows. To the right of the road is a small tidal pool with islands where ducks swim and broad mudflats where sanderlings and willets find food.

From the parking area a gate on your right leads to paths over the hillsides. From the vantage point of the modest elevation of the park you can see the Santa Cruz Mountains from San Bruno Mountain down to Mt. Umunhum.

To the north is an expanse of marsh and Bay. The salt ponds that once reflected the tall pyramids of salt at Redwood City are now drained and prepared for commercial or housing uses. West are the curves of West Point Slough marking the boundary of Greco Island, one of the largest areas of natural marsh in the South Bay.

A walk along the paths through the park is enlivened by a unique garden of "word rock poems." Read the sign at the main entrance for keys to the symbolism of the clusters of rocks you pass. Put in place by the Menlo Park Environmental and Beautification Committee in collaboration with artist Susan Dunlap, "the rocks are carefully selected to support and translate the true meaning of each word."

A walk eastward leads to a saddle, but continue over the hill beyond. If you go north through the saddle, your senses will be assailed by occasional rumblings and whiffs of gas from a methane-recovery plant operating on the site of the former sewage-treatment plant. However, this operation is temporary, a part of the process of creating a park from the dump. Meanwhile some of the profits from the operation go toward completion of the park.

In addition to paths over the hills, the 2-mile trail around the park by the slough is a popular route for runners, who can enjoy a glimpse of marsh life along the way.

SEE MAP ON PAGE 289

THE BAY TRAIL FROM MARSH ROAD TO DUMBARTON BRIDGE

Trails by marsh, slough, and Bay for birdwatching, walks, and jogging.

Distance: Bayfront Trail: 5 miles round trip; Ravenswood Trail 4-mile loop

Time: Bayfront Trail: 1½–2 hours; Ravenswood Trail: 1½ hours

This trip combines two trails—the 2.5-mile Bayfront Trail, which runs along the marshlands next to the Bayfront Expressway and around the perimeter of the Sun Microsystems complex to the University Avenue/Highway 84 junction, and the Ravenswood Trail, which makes a 4-mile loop northeast from that junction following Ravenswood Slough, circles a salt pond to the Bay's edge, then returns to a trail along Highway 84 that skirts around a fenced utility substation and firefighters training center and leads back to the University Avenue junction. During the fall hunting season some sections of this trail are open only to hunters.

Popular with noontime runners from nearby offices and with those who want a longer run than the 2-mile path around Bayfront Park, this long stretch of Bay Trail is also an important link to bicycle lanes across the Dumbarton Bridge and to trails in the Don Edwards San Francisco Bay National Wildlife Refuge. A freeway overpass from the DESFBNWR leads to Coyote Hills Park of the East Bay Regional Parks District. A bicycle trail from there goes all the way to Niles Canyon.

Negotiations have long been under way to close two gaps in the Bay Trail route south of the Highway 84 approach to the Dumbarton Bridge: the first is between the existing trails in the north and south sections of Ravenswood Open Space Preserve; the second gap is between the southern Ravenswood Preserve entrance at Bay Road and the existing surfaced trail from Palo Alto that ends just north of Runnymede Street. When these gaps are closed, there will be a continuous trail from Menlo Park's Bayfront Park to Mountain View's Shoreline Park.

The first leg of this Bay Trail route south of Highway 84 is an existing 0.5-mile levee trail running south in the northern section of the Ravenswood Open Space Preserve to the preserve boundary. Bay views east and the sight of birds on the salt ponds and mudflats are your rewards for this short trip. It can be reached from access (1) at the Ravenswood Pier, page 288 (the pier itself is closed).

Until the expected trail connections are completed south from Highway 84, the best Bay Trail access is from the second leg of the route at Bay Road in the southern section of the Ravenswood Open Space Preserve, described in the next trip.

SEE MAP
ON PAGE
289

A WALK NORTH IN RAVENSWOOD OPEN SPACE PRESERVE AROUND A RESTORED MARSH

On paths and boardwalks past tidal marsh, open water, and a slough you have the opportunity to examine the variety of bird life.

Distance: 2.4 miles round trip

Time: 1 hour

To reach this preserve see directions for access (2) page 288. At Ravenswood Open Space Preserve a small viewing plaza and bench near the parking lot overlook the channel of a slough. From the plaza you look across the Bay toward the narrows where the Dumbarton Bridge and an abandoned railroad bridge cross to Fremont. The north side of historic Cooley Landing is approximately the original shoreline. Early settlers envisioned that it would become the South Bay's leading port when scow schooners carried wheat and hay to San Francisco from what was called Ravenswood Wharf. Lester Cooley purchased it in 1863 and renamed it Cooley's Landing. The grain warehouse and brick plant he built nearby failed in the 1880s when Redwood City developed its wharves farther north. North across the water is Coyote Hills Park of the East Bay Regional Parks District.

The plaza is a good point for starting the trip by the salt pond on the north side of the slough. Cross the bridge over the slough and follow the levee path straight ahead. The slough follows around the bend in the levee. Bayward is one of the many salt ponds that ring the South Bay. Under auspices of the Coastal Conservancy and MROSD, the outer levee was breached and now the tides flood the pond, restoring it to a tidal marsh. This surfaced path for bicycle riding continues as far as a bench and viewing platform on the levee.

The viewing platform is a good vantage point from which to watch ducks and other water birds dabble or dive for food. At low tide when mudflats rim the marsh, look for the long-billed and long-legged shorebirds that find crabs, snails and mollusks in the shallows. When you have identified (or just enjoyed watching) the bird life, return along the edge of the slough to the bridge where you started.

WALK OR BIKE TO PALO ALTO FROM RAVENSWOOD OPEN SPACE PRESERVE

Enjoy the panoramic views over this great expanse of restored tidal marsh.

Distance: 2 miles round trip

Time: 1 hour

One outstanding view of marsh and Bay is from the paths along the marshes of Laumeister and Faber tracts. These lands, purchased by Palo Alto in the 1960s, were restored by breaching the levees. The expanse of cordgrass, at first glance appearing unbroken to the Bay's edge, is in fact a network of small, meandering sloughs. At low tide these ribbons of mud are alive with snails, mollusks, and worms. Incoming tides bring nourishing sediments to plants of the marsh. Cordgrass, an air purifier, removes much carbon dioxide and gives off much oxygen.

The marsh is home to many small and inconspicuous birds and animals. You may not see the shy and endangered harvest mouse, but keep an eye out for the chicken-sized but well-camouflaged clapper rail.

Marsh inhabitants that you can spot even at a distance, of course, are the common egret, 3 feet tall, and the smaller snowy egret. Happily their numbers are increasing here. Once nearly extinct, they are now common sights, thanks to the Audubon Society, which campaigned for their survival after they were nearly hunted out of existence for their beautiful nuptial feathers.

From Bay Road to just north of Runnymede Street there was no official trail, but Palo Alto paved the old 0.4-mile levee and this is now a surfaced trail. The path down the marsh makes a slight bend at Runnymede Street, then goes straight toward San Francisquito Creek, the San Mateo County boundary. You will see the row of trees bordering the channel of the creek out to the Bay. The trail crosses the creek, then continues at the edge of Palo Alto's Golf Course to Geng Road. There is parking here, and a connection to Palo Alto's long Baylands Trail, on which you can bicycle all the way to Mountain View's Shoreline.

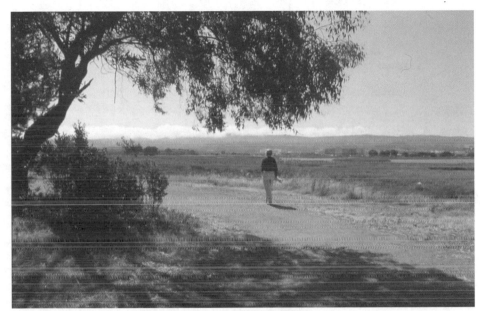

The Bay Trail offers wide views of marsh and creek in San Bruno

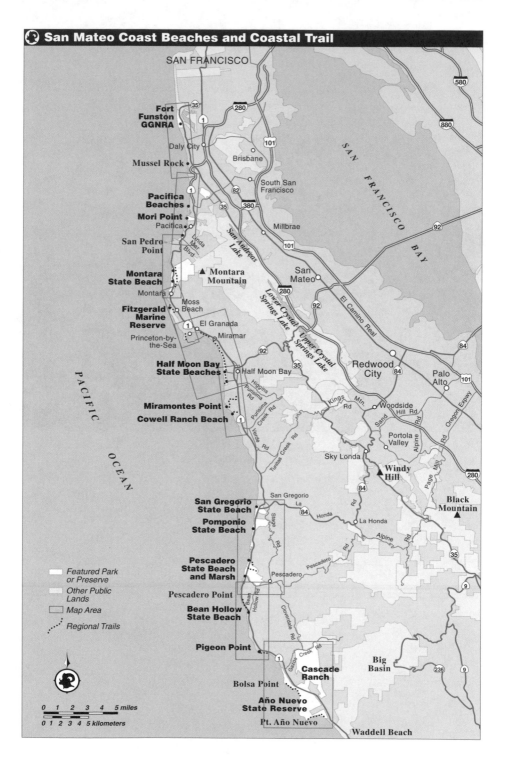

⊘ San Mateo Coast Beaches and Coastal Trail

SAN FRANCISCO

Fort
Funston
GGNRA

Daly City

Mussel Rock •

Brisbane

South San
Francisco

Millbrae

SAN

FRANCISCO

BAY

580

880

92

Pacifica
Beaches

Mori Point

Pacifica

San Pedro
Point

San Andreas Lake

San
Mateo

Lynda
Mar
Blvd

▲ Montara
Mountain

Montara
State Beach

Montara

Moss
Beach

Lower Crystal Springs Lake

El Camino Real

Fitzgerald
Marine
Reserve

El Granada

Upper Crystal Springs Lake

Princeton-by-
the-Sea

Miramar

92

35

Redwood
City

Palo
Alto

Half Moon Bay
State Beaches

Half Moon Bay

Higgins

Purisima
Rd

Kings
Rd

Mtn.

Woodside
Hill Rd

84

101

Miramontes Point

Cowell Ranch Beach

Purisima
Creek Rd

Verde
Rd

Tunitas Creek Rd

Sand

Portola
Valley

Alpine

Rd

Oregon Expwy

Sky Londa

▲ Windy
Hill

280

PACIFIC

OCEAN

San Gregorio

La

Black
Mountain ▲

San Gregorio
State Beach

Pomponio
State Beach

84

Honda

Rd

La Honda

Stage
Rd

Alpine

Rd

Pescadero
State Beach
and Marsh

Pescadero

Pescadero

35

9

Pescadero Point

Bean
Hollow
Rd

Cloverdale
Rd

Bean Hollow
State Beach

Pigeon Point

Gazos
Creek Rd

Big
Basin

236

9

Bolsa Point

Cascade
Ranch

Año Nuevo
State Reserve

Pt. Año Nuevo

Waddell Beach

Featured Park
or Preserve

Other Public
Lands

Map Area

Regional Trails

0 1 2 3 4   5 miles

0 1 2 3 4 5 kilometers

❖ San Mateo Coast Beaches ❖ and Coastal Trail

Extending more than 50 miles from San Francisco south to Santa Cruz County, this dramatic shoreline is dotted with sandy beaches, accented with rocky points, and indented by several relatively quiet bays. Along the entire southeast-trending coastline runs the Pacific Coast Highway—Highway 1—almost always in view of the sea and never more than two miles inland. This route is justly famous for its magnificent views of the surf and for its ready access to beaches and bluffs..

Historically, the Spanish Franciscan missionaries used the Coastside for grazing cattle; few crops were grown. After independence from Spain in 1821 lands belonging to the missions of Dolores in San Francisco and Santa Cruz on the coast were divided into private ranchos, the names of which still lie on the land. Some of these Mexican ranchos became towns (San Gregorio and Pescadero, for example), others became state parks (Butano and Año Nuevo), but the leisurely life of the rancheros did not last long. By 1843, Americans were challenging the Mexican authority. They soon took over the government and the land, by fair means or foul, and more intensive agriculture replaced the grazing.

Because this coast is situated across the Santa Cruz Mountains from the center of Bay Area population, and because its agriculture is profitable, most of the Coastside is sparsely developed. However, with increasing Bay Area population, housing is beginning to fill open lands, particularly in the Half Moon Bay area. The public is fortunate that so many miles of coastline offer uninterrupted ocean views and a great many beaches are open to the public. Many recent land acquisitions for open space significantly preserve this magnificent coast.

The California Coastal Trail, one of four long trails in San Mateo County, is proposed to extend from Fort Funston on the county boundary with San Francisco to Año Nuevo, close to the Santa Cruz County boundary. Here is an opportunity to walk, or ride a bicycle or a horse within sight and sound of the sea. The long-term goal of this trail is to provide a continuous route along the California coast, connecting beaches and recreation sites in 15 counties on the bluffs or rocky shores, over the sand dunes, or where necessary, inland from Highway 1 along local, lightly traveled streets. The Coastal Trail, part of the adopted San Mateo County Trails Plan, is identified in the statewide trails plan; it is part of the Joint Access Program of the State Coastal Conservancy and the California Coastal Commission.

A nonprofit organization based in Sonoma County, Coastwalk, is dedicated to introducing the public to this spectacular shore and to completing the Coastal Trail along its 1100 miles from the Oregon border to Mexico. Already long stretches of this trail exist for multi-day hikes; there are many opportunities for shorter day-hikes. Coastwalk schedules day or week-long hikes along one or more coast counties each summer. Hikers carry their personal belongings, but their camping gear and a hearty meal await them at day's end.

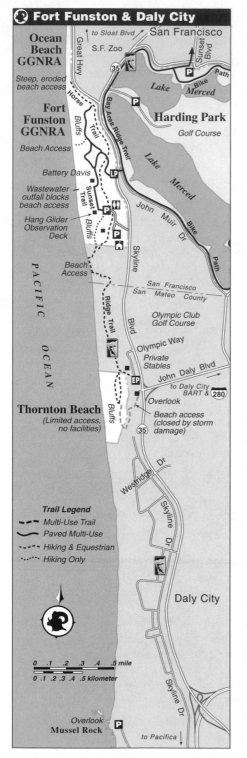

Fort Funston & Daly City

to Sloat Blvd — San Francisco

Ocean Beach GGNRA
Steep, eroded beach access

S.F. Zoo

35

Great Hwy

Sunset Blvd

Bike Path

Lake Merced

Fort Funston GGNRA
Beach Access

Horse

Bay Area Ridge Trail

Bluffs Trail

Harding Park
Golf Course

Battery Davis

Lake Merced

Sunset Trail

Wastewater outfall blocks beach access

Hang Glider Observation Deck

Bluffs

John Muir Dr

Bike Path

Skyline

Beach Access

P A C I F I C

Ridge Trail

San Francisco
San Mateo County

Olympic Club Golf Course

Blvd

Olympic Way

Private Stables

John Daly Blvd

O C E A N

Bluffs

EP

to Daly City
BART & 280

Thornton Beach
(Limited access, no facilities)

Overlook

Beach access
(closed by storm damage)

35

Westridge Dr

Skyline Dr

Trail Legend
‑‑ Multi-Use Trail
～ Paved Multi-Use
‑‑‑ Hiking & Equestrian
···· Hiking Only

0 .1 .2 .3 .4 .5 mile
0 .1 .2 .3 .4 .5 kilometer

Daly City

Skyline Dr

Overlook
Mussel Rock

to Pacifica

In San Mateo County, the State of California, the county, and the cities of Daly City, Pacifica, and Half Moon Bay own and operate beaches for all to enjoy. A few beaches are privately owned or operated. All are accessible from Highway 1, either by trail, from a roadside pullout, or from a parking area. Most public beaches charge a modest parking fee and many have self-registration kiosks to accept fees. Camping is available at the Half Moon Bay State Beaches, Butano State Park, and the privately operated Costanoa. Montara Lighthouse Hostel and Pigeon Point Lighthouse, operated by the nonprofit Hostelling International, offer inexpensive lodging in beautiful settings.

In addition to the public agencies who have secured beaches and coastside lands west of Highway 1, private, nonprofit organizations and land trusts are active in buying lands that may be lost to the public domain. Cowell Ranch State Beach is a case in point (see page 314). Another nonprofit group is the Pacifica Land Trust, which purchased the Pedro Point Headlands that soon will be open for day use.

The California Coastal Conservancy, brought into being by the Coastal Act of 1976 and funded by state bonds, works to aid local governments in the planning, development, and funding for coastal access and land acquisition. This legislation limited coastal development west of Highway 1 to facilities that are visitor-serving and required that public access is available where development is allowed.

On clear days the view of the intense blue sea and white-crested waves, stretches far beyond the shore. Onshore, sandpipers, marbled godwits, and willets search for unwary crabs and clams. Grebes paddling in the water duck below the surface and terns and pelicans dive from above for fish. Offshore is a parade of ships of all sizes. On foggy days the scene changes—it becomes more closed in, the sea and sky are leaden, and the air is damp.

Nevertheless, a vigorous walk along the strand or on a bluff-top trail can bring a sense of solitude and peace. On a stormy day the sight and sound of huge waves crashing on the shore reminds one of the immense power of the sea ceaselessly eating away at the bluffs.

It is inadvisable to climb on the rocky points just offshore from the strand. Rogue waves or incoming tide breakers can knock a person into the crashing surf.

Thoughtless use of the fragile coastal dunes can quickly degrade native plant species that hold the sand in place. Then, when the natural mechanism for stabilizing the dunes is lost or disturbed, sand blows, dunes shift and sand is lost to the beaches. Numerous bird species depend on the dunes for nesting. The snowy plover's existence is currently threatened and almost all San Mateo coast beaches are closed to dogs. Visitors should not walk on the dunes nor disturb the plants.

Described here are 33 beaches and the trails that traverse them and one trail on the east side of Highway 1 that climbs a steep ridge to the Chalks in Big Basin Redwoods State Park.

Look for the Coastal Access signs.

✦ Fort Funston & Daly City ✦

Thornton Beach, slated to become part of the Golden Gate National Recreation Area, is a remnant of a once-popular state beach. There is no official access from the former park's entrance off Skyline Boulevard in Daly City, but limited access is available on a trail from the horse stables on Olympic Way north of the old park entrance. This half-mile collection of sand dunes below the bluffs is flanked on the north by Fort Funston and at very low tides by narrow, sandy beaches extending south to Mussel Rock. A segment of the Bay Area Ridge Trail and the Coastal Trail follows a 1.2-mile sandy trail up and down the dunes from Fort Funston in San Francisco south to Thornton Beach. Both trips begin from Fort Funston in San Francisco only, thus making it a 2.4-mile round trip.

Jurisdiction: GGNRA (operates the **Fort Funston** facility): 415-239-2366

Facilities: Native plant nursery; viewing deck with benches in protected nooks; a hang-glider launching site; historic features of past wars; trails; picnic tables; water; phone; restrooms; parking

Rules: Fort Funston is open from sunrise to sunset; dogs must be on leash or under voice control and owners must pick up pet litter

Maps: USGS topo *San Francisco South*

How to Get There: Fort Funston: from the north, take Hwy 35 (Skyline Blvd.) to Lake Merced and after passing John Muir Dr., go 0.1 mile, and turn right (west) into Fort Funston. At fork in road, bear right and continue to extensive parking area. From the south, take Hwy 35 (Skyline Blvd.) north to John Muir Dr., make a U-turn at the signal and go south on Skyline Blvd. 0.1 mile, turn right (west) into Fort Funston, and then following remaining directions going south.

SEE MAP
ON PAGE
296

A ROUND TRIP ALONG THE STRAND

This trip is best taken at low tide when the strand is adequate for casual walking. The ceaseless wave action continues to erode the coastal bluffs.

Distance: 2.4 miles

Time: 1+ hour

Elevation Change: Level after 200′ descent and subsequent ascent

From the bluffs at Fort Funston, stairs and a sand-ladder lead down to the beach where the trail takes off south. Overhead, hang-gliders and para-gliders join pelicans and seagulls as they soar with the winds. Around you on the dunes in spring and summer is a restored native garden of wildflowers in many hues—crimson Indian paintbrush, yellow, gray-leaved lizardtail, purple sand verbena, and lavender sea daisies. When the tide is out, you can take a stroll beside the sea to find shells of many shapes, crabs skittering at the edge of an oncoming wave, and scattered flotsam and jetsam brought in on the tide.

When you reach a long, high dune paralleling the shore, you rise to its crest to find windswept Monterey pines and a couple of picnic tables in its lee. These are all that remain from the days when Thornton Beach had a fine entrance road down to picnic areas and camping sites along the shore. Heavy storms battering the coast in the 1980s and the run-off from city streets eroding the bluffs marked the demise of this beach.

Here is the place to turn around and head north to Fort Funston and its bluff-top viewing deck. From this deck you can look north to Point Reyes, west to the Farallons, and south to San Pedro Point in Pacifica. Almost the entire expanse of sandy beaches that you see in either direction is in the public domain.

Daly City's **Ocean Beach**, is only accessible from the parking area at Mussel Rock, situated at the north end of Westline Dr. The trail is steep in places and the beach best used at low tide. The rocky islets off the coast are hazardous to get to and subject to dangerous and unexpected rogue wave action. Signs warn of these hazards. Do not attempt to reach them.

◆ Pacifica Beaches ◆

Curving beaches between rocky points adjacent to Highway 1 beckon visitors to sandy coves and rolling surf. The northernmost beach is Pacific Manor Beach, where a COASTAL ACCESS sign on Palmetto Avenue directs visitors to a path around two apartment complexes leading to stairs down to the strand. Muni buses serve this area.

Farther south are Sharp Park Beach, Mori Point, Rockaway Beach, and the Pacifica State Beaches. The State of California and the city of Pacifica cooperated to connect these beaches by walks and trails to form the continuous 7-mile waterfront experience for coastal enthusiasts described here. The Coastal Trail follows the

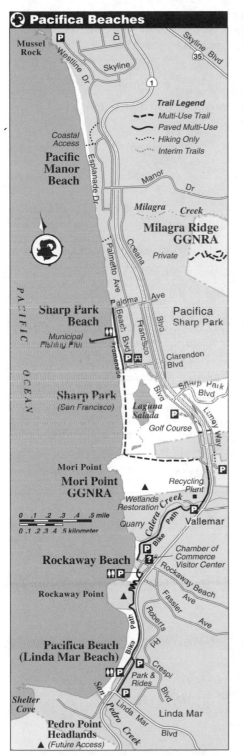

shore south from Paloma Avenue to the proposed connection over the Pedro Point Headlands to the Devils Slide Highway right-of-way.

The Golden Gate National Recreation Area, following a study of Pacifica's recreational needs, worked with the National Oceanic and Atmospheric Administration, the Pacifica Chamber of Commerce, and the city of Pacifica to open a joint Visitor Information Center in Pacifica. It is located at 225 Rockaway Beach Avenue, Suite 1. Maritime displays, maps, trail guides (including this one) and nature books, and tourist information are offered at the center, which is open daily.

Jurisdiction: City of Pacifica: 650-738-7380

Facilities: Paved paths; benches; picnic areas; restrooms; fishing pier; parking, golf course; fee

Rules: Trails are for walkers and bicycle riders; dogs on leash

Maps: USGS topo *San Francisco South*

How to Get There: Sharp Park District: From Hwy 1 take Paloma off ramps, turn west on Paloma to streetside parking.

SANDY SOJOURNS IN PACIFICA

A public beach and ocean front trail stretches for a mile along Pacifica's Sharp Park district.

From Paloma Avenue south to Clarendon Road, the wide, paved 0.5-mile trail for hikers, wheelchair users, and bicyclists runs behind a sturdy sea wall bolstered with huge boulders. After the trail passes the Pacifica pier, a generous landscaped border of lawn separates Beach Boulevard from the trail. Occasional picnic tables and barbecues set on little knolls, benches, and tall, square columns topped with attractive light fixtures invite visitors and residents to enjoy this beach and open space.

Beyond Clarendon Road, where there is limited street parking, the 0.5-mile trail rises to the top of a bulwark of boulders topped with loose earth, meant to protect the Sharp Park Golf Course from the ravages of winter storms. This public course built around Laguna Salada (Spanish for salty) and several other lagoons, fills the land back to Highway 1 and extends east toward the GGNRA lands on Sweeney Ridge. The elevated trail overlooking the ocean continues past the golf course to the north side of Mori Point.

MORI POINT

Jurisdiction: Golden Gate National Recreation Area

Facilities: Undeveloped except for informal hiking trails

Rules: No dogs, bikes, camping, or fires

Maps: USGS topo *San Francisco South*

How to Get There: Take Hwy 1 to Sharp Park Rd. take exit to Francisco Boulevard (frontage road) and go south continue on Bradford Way to parking on Mori Point Road. From Clarendon Rd. in Pacifica (see above), Walk along the trail by the ocean to Mori Point trails

When the Golden Gate National Recreation Area (GGNRA) acquired this point that rises some 200 feet above the surrounding coastal beaches, they fulfilled a longtime dream. Community activists in Pacifica, nonprofit organizations, government agencies, and elected officials worked for 18 years to secure 105 acres on this rugged ridge for the public domain. Its rocky promontory offers views of the coast from Point San Pedro in the near south to Point Reyes in the distant north. Glimpses of its rocky headlands battered by breakers rolling in from the Pacific

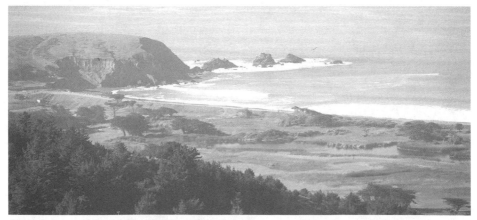

Mori Point seen from Milagra Ridge on a clear day

remind one of the power of the sea. Many native species live on its slopes and in the marshes below the ridge along the Laguna Salada and Calera Creek.

Presently hikers can follow several informal trails that lead to the summit of the ridge's two knobs and another that contours above its wave-washed cove. Meanwhile, volunteers are helping lay out a trail system that will consolidate these trails, protect its native species and take advantage of the spectacular views.

The Coastal Trail for hikers and bicyclists continues south around Mori Point by following Mori Point Road west out to Highway 1. Here a 0.3-mile, paved sidewalk on the west side of the highway continues to a paved, 0.4-mile off-road multi-use trail. The landscaped entrance to this trail is near the gates to the Wetlands Restoration Area, which recycles water from the Calera Creek Recycling Plant. This very popular trail skirts marshy Calera (Spanish for limestone) Creek on the south-eastern side of Mori Point, where a limestone quarry once operated.

ROCKAWAY BEACH

A small swimming and surfing beach in the lee of Mori Point.

Jurisdiction: City of Pacifica

Facilities: Swimming beach; grassy seating area; picnic tables; restrooms; nearby shops and restaurants

Rules: No beach fires; no motorized vehicles on beach

Maps: USGS topo Montara Mountain

How to Get There: From Hwy 1 take Rockaway Beach Ave. west and proceed to off-street parking both north and south of this street

Around Mori Point and the deserted quarry is the **Rockaway Beach** section of Pacifica. At the mouth of small streams at each end of this avenue are little coves set between two rocky points. North of the avenue are limited parking and a short section of paved ocean front trail fenced with nautical rope. South of the avenue is a swimming and surfing beach protected from the winds by the bulk of Mori Point.

PACIFICA STATE BEACH

A zigzag path climbs the ridge south of Rockaway Beach and continues along the wide, sandy beach.

Jurisdiction: State of California Parks

Facilities: Beautiful strand and surfing beach, parking, restrooms, and nearby restaurants, markets, hotels and motels

Rules: Dogs on leash, parking in designated areas

Maps: USGS topo *Montara Mountain*

How to Get There: Take Hwy 1 to parking areas at Linda Mar Blvd and Crespi Dr.

This 1.5-mile-long, wide, sandy beach with dunes anchored by beach grass and ice plant at its north end extends south to the cove where Pedro Point juts west into the Pacific Ocean. This a favorite surfing beach, where the black-wet-suited surfers bobbing over swells and gliding down waves look like seals at play. On clear days, the sea sparkles and waves crash on the shore, seagulls wheel over the picnic tables, and children search for shells and make sand castles.

At Crespi Boulevard the paved trail crosses to the east side of Highway 1, but you can follow the strand all the way to the cove at Pedro Point. A new 1.5-mile connection to the Devils Slide section of Highway 1 will take hikers and bicyclists over the Pedro Point Headlands. When the Devils Slide Tunnel is built, the Coastal Trail will follow old Highway 1 and former routes across the mountain to Gray Whale Cove. Here it will join the existing segment, Gray Whale Cove Trail in McNee Ranch State Park.

◆ Pacifica to Montara ◆

GRAY WHALE COVE STATE BEACH

This one-time clothing-optional state beach is again open to the general public.

Jurisdiction: State of California Parks: 650-726-8819

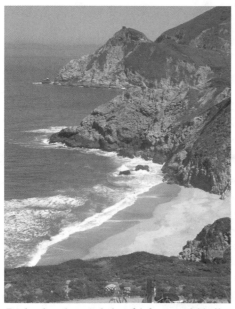

Pocket beaches sit below high coastal bluffs

Facilities: Stairs to beach, restrooms, small, sheltered coves

Rules: Dogs on leash only; no fires; open from 8 A.M. to dusk

Maps: USGS topo *Montara Mountain*

How to Get There: From Hwy 1 in Pacifica drive south to parking area on east side of the highway at Gray Whale Cove, or continue south to plentiful parking at Montara State Beach. Take the Gray Whale Cove Trail north and cross the highway to the beach entrance. From Hwy 1 in Half Moon Bay drive north to parking at Montara State Beach or Gray Whale Cove parking parking area is situated on the east side of Highway 1. After carefully crossing the highway to the blufftop, you will find a path on your right (north) that leads to sturdy stairs down to the beach (an abandoned road goes off left under some wind-sculpted cypress trees, but it ends abruptly about eight feet above the sand).

Here are three small coves hemmed in by sheer-sided cliffs. The southern two join by coastal strand, except at very high tide. The third, only accessible at very low tide is the northernmost. Each offers golden sands and protection from coastal breezes at the base of the steep cliffs.

A springtime treat is the beautiful display of wildflowers that lavishly decorate the hill beside the stairs to the beach: purple lupines, golden poppies, deep blue larkspur, white pearly everlasting, pink maritime daisy, purple iris, ferns, lush cow's parsnip, tall rusty-flowered bee plant, a profusion of pink clarkia, and fragrant sage.

Up a few steps from the Gray Whale Cove parking area is the mile-long **Gray Whale Cove Trail**, which contours along the ridge south to the McNee Ranch State Park entrance. Slightly north and below the highway is the infamous Devils Slide, which persists in falling off into the sea, taking parts of Highway 1 with it.

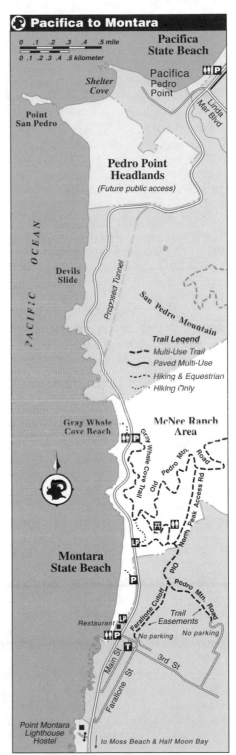

MONTARA STATE BEACH

Walk, run, or build sand castles on this long stretch of public beach.

Jurisdiction: State of California Parks: 650-726-8819
Facilities: Stairs to beach from parking on west side of Hwy 1 across from McNee Ranch entrance; parking (available until 5 P.M.); restrooms and water at south end of beach
Rules: Open dawn to dusk, dogs on leash, no fires
Maps: Map on page 303 USGS topo *Montara Mountain*
How to Get There: Take Hwy 1 south about 6 miles from Pacific or north 8 miles from Half Moon Bay to parking on west side of Hwy 1, as above.

Just south of Gray Whale Cove and separated from it by a ragged, rocky point is this lovely, mile-long, wide beach of golden sand and rolling surf. From the small, unpaved north parking area on the west side of Highway 1 there are steps down the side of a ravine to the beach where Martini Creek drops into the sea. Long walks along this broad strand, strewn with bits of sea plants and creatures tossed on shore by the waves, bring views of the rocky points both north and south.

Brooding over this lovely coastside is the 1898-foot Montara Mountain. Most of the mountain is in the public domain as McNee Ranch State Park. At its northern base lies San Pedro Valley County Park and adjacent to the south lies a large holding of the Peninsula Open Space Trust.

❖ Fitzgerald Marine Reserve ❖

Observe numerous specimens of marine life, walk its clifftop trail, and visit its white-sand beach.

Jurisdiction: County of San Mateo
Facilities: Parking and restrooms, trail to tidepools, sandy beach and clifftop viewing site
Rules: Visitors are asked to enjoy observing the marine life, but take no specimens. This is a very fragile environment. No dogs or horses allowed on beach.
Maps: USGS topo *Montara Mountain*. Map and excellent reference book: *Natural History of the Fitzgerald Marine Reserve* by Friends of Fitzgerald Marine Life Refuge
How To Get There: Go north from Half Moon Bay about 6 miles, take California Avenue west to North Lake Street and turn right. There is parking for 42 cars and an additional area accommodates 20 cars along North Lake Street.

This San Mateo County Marine Reserve in Moss Beach extends along the Coast for three miles and out into the ocean for 1000 feet, from north of California Avenue south to Pillar Point. Established in 1969 at the urging of then Supervisor James V. Fitzgerald, it is now a San Mateo County Reserve affiliated with the State of California Department of Fish and Game. The Reserve is open from sunrise to sunset and docent trips are offered under the auspices of San Mateo County's Coyote Point Museum. After the required hearings on the Fitzgerald Master Plan and EIR in 2004, the county plans to expand the visitor center to offer more interpretive talks and displays and to increase the parking area capacity.

From the visitor center and parking area a path descends beside San Vicente Creek to the beach and tidepools. At low tide when the rocky shale shelf is exposed, visitors can carefully walk on it to observe the complex, but fragile marine community in the pools and on the rocks. The area between high and low tide is home to many endangered species and to a great variety of seaweed, crabs, sponges, sea anemones, starfish, and fish. An interpretive brochure available at the reserve office explains the tidal zones and identifies one marine animal that lives in each. Pictures of marine animals help you place them by their general characteristics in their categories or *Phyla*. Try grouping them by stinging tentacles, jointed legs, spiny skin, soft body inside a shell, etc.

County marine biologists are studying roped-off test plots on the rocks to determine the health of this reserve. By counting the species in a square-meter test and a control plot, researchers expect to identify how the reserve's marine life is regenerating from past overuse. Begun in 1994, these studies continue today. Variables affecting marine life are wave conditions and human visitation. Although biologists are noticing an improvement in visitor behavior—they observe, photograph, or draw, but don't take specimens—this fragile environment is easily damaged.

Offshore, on Nye's Rock is a colony of 300 harbor seals. Visitors often hear their barking and see them on the rocks or swimming in the lagoon.

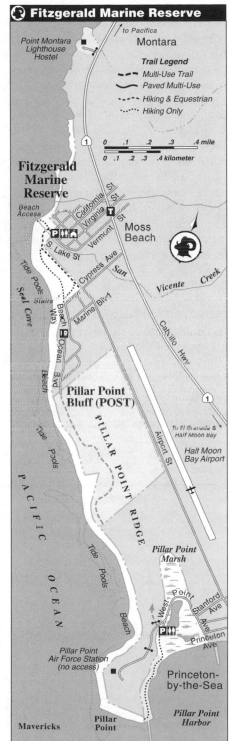

When the tide is out, the sandy beach is accessible for strolls along the water, but visitors should be mindful that high tides almost obliterate the beach. Check the tide tables posted at the visitor center or those published daily in local newspapers for tide and weather information. Photos from 1911 show a large sand dune situated between the ocean and the present shoreline. It is thought that cliff modifications and breakwaters constructed along the coast have caused this change.

When you have checked out the tidepools and coastal strand, try a 0.5-mile bluff-top walk south from the visitor center. Until the bridge over San Vicente Creek, recently washed out in a winter storm, is repaired, take the foot trail from the corner of California Avenue and North Lake Street uphill through coastal shrubs to reach the Monterey cypress grove on the bluff. From there you can walk right (north) to the flat blufftop where spring wildflowers bloom and a wide view of the coast spreads before you.

From here at low tide look just north of the main entry trail for a geologic syncline identified by several exposed concentric rings of Pleistocene shale rock grouped around some large table rocks. Earth movements along the Seal Cove Fault that enters the sea here, a part of the San Andreas Fault complex, lifted the coastline up against Montara Mountain. To the northeast you can see the long sweep of this mountain forming a backdrop for this coastal area. At high tide large combers roll in to inundate and continually batter all these rocky protrusions dating from the Pleistocene era, some 7–10 million years ago.

After you have oriented yourself on the bluffs, walk south into the cypress grove and follow the trail as it meanders through the trees. The first inhabitants of this coast, an ancient people dating back an estimated 6000 years, left recently discovered middens or burial grounds. Later peoples, the Ohlones, came to the Coast from the Bayside to fish and hunt, but apparently did not live here. Now, more than 135,000 people come each year to wander the bluffs, enjoy the views, and explore the marine life in the tidepools. About 20% of these visitors are school children.

Continuing south through the trees, the trail dips down to the former lands of Rev. Arthur Smith of Oakland, where three palm trees and a few remnants of foundations mark the location of his large, Victorian summer residence. A fence just beyond the wooden steps that lead down to Seal Cove Beach marks the end of the trail. Visit to this fine-sand beach on a hot summer day will for wide views of blue sea south to Pillar Point and north to Point San Pedro, and the sight of gulls wheeling, terns diving, and shorebirds picking the sand for worms. Return along the bluff for different views or follow a trail east to an opening in the fence and traverse the trail along the course of the Seal Cove Fault back to the visitor center.

POST has recently announced its purchase of the 119 acres known as Pillar Point Bluff north of Half Moon Bay. Its views of the rocky coastline extend south to where expert surfers ride huge waves in the annual Mavericks Surf Contest. Northeast is Montara Mountain rising above the coastal plain. POST plans to fix the erosion problems and remove pampas grass. POST will build a 1-mile section of the Coastal Trail with a grant from the Coastal Conservancy. This trail will replace a web of informal trails that cross the bluff. To reach the site, walk south from Fitzgerald Marine Reserve, or from the public parking area at the Seal Cove cul-de-sac, on Beach Way and continue on Ocean Boulevard to Bernal Ave. At this writing informal trails wander south on the bluff past a communications tower and continue downhill on a wide, paved road to the Pillar Point Marsh parking area. A Coastal Access parking area on the bluff at Cypress Street near the Moss Beach Distillery can be reached from Highway 1.

SEE MAP ON PAGE 305

PILLAR POINT MARSH

Observe many species of birds in the marsh and surfers riding wild waves around the point.

Jurisdiction: San Mateo County: 650-363-4020

Facilities: Marsh for bird watching; graveled trail to marsh and west breakwater; parking area by marsh

Rules: Do not enter the marsh; no dogs, camping, or beach fires

How to Get There: Take Hwy 1 north from Half Moon Bay or south from Pacifica to Princeton, take Capistrano Road west to Prospect Way and turn left. Go right on Broadway and immediately turn left on Harvard Avenue. At the end of Harvard, turn right on West Point and go 0.5 mile to the marsh parking area.

Pillar Point's 175-foot ridge with its antenna is the dominant feature of the middle coastline of San Mateo County. On its northwest side is the Fitzgerald Marine Reserve, on its heights is a United States Air Force tracking station, and in the sheltering arm of its southwest side are the Pillar Point Marsh and Pillar Point Harbor.

The 35-acre freshwater Pillar Point Marsh nestled within the protective arm of the Pillar Point promontory is now flourishing after years of neglect. Fed by a clear creek flowing through willow trees and tall grasses, this marsh is a resting place for migratory birds winging along the Pacific Flyway and for many species of year-round resident birds. At any time of year, even the casual visitor will see snowy-white egrets patiently watching for a meal of frogs or other marsh-dwellers. Especially in spring, red-wing blackbirds trill their mating calls from perches on cattails and flash their red shoulder patches as they fly low across the marsh.

A graveled trail edges the west side of the marsh and continues along the base of Pillar Point to the west breakwater. En route you can scan the relatively calm harbor for terns and pelicans diving for unwary fish or see marbled godwits and sandpipers searching for clams in the shallow, quiet water of the harbor's shore. Bring your binoculars and a bird book to identify these and many other birds as you rest on one of the benches along the route. From the west breakwater, you can walk on the beach around the bluff to see huge combers send saltwater spray skyward as they collide with Sail Rock. Watching experienced surfers ride these waves past rocky protrusions is a fascinating culmination of your walk.

On your return to the marsh, you can walk east on its sandy beach almost to the Romeo Pier, a private loading dock for the fishing industry. A beautiful northwest backdrop for this moon-shaped harbor is the long arm of Montara Mountain. At extremely low tide, the sandy beach and the former, but now submerged, Ocean Boulevard are completely exposed and you can walk all the way to Broadway at the mouth of Denniston Creek in Princeton.

PILLAR POINT HARBOR

See the fishermen unload their catch and watch the seagulls try for a bite.

Jurisdiction: San Mateo County Harbor District

Rules: Apply to the Harbor District for moorage.

Facilities: Harbor for commercial and pleasure craft; boat launching ramp; public fishing pier; benches along the quay; RV park; restrooms; parking

Maps: USGS topo *Montara Mountain*

How to Get There: Go north from Half Moon Bay or south from Pacifica to Capistrano Rd. turn southwest toward the water and park in several public areas by the harbor.

For many years fishermen and farmers on the Coastside struggled to get their fish and produce to market in San Francisco from the small communities west of the Santa Cruz Mountains. Repeatedly they petitioned the county supervisors and the national government to help build a safe harbor. Finally, after World War II, Pillar Point was designated as a harbor to be implemented by the Army Corps of Engineers and managed by San Mateo County Harbor District.

When the harbor was completed in 1961, it quickly was discerned that the great outer arms of the breakwater were insufficient to deflect the strong winter storms coming in past Pillar Point. A long west arm was added to the breakwater, but still the inner harbor was too exposed. After the addition of an interior breakwater in 1982, the small-boat anchorage is safe now and filled with local fishing vessels and pleasure craft.

Today restaurants and a few motels offer visitors the opportunity to linger here for few hours or days, observe the visitors and birds from quayside benches, try a bit of fishing, or watch the pleasure craft ply the waters.

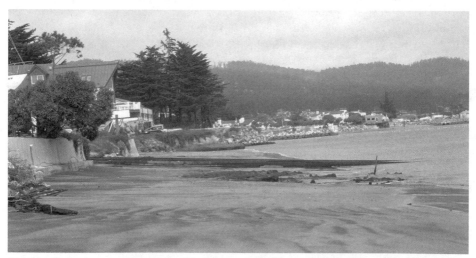

Try a walk on the strand when the tide is out at Pillar Point Harbor

◆ Half Moon Bay State Beaches ◆

Walk the strand or try the paved, 3-mile Coastal Trail on foot, bike or horse past four state beaches.

Jurisdiction: State of California Parks: 650-726-8819

Facilities: Visitor Center at Francis Beach; 4-mile paved trail and parallel horse trail to Venice Beach; day-use picnic areas; parking areas; restrooms; camping sites

Rules: Trails open in daylight hours; no dogs on beach but allowed on trails and in picnic and camping areas on 6-foot leash; please refrain from removing shells, driftwood, and other natural features; fireworks are prohibited; horses restricted to a separate trail running from Francis to Roosevelt Beach and not allowed on beach at any time

Maps: USGS topo *Half Moon Bay*

How to Get There: From Hwy 1 in Half Moon Bay go south to Kelly Avenue, turn west and go 0.5 mile to parking at Francis Beach.

The paved Coastal Trail, locally known as the Coastside Trail, runs for almost three miles through the California State Beaches at Half Moon Bay to join the trail at Mirada Surf. On it you can walk, bike, or ride a horse within sight and sound of the sea. Laid out east of the parking areas and campsites and behind the dunes, it crosses two major Coastside streams and several intermittent rivulets. At all beaches there is a fee for day-use at convenient, recently renovated parking areas, camping, and restroom facilities.

Since parking is plentiful at **Francis Beach** off of Kelly Avenue in Half Moon Bay, this trip is written south to north. Pick up the Coastside Trail just east of the parking and campground areas and head north under a sheltering row of Monterey cypress trees. In this park a low chain-link fence separates the bicycling and hiking trail from the horse trail. Equestrians access the trail from Kelly Avenue, not from the park.

At the end of the campground swing left around the park maintenance area, note a trail to the beach between the sand dunes and soon another on the right leading to a creek crossing for horses. When you step onto the metal bridge spanning Pilarcitos Creek, look for a bronze plaque honoring John Hernandez, a Half Moon Bay resident, who was instrumental in developing this Coastside Trail and the Seymour Bridge at Blufftop Coastal Park (formerly Poplar Beach). From the Hernandez bridge you can see the swollen creek rushing to the ocean after winter storms or a smaller creek lazily meandering through the willows that crowd its banks. The dunes here are roped off and posted as Snowy Plover habitat. Visitors should stay away from the nesting sites of these small, threatened birds. No dogs are allowed on any of these beaches.

Continuing north you pass fields of yellow lupine, low-growing coyote bush, bright orange poppies, and yellow mustard and oxalis. Here a split-rail fence separates the horse trail from the many walkers and bicyclists who use this trail. Soon you reach **Venice Beach**, accessible from Highway 1 on Venice Boulevard, where there is ample parking, camping, and restrooms.

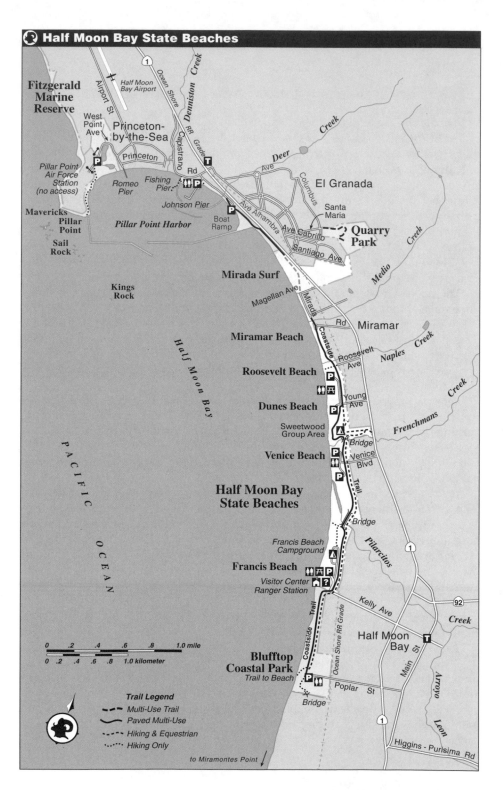

Half Moon Bay State Beaches

Fitzgerald Marine Reserve

Half Moon Bay Airport

Princeton-by-the-Sea

Princeton

West Point Ave

Pillar Point Air Force Station (no access)

Romeo Pier

Fishing Pier

Johnson Pier

Mavericks
Pillar Point

Sail Rock

Kings Rock

Pillar Point Harbor

Boat Ramp

El Granada

Santa Maria

Quarry Park

Mirada Surf

Magellan Ave

Miramar Beach

Miramar

Roosevelt Beach

Roosevelt Ave

Naples Creek

Dunes Beach

Young Ave

Sweetwood Group Area

Frenchmans Creek

Venice Beach

Venice Blvd

Bridge

Half Moon Bay State Beaches

Francis Beach Campground

Francis Beach

Visitor Center
Ranger Station

Pilarcitos

Half Moon Bay

Kelly Ave

PACIFIC OCEAN

0   .2   .4   .6   .8   1.0 mile
0   .2   .4   .6   .8   1.0 kilometer

Blufftop Coastal Park
Trail to Beach

Poplar St

Bridge

Coastside Trail

Ocean Shore RR Grade

Higgins - Purisima Rd

Arroyo Leon

Trail Legend
Multi-Use Trail
Paved Multi-Use
Hiking & Equestrian
Hiking Only

to Miramontes Point

Wherever a creek flows into the sea, the dunes are lower, and views from the trail expand. You can usually find a little path out to the bluffs or down to the beach to fully experience the continuous crashing of waves on the shore, seagulls wheeling overhead, and salty ocean breezes blowing in your face. Especially in winter you will find numerous shorebirds searching the shore for clams. Shell and driftwood hunting are also best in winter after heavy storms.

After passing the stables at Sea Horse Ranch, you cross another metal bridge spanning Frenchman's Creek and reach a lovely meadow protected by a semi-circle of venerable Monterey cypress and Monterey pines. These trees, sculpted by years of onshore winds, once sheltered a seaside home. Today picnic tables, barbecues, and restrooms nestle among the trees. Take the narrow path along the high north bank of Frenchman's Creek to find a few benches and bluff-top trail with dramatic views of seagoing vessels, sailboats, and fishing boats not too far offshore.

Although you can follow the narrow trail along the cliffs, the Coastside Trail continues from the east end of the meadow to **Dunes Beach**. Here an extensive parking area is accessible from Highway 1 via Young Avenue. From the bluffs here your views extend north to prominent Pillar Point and south along the curve of the shoreline to Miramontes Point. Easily distinguished by its radar screen and white government buildings atop a mesa, Pillar Point shelters with the curve of its south side the Pillar Point Harbor for small craft, with breakwater and lighthouse. Here too, is the waterfront interpretive trail at Pillar Point Marsh and a cluster of marine-related buildings and restaurants.

Continuing to the northernmost parking area on this trail at **Roosevelt Beach**, accessible from Highway 1 north of Half Moon Bay via Roosevelt Boulevard you find high dunes, partially planted with dune grass and a well-defined trail to the beach. A small creek, locally known as Naples Creek, meanders along Naples Beach and empties into the bay. From here it is less than 0.5 mile to the end of the separated trail. On your way you pass a group of brown-shingled condominiums on the bluff-top and emerge at the outflow of Arroyo del Medio. In severe storms of recent years old Highway 1 was washed out, but San Mateo County built a new 10-foot wide, non-motorized bridge across the sheer-sided creekbed. The Coastside Trail officially ends here, although you can walk farther north along oceanfront streets for several blocks. When the Coastal Trail through Mirada Surf is completed, you will be able to go north another 0.4 mile to reach existing trails in the Princeton area.

SEE MAP
ON PAGE
310

MIRADA SURF

Watch surfers wait for the perfect wave or walk the Coastal Trail in this newest public beachfront property.

Jurisdiction: San Mateo County: 650-363-4020

Facilities: A link in the Coastal Trail (trail not completed); restrooms and benches to be completed soon

Rules: Dogs on leash; no horses on trail or beach

Maps: USGS topo *Half Moon Bay*

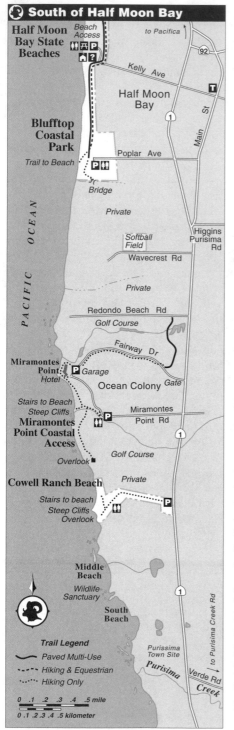

How to Get There: Go north from Half Moon Bay or south from Pacific to parking off of Capistrano Rd. in Princeton and walk south on the Coastal Trail.

In August 2003 the San Mateo County Parks and Recreation Foundation, with generous grants from the Coastal Conservancy and the Land and Water Conservation Fund, completed its acquisition of the beautiful 49-acre coastal property in El Granada known as Mirada Surf. The western 15-acre parcel lies along the surf just south of Pillar Point Harbor and extends back from the sea to Highway 1. San Mateo County with Coastal Conservancy funds then retained a design and planning team to complete the missing link in the Coastal Trail from the Pillar Point Harbor south to the existing trail along the Half Moon Bay State Beaches. An uninterrupted view of the sea and the surf beyond the rock retaining wall are highlights of this stretch of coastal San Mateo County. Watching surfers wait on their boards for the perfect wave and then glide down its foamy break will add to the pleasure of a trip on this soon-to-be built trail.

BLUFFTOP COASTAL PARK

Coastal bluffs offer flowery meadows in spring and wide sea views whenever the fog clears.

Jurisdicion: City of Half Moon Bay

Facilities: Paved path, the Coastal Trail, to Seymour Bridge; large parking area; portable restrooms

Rules: Dogs on leash; no dogs or horses on beach

Maps: USGS topo *Half Moon Bay*

How To Get There: In the city of Half Moon Bay go 0.8 mile south from the Hwy 1/92 junction, turn right on Poplar Street, go four blocks to paved parking lot at the end of the street.

South from the Half Moon Bay State Beaches at Kelly Avenue the coastal terraces and sandy beaches extend approximately 2 miles to the end of Redondo Beach Road. Continuing from Kelly Avenue on foot or horseback, you enter the city of Half Moon Bay's Blufftop Coastal Park (former Poplar County Park lands). In the park you can wander on an 0.8-mile paved trail with uninterrupted views of the ocean through tall grass dotted with spring wildflowers and introduced mustard. The trail presently ends at the Seymour Bridge spanning a Monterey cypress-lined arroyo near the park's southern boundary.

Barbara VanderWerf notes in her charming book *The Coastside Trail Guidebook* that the crumbling concrete rings you pass along the trail are remnants of a World War II practice range on which guns were mounted to aim at targets at sea.

If you want to walk on the beach, look for the trail near the parking area that leads down to the beach. You can go north or south from here for a stroll or brisk walk. Except at very high tides, is quite possible to go south all the way to the rounded (*redondo* in Spanish) points seen on the topo maps at the end of Redondo Beach Boulevard. Beyond here the surf washes close to shore and crashes against the rocks at the foot of the cliffs. Serious erosion at the mouth of an intermittent creek here makes cliff access hazardous, so retrace you steps northward.

Look for the house with wide roof overhang on Railroad Avenue south of Poplar. Once the depot for the Ocean Shore Railroad, it is now a private home. This railroad, which ran from 1907 until 1920, was planned to extend from San Francisco to Santa Cruz. But the tracks never bridged the gap between Tunitas Creek, 8 miles south of Half Moon Bay, and Davenport Landing. However, passengers took a scenic ride in a Stanley Steamer across the unfinished section. On several beaches remnants of this historic route are visible.

MIRAMONTES POINT COASTAL ACCESS

Visit a pocket beach and walk the mile-long trail.

Jurisdiction: State of California Parks and Recreation: 650-726-8819

Facilities: wide paved paths for golf carts and walkers; parking for 25 cars in hotel garage for Coastal Trail users; beach access; overlook; restrooms; hotel; golf course

Rules: stay on the trail; no camping or beach fires

How to Get There: From the Hwy 1/92 junction in Half Moon Bay, drive south less than 1 mile, turn right (west) on Miramontes Point Road, and continue to Coastal Access parking area on left or drive to the entrance kiosk and get parking pass for garage.

At this writing, access to the Coastal Trail starts on the bluff midway in its course through this private property of hotel, swimming pool, spa, and well-kept golf courses and golf cart paths. The Coastal Trail follows these paths both north and south beside the course. You can descend to a small cove below high cliffs or walk its surfaced paths in the sight and sound of the sea.

From the Coastal Access parking area or from the garage, step onto the surfaced path and walk toward the water. The path from the Coastal Access parking area descends gradually toward the beach, passing on the left the southern leg of the Coastal Trail. Continue a few steps farther on the path to the beach stairs. At the foot of the stairs lies a small beach between two rocky points. In summer feeding seals venture close to shore; offshore other adventurers in small craft ply the waters in search of fish.

When you return to the top of the stairs, take a few steps toward the hills and turn right onto a sturdy bridge over a creek canyon shaded by tall cypress trees. Beyond the bridge, you follow the path south past golf course tees on the ocean side and rolling greens and fairways on the other. The writers saw killdeer on the greens and a great blue heron stalking frogs or snakes beside the trail. This leg of the trail ends at an overlook with views of the distant horizon, Pillar Point north, and to the south the stairs leading to Cowell Ranch State Beach. Someday the Coastal Trail will bridge the approximate half-mile of intervening land.

Returning to the hotel in the center of the property, follow the Coastal Trail in front of the spacious lawns and terraces and around its north side. The path continues beside Fairway Drive, then crosses to the north side and over a bridge leading to the property's boundary fence. Here in a row of tall cypress will soon be a gate that opens onto another trail headed for Redondo Beach Road. For now, retrace yours steps to your parking area, either the garage or the Coastal Access lot.

COWELL RANCH STATE BEACH

A charming little cove under high cliffs invites the hardy to descend a long flight of stairs to enjoy sea and sand.

Jurisdiction: State of California

Facilities: Off-street parking on west side of Hwy 1; restroom (accessible for the physically limited); and paved trail to overlook; viewing platform with scope to train on seals; benches along trail and at view site; stairs to beach; explanatory plaques at parking area along Hwy 1

Rules: Open 8 A.M. to sunset; stay on the trail; no dogs on beach; no fires or camping

Maps: USGS topo *Half Moon Bay*

How to Get There: From Hwy1/92 junction in Half Moon Bay go south about 1 mile to a well-marked entrance on west side of road, just south of city limits.

This picturesque State of California beach was acquired and developed as part of a larger purchase by the Peninsula Open Space Trust. At the well-marked entrance you will find an interpretive signboard. On one side of the sign are details of the POST acquisition; the other side tells the history of the land, from Native American habitation through whalers to settlers of European descent.

A wide, half-mile-long, level, graveled path from the parking area (and accessible to the physically limited) traverses the coastal terrace out to the cliff overlooking the sea. Along the path are benches of recycled material and more interpretive signs. To the south are fenced agricultural fields. In one place the fence is interrupted by a delightful, though now somewhat rusted, wrought-iron gate decorated with a humpbacked whale design.

At the cliff end of the path is a circular vista point, surrounded by a wooden railing, where there are more interpretive signs, a telescope, benches and another restroom. From this point are splendid views of the Coast, with the long arm and radar tower of Pillar Point prominent in the north. Immediately south of the point is a protected harbor-seal breeding ground—the rocks offshore and the beach are off-limits to humans. Read the interpretive signs to learn the story of these large mammals.

From the vista point a long flight of steps leads north to a small, curving, golden sand beach. Tucked up against the tall cliffs, it is one of the more protected beaches along the San Mateo Coast. (Note: Severe winter storms often damage the lower 4 or 5 steps, which make it difficult to reach the beach.) This beach is home to the western snowy plover, a protected species.

In 1987 POST bought 1197 acres of the former Cowell Foundation lands on the east and west side of Highway 1, just south of the Half Moon Bay city limits. In 1989 Post transferred the land to the Coastal Conservancy, which then sold the acreage to local farmers. Attached to the sale were conservation easements that

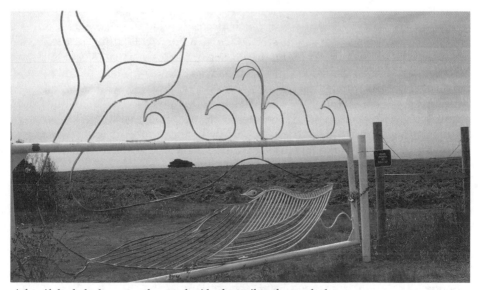

A fanciful whale decorates the gate beside the trail to the overlook

protect the land from development in perpetuity. Easements on the blufftops to be used for a future Coastal Trail, also donated by POST, will be activated when money for fencing and appropriate trail construction is available.

POST also donated to the Coastal Conservancy the 5-acre historic Purissima (early spelling) Townsite, situated on the northeast corner of present-day Purisima Creek Road and Highway 1. Only the foundations of the former Dobbel mansion remain on the southeast corner of Purisima Creek Road, but a double row of cypress trees defines the curving driveway. The site can be identified by Monterey cypresses and pines bordering its frontage on Highway 1, but brambles and vinca have taken over the land.

◆ San Gregorio to Pescadero ◆

SAN GREGORIO AND POMPONIO STATE BEACHES

Jurisdiction: State of California

Facilities: Parking, restrooms; long sandy beaches

Rules: Open 8 A.M. to sunset; no dogs on beach; do not remove sea specimens or driftwood; no fires on beach

Maps: USGS topo *San Gregorio*

How to Get There: Take Hwy 1 or Hwy 84 (La Honda Rd.) to the junction of these two roads, go south less than ¼ mile on Hwy 1 to park entrance on west side of road.

These two beaches are popular destinations for daytime visitors from the Bayside. San Gregorio has a self-service fee structure (called an "iron ranger") when the ranger isn't present. This beach encompasses estuary of San Gregorio Creek at the point where it runs into the ocean. The State of California owns these estuarine lands on both sides of the creek east of Highway 1, while the Peninsula Open Space Trust has conservation easements or ownership of lands on the north, south, and east of San Gregorio State Beach stretching almost to the town of San Gregorio. These lands someday may provide valuable trail links to the coast.

San Gregorio's large beach, with a cave under the cliff at its north side, tempts the visitor to walk south for long distances. Swimming here is not advisable, due to the strong undertow, which has been known to pull people out to sea. Driftwood and all sorts of interesting detrita lie at the tide line; flocks of sandpipers skitter in and out of the waves' edge. There is always something interesting to find or to watch at this wide and beautiful beach.

On the grassy strip beside the parking area is a historic marker noting that Captain Gaspar de Portolá and his party of Spanish explorers camped here for three days in October 1769. Although they missed the object of their search—Monterey Bay—they later found San Francisco Bay.

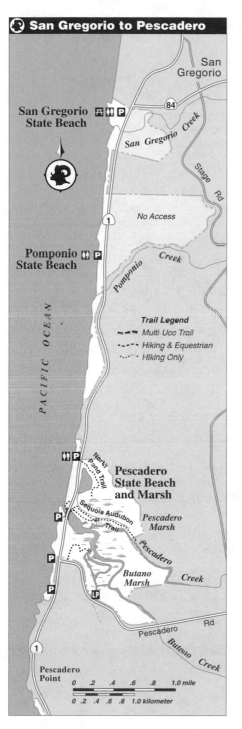

San Gregorio to Pescadero

POMPONIO STATE BEACH

A smaller beach than San Gregorio invites you to explore its strand and enjoy the invigorating sea breezes.

Jurisdiction: State of California

Facilities: Small parking lot; picnic tables; barbecues; restrooms

Rules: No dogs, beach fires, horses, or camping are allowed

Maps: USGS topo *San Gregorio*

How to Get There: Follow instructions for San Gregorio Beach and continue almost 3 miles south to park entrance on west side of road.

This beach is about 1.5 miles to the south, and could be called a part of San Gregorio Beach, since their sands are contiguous. A walk between the two would be an exhilarating experience when the surf is calm, the tide is low, and the clouds are scudding fast from the west. The visitor facilities are situated on the north side of Pomponio Creek at the beach's southern end. To reach the strand you climb up a sand dune and descend to the wide beach where the western snowy plover, a threatened species, is a year-round resident. Since the plover nests in the dune grass, visitors are asked to stay away from these sandy hillocks.

PESCADERO STATE BEACH AND PESCADERO MARSH

Jurisdiction: State of California, Department of Parks and Recreation: 650-879-2170

Facilities: Beach for sunbathing; fishing; trails for nature study; as of this writing, there are no docent-led hikes through the marsh

Maps: State parks brochures *San Mateo Coast State Beaches* and *Pescadero Marsh Natural Preserve,* USGS topo *San Gregorio*

Rules: Open 8 A.M. to sunset; trails for hikers only; hunting and dogs not allowed in preserve; no dogs on beach; no beach fires, camping, or motorized vehicles; boats not allowed in sloughs during nesting season, March through August

How to Get There: Take Hwy 1 south from Half Moon Bay for 17 miles. The state beach has three parking lots, all on ocean side of Hwy 1: (1) north of Pescadero Creek Bridge, (2), and (3) south of bridge, all with restrooms. Parking lot 1 has a few picnic tables and barbecues.

Near the town of Pescadero (Spanish for the fishing place) are Pescadero Beach and Marsh, welcome resources for the recreationist and the nature lover. Pescadero State Beach's 2 miles of sandy beach, coves, dunes and rocky outcroppings lie on the west, or ocean, side of Highway 1, and its 500 acres of marsh preserve are on the east side. The estuary of Butano and Pescadero creeks is a protected habitat for both migrating and resident birds and fish.

In the early years of this century, European farmers who had settled in Pescadero drained much of the original marsh and used the area for agriculture. Owned by the Nunziatti family, the marshy areas remaining were managed after World War II by Tom Phipps as a hunting club. Migrating birds were the quarry, as well as ducks and Asian pheasants raised specifically for hunting.

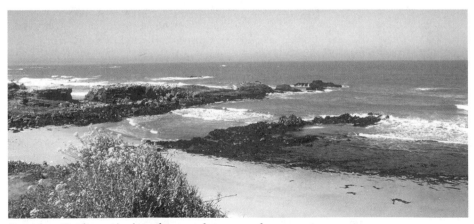

Pescadero Creek empties into the ocean between rocky ramparts

In the 1960s, members of the Sequoia Audubon Society realized what a valuable habitat the marshland was and raised money to buy part of the land from the Nunziatti family. During the early 1970s the state parks acquired this nucleus of Pescadero Marsh, and continued acquisition until today. The state now owns 90% of the original marshland.

POST negotiated conservation easements on farming lands to the east. Ongoing marsh restoration efforts, managed by the state parks, aim to improve the habitat and protect native species. One trail, named for the Sequoia Aubudon Society, honors their efforts to preserve the marsh. Pescadero Marsh, one of the premier birding spots in the county, is the only sizable estuarine marsh between Bolinas Lagoon and Elkhorn Slough.

SEQUOIA AUDUBON TRAIL

SEE MAP ON PAGE 317

Follow Pescadero Creek upstream to the end of the preserve.

Distance: 2.5 miles round trip

Time: 1½ hours

Park at the first lot south of the creek on the west side of the highway. Cross the highway bridge on a safe sidewalk on the west side, then go left down to the beach and under the bridge to reach the Sequoia Audubon Trail. On the dunes note that native dune grass planted to replace the invasive foreign ice plant is doing well.

At a junction with a trail leading straight ahead, on which you will return, you reach a signboard, which has information about spawning steelhead and advisories to boaters. From here go right on the somewhat obscured and unmarked Sequoia Audubon Trail at the base of a high sand hill, passing on your right an unsigned track leading to a shingled beach on Pescadero Creek itself. This estuary with calm waters and small beach might be a safe and pleasant place to swim on a hot day, avoiding the dangerous cold undertow of the ocean beach itself.

The main Sequoia Audubon Trail soon reaches another junction, where on the left there is a bridge over a slough and a viewing platform. This area of the marsh is being managed by state scientists so that various sloughs, dikes, and tidal gates keep water in the marsh and the pond for a longer period. Here you may see egrets feeding, herons stalking their prey, or a pair of cinnamon teal ducks paddling through the water.

This trip continues straight (east) on the Sequoia Audubon Trail along a levee next to the slough. You are several hundred feet north of the main Pescadero Creek at this point. Along the way pass a huge, sprawling eucalyptus whose branches crawl along the ground, inviting climbers of all ages. Soon you reach a bench near the creek where you can view the marsh extending to the south. Look for some wood-rat nests in the thick willows, and for more benches by Pescadero Creek.

After about a mile, retrace your steps from the far end of the Sequoia Audubon Trail to the viewing platform and bridge that you passed earlier. Here take the right-hand trail going northwest. You will see bushes of twinberry, a member of the honeysuckle family, which has reddish-yellow flowers in spring and black berries

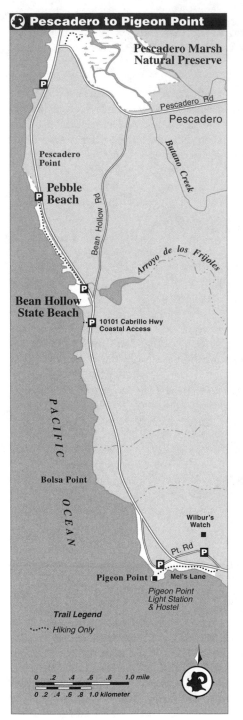

Pescadero to Pigeon Point

Pescadero Marsh
Natural Preserve

Pescadero Rd

Pescadero

Pescadero
Point

Pebble
Beach

Butano Creek

Bean Hollow Rd

Arroyo de los Frijoles

Bean Hollow
State Beach

10101 Cabrillo Hwy
Coastal Access

PACIFIC

Bolsa Point

OCEAN

Wilbur's
Watch

Pt. Rd

Pigeon Point   Mel's Lane

Pigeon Point
Light Station
& Hostel

Trail Legend

········ Hiking Only

0   .2   .4   .6   .8   1.0 mile

0 .2 .4 .6 .8 1.0 kilometer

in fall. In damp areas there is yellow cinquefoil, a rose family relative with feathery leaves. Shortly you find two viewing benches, where you turn left (south) to return to the signboard, go under the bridge and on to the parking area.

NORTH POND TRAIL

Explore the quiet, east side of a restored marsh.

Distance: 1 mile round trip

Time: ¾ hour

Map: See map on page 317

Access to the North Pond Trail is somewhat hazardous. Park at the northernmost Pescadero Beach parking lot and scurry carefully across the highway. Traffic is fast and dangerous. This trail goes around the north and east sides of North Pond, reaching a small slough on the south side. You rise higher on the North Pond Trail, and get a splendid vista of the entire marsh, the two tributary creeks, the pond with its resident and migrating birds and the ocean to the west. Binoculars and bird books are essentials for this hike. Here you get a feeling for what the Coastside looked like before the Europeans arrived. The Pescadero Marsh is a special place, thanks to the foresighted members of the Audubon Society for their restoration work.

On this trip, you must return the way you came.

❖ Pescadero to Pigeon Point ❖

Just half a mile south of the Pescadero State Beach parking area, two narrow paths thread through ice plant, coyote bush, and seasonal wildflowers to small sandy beaches and acres of rocky surf. At very low tide some sea water remains in crevices and pools of many sizes in which sea anemones, small crabs, star fish, and myriad mollusks await the incoming tide. The sea life is delicate and perfectly balanced to survive when there is little or no water at low tide. Look, learn about the marine life, but do not take any specimens of creatures, plants, shells, or rocks.

At low tide the outcrops of tilted gray rock expose vertical striations in gradations of light gray to black. You can walk from the trail at the north end of the beach at the water's edge to the trail at the south end, except at extremely high tides. There are no parking areas, restrooms or picnic tables. Parking is possible at the side of Highway 1. No dogs, horses, motorized vehicles, taking of plants or sea life, camping, or beach fires are allowed.

PEBBLE BEACH AND BEAN HOLLOW STATE BEACHES

Stroll a winding path between these beaches on a rocky, wave-swept coast.

Jurisdiction: State of California

Facilities: A few picnic tables and barbecues; parking; restrooms

Rules: Open 8 A.M. to sunset; no dogs on trail, but are allowed on Bean Hollow beach; no horses, beach fires, or motorized vehicles; refrain from removing shells, wood, and plants

Distance: 1 mile

Time: ½ hour

Pebble Beach, part of Bean Hollow State Beach and two miles south of Pescadero Creek, has long been popular because of the unusual shiny pebbles that coat its strand. This was a popular destination in the 19th century when Pescadero had a brief fame as a summer resort. Visitors from San Francisco and the San Mateo County Bayside would stay at hotels in the little town of Pescadero and, according to a tourist guide of the time, collect pebbles from the beach. The guide noted: "Near the town is the famous Pebble Beach where agates, opals, jaspers, and carnelians, of almost every conceivable color, are found in great abundance, with a natural polish imparted by the action of the waves."

At Pebble Beach now, instead of nearby large hotels, is a parking lot with restrooms, and steps leading down to the small but beautiful beach. Collecting pebbles is no longer permitted, nor should one disturb the nearby tidepools or the interesting honeycomb-shaped rocks on the beach. But somewhat sheltered by the rocky points at each end, this beach is a protected place to splash in the shallow water at low tide.

Leading south from Pebble Beach is a narrow foot trail which meanders 1 mile south to Bean Hollow Beach through low-growing coastal-scrub vegetation. Check the information placards at the kiosk by the trail entrance for photos and descriptions of flowers and features along the trail. The spring wildflowers blooming along this trail are magnificent. The trail runs within sight and sound of Highway 1, thereby somewhat diminishing its feeling of wildness, but if you look seaward, the coastal bluffs and offshore rocks lead your eye out to the ocean. Here you may see fishing boats hovering offshore or large container ships sailing along the horizon. At low tide on warm days you may see the gray forms of harbor seals sunning themselves on the exposed rocks. If you are lucky, you may spot the spray of passing whales during their annual, December-to-March migration along the coast.

There are no beaches along this stretch of trail, but the tidally exposed rocks are used extensively by fishermen. From an occasional small pullout along the highway a fisherman's footpath runs down to the rocks above the sea. Your trail crosses many small arroyos on wooden bridges.

At **Bean Hollow State Beach**, your trail descends the bank to the sand and crosses this small, sheltered beach to the south side, where on the bluff you find another parking lot with restrooms, some picnic tables, and barbecues. This is one of the few state beaches where dogs on leash are allowed. A one-hour round trip on this trail would be pleasant, or you can divide your party, one member driving south to pick you up at the next beach. On a clear warm day the sandy beaches on either side of the parking area are ideal for children's sand play, sun bathing, or family picnics.

COASTAL ACCESS AT 10101 HIGHWAY 1

About one mile south of Bean Hollow on a western bend in the highway look west for a small sign marked 10101—the entrance to another Coastal Access point. Take this short road to a small parking area and the trail entrance at 10257 Cabrillo Highway, a few paces north at the end of a tall wooden fence. The 10-foot wide trail passes between a barbed wire fence and the side yard of a private home. Stay within the trail easement and continue to an overlook above a rocky point. Looking north you see the rugged, beautiful coastline topped by marine terraces, indented by small coves and waves rolling from hundreds of miles out in the Pacific Ocean. Just below is a tiny, craggy, private beach set off by a barbed wire fence and a broad, flat marine rock terrace. The pock-marked surface is wave-scoured and totally inundated at high tide and a favorite site for seabirds to congregate.

PIGEON POINT
LIGHT STATION

The Peninsula Open Space Trust is working with California State Parks to acquire this historic lighthouse on the south San Mateo County coast. Presently closed to visitors due to structural difficulties, Peninsula Open Space Trust and the state will see that this significant site is preserved. Just east of the lighthouse property the cliffs above Whalers Cove offer a magnificent view of rugged coastline, outlying rocks and crashing surf. Here POST plans a public seating area and a one-mile link in the Coastal Trail to be named Mel's Lane in honor of Mel Lane, former publisher of Sunset magazine.

Across the highway and a little south on Pigeon Point Road, POST built a one-mile trail that zigzags up the hillside to an overlook named Wilbur's Watch. Honoring Colburn Wilbur, retired execu-

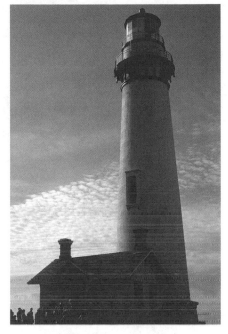

Pigeon Point Light Station

tive director of the David and Lucile Packard Foundation, the overlook offers views of the incredible coves and rocky coast on either side of Pigeon Point from Año Nuevo to Bolsa Point. Benches, an interpretive sign, and a mounted telescope at the overlook add to the pleasure of your climb to Wilbur's Watch. The trail and an eight-car parking area are open during daylight hours. Turn east from Highway 1 on Pigeon Point Road and continue to the parking area on the road's uphill side.

◆ Año Nuevo State Reserve and Coastal Access ◆

Best known for its northern elephant seal rookery, this interesting unit of the state park system has extremely varied natural features as well as human history that will fascinate all visitors. The State of California purchased Año Nuevo Island and a strip of adjacent mainland in 1958 to create the reserve, which now has been expanded to include over 4000 acres of coastal mountains, bluffs, dunes, and beaches. The section of the reserve where the elephant seals breed is restricted to public access by guided tours (from December 1 to March 31) or by permit (from April 1 to November 30). Park rangers and docents are in the reserve to assist visitors in the restricted area. No access is allowed to Año Nuevo Island.

Named for the new year in 1603 by the party of Spanish explorer Sebastián Vizcaíno, who sailed past at that season, this coastal area had long been inhabited by Native Americans who hunted, fished, and gathered shellfish from the sea.

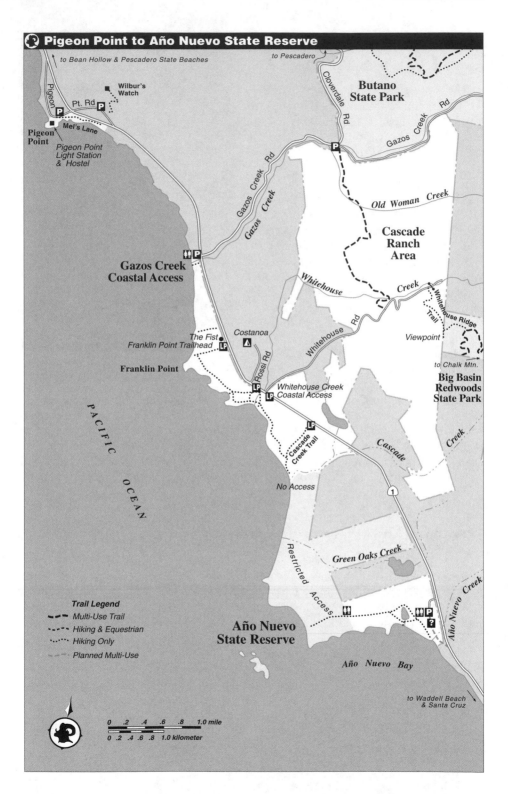

Pigeon Point to Año Nuevo State Reserve

to Bean Hollow & Pescadero State Beaches

to Pescadero

Pigeon Pt. Rd

Wilbur's Watch

Cloverdale Rd

Butano State Park

Gazos Creek Rd

Pigeon Point

Mel's Lane

Pigeon Point Light Station & Hostel

Gazos Creek Rd

Gazos Creek

Old Woman Creek

Cascade Ranch Area

Gazos Creek Coastal Access

Whitehouse   Creek

Whitehouse Ridge Trail

Costanoa

The Fist
Franklin Point Trailhead

Whitehouse Rd

Viewpoint

to Chalk Mtn.

Franklin Point

Rossi Rd

Whitehouse Creek Coastal Access

Big Basin Redwoods State Park

Cascade Creek Trail

Cascade   Creek

No Access

1

P A C I F I C   O C E A N

Restricted Access

Green Oaks Creek

Año Nuevo Creek

Trail Legend
– Multi-Use Trail
--- Hiking & Equestrian
····· Hiking Only
– – Planned Multi-Use

Año Nuevo State Reserve

Año Nuevo Bay

to Waddell Beach & Santa Cruz

0   .2   .4   .6   .8   1.0 mile
0 .2 .4 .6 .8 1.0 kilometer

After the founding of Mission Santa Cruz 19 miles to the south, the natives were greatly reduced in numbers due to their contact with Europeans. The Año Nuevo lands were used for pasturage, then became part of a private Mexican rancho in 1842, and eventually some of the land was purchased by the Steele brothers, who operated a dairy farm at Año Nuevo. Some of the park buildings, including the visitor center, a former barn, are relics of this period.

Lands on the northeast side of Highway 1 that are part of Año Nuevo State Reserve, formerly Cascade Ranch, are now open for trail use. Take Gazos Creek Road east to the intersection of Gazos Creek and Cloverdale roads and park off-road. Two old farm roads used for ranger patrol, Old Womans Creek Road and Whitehouse Road, are open to bicyclists and equestrians. Hikers can use these roads too. In addition, hikers can take a rough trail leading south from Old Womans Creek Road to Whitehouse Road. Then they can take Whitehouse Creek Road uphill to the Whitehouse Ridge Trail, a hikers-only trail to the Chalks in Big Basin Redwoods State Park (described on page 327 below in the Whitehouse Ridge Trail section).

Old Womans Creek Road is gated against vehicle access, but Whitehouse Road is open to vehicles up to the gated private road just beyond the hikers trailhead to the Chalks.

The San Mateo Coast Natural History Association publishes an excellent booklet, which is invaluable for a visitor taking the self-guiding nature walk from April through November. *Peninsula Trails* will not attempt to replicate the information in this booklet, but describes other trails in the Año Nuevo State Reserve that visitors will enjoy.

Jurisdiction: State of California Parks and Recreation: 650-879-2025, advance reservations necessary beginning October 1: 800-444-4275

Facilities: Elephant-seal rookery; visitor center with parking; restrooms; guided walks; small pond and beach (fee); five Coastal Access points; trail in Cascade Ranch Area for hikers, bicyclists, and equestrians; hiking trail connection to Chalk Mountain in Big Basin Redwoods State Park

Maps: USGS topos *Franklin Point* and *Año Nuevo*

How to Get There: Take Highway 1 south 30 miles from Half Moon Bay or north 19 miles from Santa Cruz to main entrance station on west side of highway to meeting place for guided walks.

FIVE WALKS TO AÑO NUEVO BEACHES

There are five places along Highway 1 between the Año Nuevo main entrance and Gazos Creek that provide public access to the Coastside. About 6 miles north of the reserve is the **Cascade Creek Trail**. Here are a parking lot and a trail that crosses about a mile of grassland toward the southwest, with views of Año Nuevo Island at the end of the curving coast. There is native bunchgrass and prostrate coyote brush and in spring lovely displays of blue-eyed grass and yellow sun-cups. A row of eucalyptus and cypress trees remains from a windbreak planted years ago to shelter agricultural fields. You will note a marshy area at the delta of Cascade Creek, where once stood a dam to impound water for irrigation in the summer.

This marsh is now splendid bird habitat. Here you are at the northern border of the closed area of Año Nuevo Reserve; go anywhere you want to the north, but not to the south. A lovely, lonely beach is at the foot of the bluffs at the end of this trail, but it is covered at high tide.

A trail along the bluff goes north to the next beach access points at **Whitehouse Creek**, which are only 0.4 mile north. If you return to Highway 1 and drive, you will find two roadside parking areas here, one on the south, one on the north side of Whitehouse Creek. No house remains, but there is evidence of early settlement here—Monterey pine and eucalyptus trees and non-native gorse bushes. The southside trail crosses fields to join the Cascade Creek Trail and reaches the coastal bluffs beside the steep gulch of Whitehouse Creek.

The north-side trail winds around in the grasslands, but it is easy walking and inspires one to run and enjoy the fresh breezes and sunshine (you would not want to come here on a foggy day; the trails are too indistinct and the bluffs too sudden!). Look here for sea otters resting in the kelp beds off the rocky shore, and marvel at how the sea has carved off a rocky "sea stack" just beyond the cliff. This stack has a grassy thatch on top, remnant the coastal prairie.

About one mile farther north is the **Franklin Point Trail**. This point is named in memory of an American clipper ship, the *Sir John Franklin*. Traveling in a dense fog to San Francisco from the East Coast, it went aground on the rocks here in 1865. The trail entrance is marked by a unique wooden sculpture which resembles a fist; in fact, the rangers call it "The Fist." There actually are two small pullouts here, not far apart. The terrain here is markedly different from that of the grasslands farther south. This is an area of sand dunes with marshlands in between, all covered with dense vegetation of dune grass, coyote brush, wild strawberry, lizard tail, yarrow, and in very wet areas, lush cinquefoil plants, a yellow-flowered member of the rose family. The trail to the beach is not very well defined, and goes through some wet areas. We do not recommend leaving the trail, as the undergrowth is difficult to walk through, and susceptible to damage. This is marvelous habitat for all kinds of animals. Northern harriers, red-tailed hawks, and other raptors are continually gliding overhead looking for their next meal.

After you have walked about half a mile from the highway, you reach the dunes near Franklin Point, and can see to the north a long sandy beach stretching all the way to Gazos Creek, the north end of Año Nuevo State Reserve. Much of this beach is covered at high tide, but at low tide it is perhaps one of the least-visited and private beaches on the San Mateo Coast. It is not only humans that find this a secluded beach; when the authors visited it in March 1996 they were astonished to find on the smooth sand a set of sea-turtle tracks leading toward the ocean from a conspicuous mound of sand. A female turtle had come ashore in the night and laid her eggs, covered them with her flippers and gone back to sea! This is a rare event on this part of the California coast. The turtle probably was either a Pacific Ridley or a leatherback turtle, and it is important to make sure that there remain such quiet, protected beaches for these giant creatures to use.

The northernmost Coastal Access in Año Nuevo Reserve is at **Gazos Creek**. From here The Fist is visible about 1 mile to the south. The parking area at Gazos Creek has restrooms and steps down to the beach, and the signs say NO VEHICLES, DOGS, FIRES OR CAMPING. OPEN 8 A.M. TO SUNSET. You can walk south along the beach, looking for

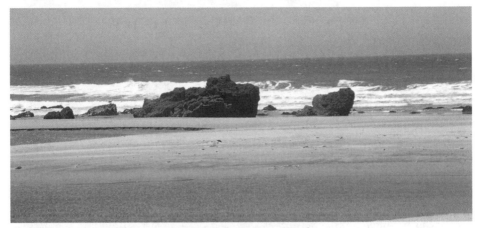

Low tide exposes a wide beach and huge rocks at Gazos Creek

lavender sand verbena, wild cucumber, and buttercups blooming in spring. A coastal trail shown on the Año Nuevo map that is purported to start from this beach on the dunes has not been maintained for many years, and one should not attempt to walk south on the beach itself except at low tide. The parking and beach access trails described above are used mainly by fishermen. Other visitors too, will find this an exhilarating way to experience the uncrowded parts of California's coast.

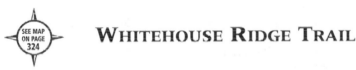

WHITEHOUSE RIDGE TRAIL

Across Highway 1 from the Coastal Access at Whitehouse Creek are Whitehouse Creek Road and the route to a foot trail that climbs the coastal mountains up to Big Basin Redwoods State Park. To get to the trailhead, turn northeast onto Whitehouse Road and follow it for about a mile through private property before reaching the Cascade Ranch section of Año Nuevo State Reserve. Continue on the dirt road winding uphill around some sharp turns with Whitehouse Creek alongside. When you reach a PRIVATE ROAD sign, park at a pull-out and look for the trail entrance in a narrow canyon on the south side of the road. This trail is open to hikers only and winds uphill around many zigzags to two look-outs from which you get tree-framed views of Pigeon Point and Año Nuevo Island. Continue uphill to a hilltop in the Chalks section of Big Basin Redwoods for uninterrupted views north, east, and south over vast forests of redwood, Douglas fir, knobcone pine, and numerous oaks. Westward is the Pacific, its crenellated shoreline revealing breakers dashing against the rocks both south and north. About a mile inland on Chalks Road is 1609-foot Chalks Mountain.

There is a private camp, lodge, and small specialty foods store just across the road from The Fist known as **Costanoa**.

Appendix 1: Trails for Different Seasons and Reasons

*Outstanding Outings

FOR THE SEASONS

SPRING—FABULOUS FLOWER FIELDS

San Bruno Mountain Park	Summit Loop Trail
Crystal Springs Trail	at Edgewood Road
*Edgewood County Park and Natural Preserve	Serpentine Loop Trail
Rancho San Antonio Preserve	High Meadow and Upper High Meadow Trails, Wildcat Loop Trail Duveneck Windmill Pasture
Monte Bello OSP	Bella Vista Trail, Adobe Creek Trail
*Black Mountain	
Russian Ridge OSP	Bay Area Ridge Trail
*Coal Mine Ridge	Ridge Rest

SHADY TRAILS FOR HOT SUMMER DAYS

*Butano State Park	Little Butano Creek Trail
*Mills Canyon Nature Area	Creekside Trail
Huddart Park	Loop Trip Through Center of the Park along McGarvey Gulch
Skyline Trail	from Wunderlich to Huddart Park
Stevens Creek Park	Creek Trail
Long Ridge OSP	Achistaca Trail
San Pedro Valley Park	Old Trout Farm Trail
Purisima Creek OSP	Redwood Trail
El Corte de Madera Preserve	Meandering the Methuselah
Edgewood Park	Sylvan Loop
Skyline Ridge Preserve	Lambert Creek Trail
Monte Bello Preserve	Stevens Creek Nature Trail
Upper Stevens Creek Park	Grizzly Flat Trail

FALL COLOR—TIME FOR CALIFORNIA GOLD

Wunderlich Park	Lower park trails
*Upper Stevens Creek Park	Alternate Trail and Table Mountain—black oaks
Coal Creek Preserve	
Upper Alpine Road Trail	
Huddart Park	Bigleaf maples along creeks
Windy Hill Loop Trail	Deciduous oaks
*Monte Bello Preserve	Canyon Trail
Pescadero Creek Park	Old Haul Road
Sam McDonald Park	Heritage Grove Trail

WINTER WALKS—FOR A BREATH OF AIR
BETWEEN SHOWERS ON SURFACED PATHS

San Andreas Trail	to Larkspur Drive
Sawyer Camp Trail	
"The Loop" through	
Portola Valley	Alpine Road Hiking, Riding and Bicycle Path and Sand Hill Road Paths
	Santa Cruz Avenue to Freeway 280
Arastradero/Foothill	
Expressway Hub Trails	
*The Bay Trails	
San Bruno Mountain Park	Bog Trail and Guadalupe Trail
*Coastal Trail	Half Moon Bay State Beaches

HOW FAR IS IT?
From Short Walks to Long Hikes

SHORT WALKS ON NEARLY LEVEL TRAILS LESS THAN FIVE MILES

All Coastal Trails	especially Half Moon Bay State Beaches
Año Nuevo State Reserve	Cascade Creek Trail
*Whitehouse Creek Trails	
San Bruno Mountain Park	Saddle Loop Trail
Junipero Serra Park	Live Oak Nature Trail
San Andreas Trail	short round trip from north end at San Bruno Ave.
Sawyer Camp Trail	short round trips from south end
Laurelwood Park	Main paved trail from Shasta Drive
"The Loop"	Alpine, Portola, Sand Hill Road trails—any segment
Arastradero Foothill	
Expressway Trails	
*Rancho San Antonio	
Park and Preserve	Trail to Deer Hollow Farm
	Rogue Valley Trail
Stevens Creek Park	Creek Trail, Mt. Eden Hiking and Riding Trails from Mt. Eden Road to Canyon Trail junction
*The Bay Trails	
San Pedro Valley Park	Weiler Ranch Road, Old Trout Farm Trail
Crystal Springs Trail	Freeway 92 to Edgewood Road
*Burleigh Murray State Park	A Hike on a Historic Ranch
Purisima Creek Redwoods	Purisima Creek Trail from west entrance—1st mile
	Redwood Trail
Skyline Ridge Preserve	Loop trip around Alpine Lake
Butano State Park	A Historic Ranch Trip
Los Altos Hills	Artemas Ginzton and Juan Prado Mesa pathways
Memorial Park	West Side Loop Trip on Creek and Homestead trails
Pescadero Creek Park	Short Walk to Pescadero Creek
Stevens Creek Park	Trails from Mt. Eden Road to Canyon Trail Junction, and Creek Trail

LONG HIKES—*Five to ten miles*

Butano State Park	Circumnavigate the Park
Sawyer Camp Trail	round trip on entire trail
Waterdog Lake, Sheep Camp and Crystal Springs trails	to Edgewood Road
Huddart Park	All-Day Hike Circling the Park
Wunderlich Park	Figure-Eight Loop Trip
Skyline Trail	
Fremont Older Preserve	to Stevens Creek Park and return on Hayfields, Ridge, and Old Canyon Trails
*Saratoga Gap	to Monte Bello Preserve Page Mill entrance
San Bruno Mountain Park	Summit Loop and East Ridge Hike
Sweeney Ridge GGNRA	Mori Ridge Trail to Discovery Site round trip Ridge Trail from Milagra Ridge to Portola Gate and return
Purisima Creek Redwoods	Loop Trip from north entrance on Whittemore Gulch or Harkins trail to west entrance and return on Purisima Creek, Soda Gulch, and Harkins Ridge trails; Bald Knob and Grabtown Gulch Trip
El Corte de Madera Preserve	Westward Ho!, Meandering the Methuselah, *Trip into Preserve's Southern Canyons
Windy Hill Preserve	Windy Hill Loop Trail, To the Top of Spring Ridge
Pescadero Creek Park	Brook Creek Loop, Tarwater Creek Basin Loop

LOOP TRIPS THROUGH SEVERAL PARKS OR PRESERVES

◆ Upper Stevens Creek Park, Monte Bello, Long Ridge and Hickory Oak preserves on Charcoal Road and Canyon, Grizzly Flat, Peters Creek, Long Ridge and Hickory Oak trails

◆ Monte Bello Preserve, Skyline Ridge, Russian Ridge and Coal Creek preserves on Stevens Creek Nature Trail, Skid Road, Bay Area Ridge trails, Coal Creek Meadows, Upper Alpine Road and Monte Bello Boundary Line Trail

◆ *Monte Bello, Skyline Ridge and Long Ridge preserves an Upper Stevens Creek Park on Stevens Creek Nature Trail, Skid Road, Bay Area Ridge Trail, Grizzly Flat and Canyon Trails

◆ Stevens Creek Park through Fremont Older Preserve on Lookout, Ridge, Old Canyon, Stevens Canyon trails

◆ *Rancho San Antonio Preserve Loop Trip on Deer Hollow, Upper Meadow Ridge and PG&E service road trails

EXPEDITIONS—*Trails combined for hikes of more than ten miles*

◆ Highway 92/Cañada Road to Wunderlich Park Skyline Boulevard entrance on Crystal Springs and Skyline trails

◆ Belmont to Wunderlich Park, a 2-day trip, with car shuttle, on Waterdog Lake, Sheep Camp, Crystal Springs trails to Huddart Park trail camp for overnight; next day, Crystal Springs, Skyline and Alambique trails to Wunderlich Park main entrance on Woodside Road

◆ San Andreas, Sawyer Camp trails round trip

◆ Skyline Trail from Huddart Park to Wunderlich Park and return

◆ Huddart Park main entrance to Purisima Creek Redwoods Preserve west entrance and return—on Dean, Crystal Springs, Skyline and Purisima Creek trails or take in reverse and overnight at Huddart Park trail camp

◆ Duveneck Windmill Pasture Area to Black Mountain in Monte Bello Preserve, Bella Vista and Canyon trails to Saratoga Gap; or take in reverse

◆ Purisima Creek Redwoods—Bald Knob and Irish Ridge Exploration

◆ Butano State Park—Circumnavigate the Park

◆ Long Ridge to Big Basin—2 or 3-day hike with overnights in Portola Redwoods and Big Basin Park

◆ Pescadero Creek Park—Butano Ridge Trail Loop

◆ Portola Redwoods to Big Basin round trip

◆ Sam McDonald to Big Basin on Towne Ridge, Brook, Pomponio, Iverson, Portola and Basin trails

DOWNHILL ALL THE WAY—*With a car shuttle*

◆ *Basin Trail from Big Basin to Portola Redwoods

◆ Waterdog Lake Trail from St. James Road to Lyall Road

◆ *Wunderlich Park, Skyline Boulevard entrance to Woodside Road entrance on Alambique Trail or Skyline, Alambique and Bear Gulch trails

◆ San Bruno Mountain Park—Either leg of Summit Loop Trail from top of mountain

◆ Junipero Serra Park from upper picnic area on Quail Loop Trail to lower picnic areas or continue to San Bruno City Park

◆ Huddart Park from Skyline Boulevard entrance on Chinquapin Trail to Miwok picnic area

◆ Windy Hill Preserve fFrom Skyline Boulevard entrances on Spring Ridge, Hamms Gulch or Razorback Ridge trails to Alpine or Portola roads

◆ Monte Bello or Coal Creek Preserves—From Page Mill Road or Skyline Boulevard on Upper Alpine Road to lower entrance gate

SPECIAL DESTINATIONS

VIEW POINTS—*Hikes to high places*

*San Bruno Mountain Park	Summit Loop Trip
Sweeney Ridge GGNRA	
Edgewood Park	Serpentine Trail
Wunderlich Park	Skyline Trail toward Mt. Hamilton
	Alambique or Bear Gulch trails to "The Meadows"
Los Trancos Preserve	Loop Trip on Francisco and Lost Creek trails
Fremont Older Preserve	Hunters Point and Maisie's Peak
Stevens Creek Park	Lookout Trail to Lookout Point
	Canyon Trail
Sheep Camp Trail	
*McNee Ranch State Park	to Montara Mountain
San Pedro Valley Park	Hazelnut Trail
El Corte de Madera Preserve	Loop Trip to Vista Point

Windy Hill Preserve   Loop Trip Around Knobs on Anniversary Trail
Russian Ridge Preserve   Trip to Borel Hill on Bay Area Ridge Trail
Monte Bello Preserve   Indian Creek Trail or Bella Vista Trail to Black Mountain
Skyline Ridge Preserve   Skyline Trail to Vista Point
Long Ridge Preserve   Over the Meadows and through the Woods
      to Long Ridge Views, and Hickory Oaks Ridge Area
*Rancho San Antonio Preserve   Upper Meadow Ridge Trail to Vista Point
      Duveneck Windmill Pasture Area–Trek to Black Mountain
Butano State Park   To an Overlook and Some Unusual Habitats
Windy Hill   Summit Hike on Anniversary Trail
*La Honda Creek Preserve   A Trip down the Meadow for a Coastside View
Purisima Creek Redwoods   Trip from North Ridge, Bald Knob Exploration
San Pedro Valley Park   Montara Mountain and Brooks Creek Falls Trail
Skyline Ridge OSP   Bay Area Ridge Trail

ALMOST WILDERNESS—*Yet so close to home*
Butano State Park   Circumnavigate the park
*El Corte de Madera Preserve   Exploring the Lawrence Creek Watershed
Huddart Park   Trails in upper park
      Skyline Trail
      Dean Trail
      Crystal Springs Trail
*Wunderlich Park   Alambique Trail in upper park
Monte Bello Preserve   Canyon Trail
Duveneck Windmill Pasture Area
Rancho San Antonio Preserve   Wildcat Loop Trail
      Rogue Valley to Upper Wildcat Canyon,
      and To the Shoulder of Black Mountain
Purisima Creek Redwoods   Trip from North Ridge to Whittemore Gulch
Portola Redwoods Park   Peters Creek Loop Trip
Pescadero Creek Park   Butano Ridge Loop Trip

CREEKSIDE TRAILS—*By pools and riffles with rocks and overhanging trees*
Mills Canyon Park
Laurelwood Park
*Huddart Park   Richards Road and Crystal Springs trails along
      West Union Creek
"The Loop"   Alpine Road Hiking, Riding and Bicycle Trail
Rancho San Antonio Preserve   Wildcat Loop Trail
Stevens Creek Park   Creek Trail
San Pedro Valley Park   Old Trout Farm Trail
Purisima Creek Redwoods   Purisima Creek Trail
      Whittemore Gulch Trail
Burleigh Murray State Park
El Corte de Madera Preserve   To Sandstone Formation and El Corte de Madera Creek
Windy Hill Preserve   Eagle Trail on Windy Hill Loop
Monte Bello Preserve   Stevens Creek Nature Trail
*Pescadero Park   To the Creek and Brooks Trail Loop
Sam McDonald Park   Forest Loop Trail Ext., Heritage Grove Trail on Alpine Creek

GLIMPSES OF 19TH CENTURY RANCHES
Orchards, vineyards, cattle grazing, milk farms and haying

◆ Año Nuevo State Reserve—Reserve visitor center a former barn

◆ Monte Bello Preserve—Indian Creek Trail or Bella Vista Trail to Morrell Ranch on Black Mountain—ranch house removed, now backpack camp on ranch site

◆ Fremont Older Preserve—Historic Older house

◆ Picchetti Ranch Open Space Preserve—Early vineyards and orchards, winery buildings preserved

◆ Rancho San Antonio Preserve—Deer Hollow Farm and former Grant Ranch house

◆ Burleigh Murray State Park—historic barn

◆ Skyline Ridge Preserve—former route from Page's Mill to Palo Alto and route to Coast

◆ Purisima Creek Redwoods, El Corte de Madera preserves, Huddart and Wunderlich county parks, Phleger Estate—sites of early logging camps

◆ Windy Hill, Long Ridge and Skyline Ridge preserves—route of early settlers farm road

MEADOWS AND HILLTOPS
For kite flying, hawk watching, peaceful picnicking

San Bruno Mountain Park	
Sweeney Ridge GGNRA	
Milagra Ridge	
Sheep Camp Trail	
Wunderlich Park	Upper Meadow on Skyline Trail
Los Trancos Preserve	Page Mill Trail
Monte Bello Preserve	Bella Vista Trail
	Adobe Creek Trail
Rancho San Antonio Park and Preserve	Wildcat Loop Trail
	Loop Trip to Upper Meadow
Fremont Older Preserve	Hunters Point
La Honda Creek Preserve	
Russian Ridge Preserve	
Pulgas Ridge Preserve	
Coal Creek Preserve	Meadow Trail
Windy Hill Preserve	Anniversary Trail, Spring Ridge Trail
Long Ridge OSP	Hickory Oak Ridge Area
Pescadero Park	Brook Trail Loop
Wunderlich Park	Upper Meadow on Skyline Trail

NATURE TRAILS AND SELF-GUIDING TRAILS

Junipero Serra Park	Live Oak Nature Trail
Huddart Park	Chickadee Trail
Rancho San Antonio Preserve	Docent trip to Deer Hollow Farm

Los Trancos Preserve Self-guiding and Docent Trips,
San Andreas Fault Trail
San Bruno Mountain Park Bog Trail
Monte Bello Preserve Stevens Creek Nature Trail
Memorial Park Tan Oak and Mt. Ellen Nature trails
Portola Redwoods Park Sequoia and Iverson trails

TRAILS ON HISTORIC ROUTES

Sawyer Camp Trail
Sheep Camp Trail
Huddart Park Richards Road Trail, Summit Springs Trail
Arastradero Bike Path
Alpine Road Hiking,
Riding, and Bicycle Trail
Upper Alpine Road
Sweeney Ridge GGNRA Portola Discovery Site of S.F. Bay
Purisima Creek Redwoods Purisima Creek Trail
Skyline Ridge Preserve Old Page Mill Road
Coastal Trail Portola Expedition route
with campsite at San Gregorio Beach
McNee Ranch Old San Pedro Mountain Road
Sawyer Camp Trail
Sheep Camp Trail

· BIRDWATCHING BY THE BAY—*By marshes and sloughs*

◆ All San Francisco Bay Trails

◆ All Coastal Trails—many species plus endangered snowy plover

◆ See *Meadows and Hilltops* above

TRAILS THROUGH FANTASTIC PENINSULA FORESTS
Once logged, now regrown

Butano State Park
Memorial Park
Pescadero County Park
Sam McDonald Park
Portola Redwoods State Park
Purisima Creek
Redwoods Preserve Purisima Creek Trail
Huddart Park
Wunderlich Park Bear Gulch Trail and Alambique-Skyline Trail Loop
El Corte de Madera Preserve Meandering the Methuselah Trail
Skyline Trail from Huddart to Wunderlich Park
Windy Hill Preserve Windy Hill Loop Trail
Hamms Gulch and Razorback Ridge trails

HIKING TRAILS OPEN FOR BICYCLISTS, EQUESTRIANS AND WHEELCHAIR USERS

FOR BICYCLISTS

On Paved Paths:

Almost all the Bay Trails
San Bruno Mountain Park
Radio Road to summit
Sweeney Ridge GGNRA   Sneath Lane
San Andreas Trail
Sawyer Camp Trail
Arastradero Hub Trails
"The Loop"
Rancho San Antonio County Park To Deer Hollow Farm

On Unpaved Service and Fire Roads:

Purisima Creek Redwoods Purisima Creek Trail
El Corte de Madera Preserve
Fremont Older Preserve All trails but footpath from Prospect Road
Windy Hill Preserve Spring Ridge Trail
Upper Alpine Road
San Pedro Valley Park Weiler Ranch Road
Skyline Ridge Preserve
Monte Bello Preserve Canyon Trail
Los Trancos Preserve Page Mill Trail
Long Ridge Preserve Hickory Oak Ridge Area
Arastradero Preserve All Trails except the Perimeter Trail

EQUESTRIAN TRAILS *(**equestrian parking)*
(Some trails closed in wet weather)

San Bruno Mountain Park
Sweeney Ridge
Crystal Springs Trail
Edgewood Park
Pulgas Ridge Preserve
Huddart Park**
Wunderlich Park**
Skyline Trail
"The Loop" Alpine, Portola and Sand Hill Road trails
Windy Hill Preserve
Monte Bello Preserve** All trails except Stevens Creek Nature Trail
Los Trancos Preserve Page Mill Trail only
Upper Alpine Road
Arastradero Preserve
Rancho San Antonio** Except Wildcat Canyon Trail
Duveneck Windmill Pasture
Fremont Older Preserve Except for Foot Trail from Prospect Road
Long Ridge Preserve Hickory Oak Ridge Area
Purisima Creek Redwoods Except for Whittemore Gulch,
Soda Gulch and Grabtown Gulch trails

El Corte de Madera Preserve
Russian Ridge Preserve

FOR WHEELCHAIR USERS—*Level, surfaced paths*

San Andreas Trail	north end
Laurelwood Park	Shasta Street entrance
Alpine Road Hiking, Riding and Bicycle Trail	(some parts)
Dwight F. Crowder Bike Path	(some parts)
Varian/Bol Park Path	
Palo Alto/Los Altos Bike Path	
Rancho San Antonio Park and Preserve	(Call MROSD for permit parking)
San Bruno Mountain	Bog Trail
Purisima Creek Redwoods	Redwood Trail
Huddart Park	Chickadee Trail
Skyline Ridge OSP	Trail around Alpine Pond
Coyote Point Recreation Area	Bathing Beach Museum and walks from Parking
The Bay Trails	Most are surfaced and almost level
Monte Bello Preserve	First part of Stevens Creek Nature Trail to Vista Point

SPECIAL OCCASIONS AND DESTINATIONS

OUTINGS WITH YOUNG CHILDREN
Try a birthday party with no crumbs on the rug.
Short walks, picnic tables, some barbecues and restrooms, kite flying

San Bruno Mountain Park	
Junipero Serra Park	
San Pedro Valley Park	
Laurelwood Park	Play equipment
Huddart Park	Play equipment
Rancho San Antonio County Park	To Deer Hollow Farm
Skyline Ridge Preserve Deck, visit Nature Center	Loop Around Alpine Pond; lunch on Nature Center (open in summer on weekends)
Purisima Creek Redwoods Preserve	Redwood Trail
Edgewood Park Day Camp Area	Take a wildflower hike with docent
Stevens Creek County Park Old Canyon Trail and Bay Tree Picnic Area	
The Bay Trails	Many picnic tables at parks along the way Sierra Point Marina Oyster Point Marina and Beach Point San Bruno Park Coyote Point Recreation Area Ryder Park

OVERNIGHT IN THE PARKS AND PRESERVES
Youth groups and backpack camps and hostels by reservation

Butano State Park	backpack camp
Half Moon Bay State Beaches	car camping
San Bruno Mountain Park	youth groups
Junipero Serra Park	youth groups
Huddart Park	youth groups and backpackers
Memorial Park	groups
*Monte Bello Preserve	backpackers on Black Mountain
Hidden Villa Hostel	(closed in summer)
Sam McDonald Park	camping for youth groups only
Hikers Hut	
Jack Brooks Horse Camp	
Portola Redwoods State Park	Campgrounds and Slate Creek Backpack Camp
Pescadero Creek County Park	Shaw Flat and Tarwater Trail Camps
*Montara Lighthouse Hostel	
Pigeon Point Light Station Hostel	

PARKS AND PRESERVES WITH MUSEUMS AND VISITOR CENTERS

Butano State Park	Nature Center
San Pedro Valley Park	
Coyote Point Recreation Area	Museum
Stevens Creek Park	
Portola Redwoods State Park	
Año Nuevo State Reserve	
Skyline Ridge OSP	Daniels Nature Center

ROUTES TO REMOTE AND ANCIENT REDWOODS

La Honda Creek Preserve	Trail to the Big Tree
Long Ridge to Portola Redwoods	Ward Road and Slate Creek Trails
Memorial Park	Tan Oak Trail
Methuselah Tree	on east side of Skyline Boulevard opposite El Corte de Madera gate CM02
Pescadero Creek Park	Brook Trail and Butano Ridge Loop Trails
*Portola Redwoods Park	Peters Creek Loop Trip, Old Tree and Slate Creek Trails
Purisima Creek Redwoods Preserve	Lower Whittemore Gulch Trail
El Corte de Madera OSP	
*Sam McDonald Park	Big Tree Trail, Heritage Grove Trail

Appendix 2: Selected Readings

Bay Area and California
Brewer, William H. *Up and Down California in 1860-1864*, Berkeley:
    University of California Press, 1974.
Brown, Alan K., *Sawpits in the Spanish Redwoods, 1787-1849*, Redwood City San Mateo
    Historical Association. 1966. Reprinted through generosity of Ken L. Fisher, San
    Mateo County, CA.
Chase, Smeaton J., *California Coast Trails*, Boston, Houghton Mifflin Co. 1913.
    Reprinted Palo Alto, Tioga Publishing Co, 1987.
Cupertino Chronicle, Cupertino: California History Center, De Anza College, Local
    History Studies, Vol. 19, 1975.
Fava, Florence M., *Los Altos Hills, A Colorful Story*, Woodside: Gilbert Richards
    Publications, 1976.
Gudde, Erwin G, *California Place Names*. 4th ed. Berkeley, University of California
    Press, 1998.
Hoover, Mildred B. and Hero Eugene Rensch, Revised by Douglas Kyle, *Historic Spots
    in California*, Stanford, CA Stanford University Press, 4th Edition, 1994.
Margolin, Malcolm, *The Ohlone Way, Indian Life in the San Francisco-Monterey Bay Area*,
    Berkeley: Heyday Books, 1978. New edition
Marinacci, Barbara and Rudy Marinacci, *California's Spanish Place-Names*. 2nd ed.
    Houston: Gulf Publishing Company, 1997.
Morrall, June, *Half Moon Bay Memories; the Coastside's Memorable Past*, El Granada:
    Moonbeam Press, 1987
Stanger, Frank M. *South From San Francisco, San Mateo County, California, Its History
    and Heritage*, San Mateo County Historical Association, 1963.
_____,*Sawmills in the Redwoods, Logging on the San Francisco Peninsula, 1889-1967*, 2nd
    printing, San Mateo: San Mateo County Historical Association, 1992.
VanderWerf, Barbara, *Montara Mountain*, El Granada: Gum Tree Land Books, 1994.

Natural History
Bakker, Elna S., *An Island Called California*, Berkeley: University of California Press,
    1971.
Conradson, Diane R., *Exploring Our Baylands*. 3rd ed. Fremont: San Francisco Bay
    Wildlife Society, 1996.
Birding at the Bottom of the Bay, Santa Clara Valley Audubon Society, Palo Alto, 2nd ed.
    1990.
Crittenden, Mabel, and Dorothy Teller, *Wildflowers of the West*, Blaine: Hancock House
    Publishers, 1992.
Little, Elbert., Nationnal Audubon Society Field Guide to North American Trees,
    Western Region. New York: Alfred A. Knopf, 1994.
Lyons, Kathleen and Mary Beth Cuneo-Lazaneo, *Plants of the Coast Redwood Region*,
    Los Altos: Looking Press, 1988.
McClintock, Elizabeth, Paul Reeberg and Walter Knight, *A Flora of the San Bruno
    Mountains*, Sacramento: California Native Plant Society, 1990.
Murie, Olaf J, *A Field Guide to Animal Tracks*, Boston: Houghton Mifflin, 3rd ed. 1990.
Pavlik, Bruce, and Pamela Muick, Sharon Johnson, and Marjorie Popper, *Oaks of
    California*, Los Olivos: Cachuma Press, Inc. and California Oak Foundation, 1991.
Peterson, Roger Tory, *A Field Guide to Western Birds*, Boston: Houghton Mifflin Co. 1990.

National Geographic Society, *Field Guide to the Birds of North America.* 3rd ed. Washington: National Geographic Society, 1999.
San Francisco Peninsula Birdwatching, San Mateo: Sequoia Audubon Society, 1996.
Sharsmith, Helen K. *Flora of the Mt. Hamilton Range of California*, American Midland Naturalist, Vol. 34, no.2, September 1945. Special reprint: Berkeley: California Native Plant Society, 1982.
Stebbins, Robert C. *A Field Guide to Western Reptiles and Amphibians of the San Francisco Bay Region*, 2nd ed. Boston, Houghton Mifflin Company, 1985.
Thomas, John Hunter, *Flora of the Santa Cruz Mountains of California*, Stanford, CA: Stanford University Press, 1961.
The Natural History of the Fitzgerald Marine Reserve, Conradson, Diane R., editor and Virginia B. Welch, Managing editor, Friends of Fitzgerald Marine Life Refuge, Moss Beach, CA.

California Natural History Guides: University of California Press, Berkeley
Carle, David, *Introduction to Water in California*
Munz, Philip A, *Introduction to California Spring Wildflowers of the Foothills, Valleys, and Coast. Revised Edition*
Hedgpeth, Joel W., *Introduction to Seashore Life of the San Francisco Bay Region and the Coast of Northern California.*
E. W. Jameson, Jr., and Hans J. Peeters, *Mammals of California. Revised Edition.*
Gilliam, Harold, *Weather of the San Francisco Bay Region.* 2nd Edition.
Robert Ornduff, Phyllis M. Faber, and Todd Keeler-Wolf, *Introduction to California Plant Life.* Revised Edition
Robert F. Heizer and Albert B. Elsasser, The Natural World of the California Indians
Steve J. Grillos, *Ferns and Fern Allies of California.*
Sharsmith, Helen K., *Spring Wildflowers of the San Francisco Bay Region.*
Schoenibert, Allan A., *A Natural History of California.*
Arthur D. Howard, *Geologic History of Middle California.*

Trail Guides
Backpacking California, Edited by Paul Backhurst, Berkeley: Wilderness Press, 2001.
California State Coastal Conservancy, *San Francisco Bay Shoreline Guide*, Berkeley: University of California Press. 1995.
Maps, San Francisco Bay Trail, San Francisco Bay Trail Project, Oakland: Association of Bay Area Governments.
Heid, Matt, *101 Hikes in Northern California*, Berkeley: Wilderness Press, 2000.
Rusmore, Jean *The Bay Area Ridge Trail, Berkeley*: Wilderness Press, 2nd edition, 2002.
Rusmore, Jean, Betsy Crowder and Frances Spangle, *South Bay Trails*, Berkeley: Wilderness Press, 3rd edition, 2000.
VanderWerf. Barbara, The Coastside Trail Book, El Granada, Gum Tree Lane Books, 2nd edition, 1995.
Granada, A Synonym for Paradise: The Ocean Shore Railroad Years
Montara Mountain.
Weintraub, David *East Bay Trails*, Berkeley: Wilderness Press, 1998.

Appendix 3: Information Sources on Parks, Preserves, Trails, and Trail Activities

PUBLIC AGENCIES

Golden Gate National Recreation Area, NPS
Fort Mason
San Francisco, CA 94123
415-561-4700

Fort Funston Ranger Station
415-239-2366
www.nps.gov/goga/

Pacifica Visitor Center
225 Rockaway Beach Avenue
Pacifica, CA 94044
650-355-4122
www.pacificachamber.com/

**Don Edward's San Francisco Bay
National Wildlife Refuge**
P.O. Box 524
Newark, CA 94560
510-792-2222
www.gypcnme.com/don%20edwards%
20wildlife%20refuge.htm

**State of California,
Department of Parks and Recreation**
800-777-0369
www.parks.ca.gov/

San Mateo Coast
See individual parks in text
650-726-8819
Reservations 800-444-7275
Backpack camps in Portola Redwoods
and Big Basin Park 831-338-8861

California State Coastal Conservancy
1330 Broadway, Suite 1100
Oakland, CA 94612
510-286-1015
www.coastalconservancy.ca.gov/

Midpeninsula Regional Open Space District
333 Distel Circle
Los Altos, CA 94022
650-691-1200
http://www.openspace.org/

**San Mateo County
Parks and Recreation Department**
County Government Center
590 Hamilton St.
Redwood City, CA 94063
650-363-4020
Reservations 650-363-4021
http://www.eparks.net/smc/county/home

**Santa Clara County
Parks and Recreation Department**
298 Garden Hill Drive
Los Gatos, CA 95031
408-355-2200
Reservations 408-355-3751
www.parkhere.org

San Mateo Coast Beaches
www.parks.ca.gov/parkindex/

Fort Funston and Thornton State Beach	415-239-2366
Pacifica City and State Beaches	650-738-7380
Montara State Beach	650-726-8819
Half Moon Bay State Beaches	650-726-8819
Cowell Ranch State Beach	650-726-8819
James V. Fitzgerald Marine Reserve	650-728-3584
Pillar Point Marsh	650-728-3584
Blufftop Coastal Park	650-726-8297
San Gregorio and Pomponio State Beaches	650-726-8819
Pescadero State Beach and Marsh	650-726-8819

Pebble Beach
and Bean Hollow Beach   **650-879-2179**

Año Nuevo State Reserve
and Coastal Access   650-879-2025

CITY PARKS DEPARTMENTS

Atherton	650-325-4457
Belmont	650-595-7441
Brisbane	650-467-6330
Burlingame	650-696-3770
Daly City	650-991-8001
East Palo Alto	650-953-3100
Foster City	650-345-5731
Half Moon Bay	650 726-8297
Los Altos Hills	961-941-7222
Menlo Park	650-858-3470
Millbrae	650-259-2360
Mountain View—	
Deer Hollow Farm	961-903 6430
Pacifica	650-738-7380
Palo Alto	650-329-2261
Portola Valley	650-851-1700
Redwood City	650-780-7250
San Bruno	650-877-8868
San Carlos	650-802-4382
San Mateo	650-377-4640
South San Francisco	650-877-0560
Woodside	650-851-6790

Bay Area Open Space Council
www.openspacecouncil.org/

TRANSPORTATION AGENCIES SERVING PARKS AND PRESERVES

BART   415-992-2278
www.bart.gov/   510-465-2278
Customer Service Hours
Monday through Saturday 6:00 A.M. to 10:00 P.M.
Sunday 8:00 A.M. to 10:00 P.M.
Local Telephone Numbers
Oakland/Berkeley/Orinda   510 465-2278

San Francisco/Daly City   415 989-2278

**South San Francisco/
San Bruno/San Mateo**   650 992-2278

Concord/Walnut Creek/
Lafayette/Antioch/Pittsburg/
Livermore   925 676-2278

Hayward/San Leandro/
Fremont/Union City/
Dublin/Pleasanton   510 441-2278

Richmond/El Cerrito   510 236-2278

BART Police	877-679-7000
Emergency	911
Non-emergency	877 679-7000
TDD	510 839-2278
Elevator Availability	510 834 LIFT
	888 235-3828
Delays and Service Updates	510 834-2100
Lost and Found	510 464-7090

**San Francisco
Municipal Railway—MUNI**
www.sfmuni.com/   415-673-6864

**Samtrans (San Mateo
County Transit District)**
www.samtrans.com/   800-660-4287

**Santa Clara County
Transportation Agency**   800-894-9908
www.vta.org/

TRANSPORTATION GUIDES

Metropolitan Transportation Commission,
Regional Transit Guide, 9th ed., Oakland:
Metropolitan Transportion Commission, 1996.
www.mtc.ca.gov/

Bay Area Open Space Council and Greenbelt
Alliance, Transit Outdoors, The Public Transit
Guide to San Francisco Bay Area Regional
Parks, San Francisco: Greenbelt Alliance, 1995.
www.openspacecouncil.org/OSC/

ORGANIZATIONS SPONSORING GROUP HIKES, BICYCLE AND HORSEBACK RIDES, INTERPRETIVE TRIPS, TRAIL MAINTENANCE DAYS

Many public agencies offer docent-led nature walks and occasional trail maintenance days. Consult the agency near you from the above list. In addition, local and statewide nonprofit groups sponsor outdoor trips for environmental education and enjoyment, such as the following groups:

Hostelling International
Santa Clara Valley Chapter   408-293-3787
www.hiayh.org/

San Francisco Chapter   415-771-7277
www.norcalhostels.org

Juan Bautista de Anza Trail   415-744-3968
http://www.nps.gov/juba/

Audubon Society—Bird walks
Sequoia Chapter   650-529-1454
http://www.sequoia-audubon.org
Santa Clara Valley Chapter   408-252-3747
www.scvas.org

Bay Area Orienteering Club   408-255-8018
http://www.baoc.org/

Bay Area Ridge Trail Council
Quarterly Outings Calendar
of guided trips   415-561-2595
http://ridgetrail.org/index.htm

San Francisco Bay Trail   510-464-7935
http://baytrail.abag.ca.gov/

Bicycle Groups, e.g. California Association of Bicycle Organizations, East Bay Bicycle Coalition, ROMP, Western Wheelers

California Native Plant Society
Santa Clara Valley Chapter   650-856-2636
www.stanford.edu/~rawlings/blazcon.htm

San Mateo County Chapter   650-948-1829
                                 800-325-2843

Coastwalk   707-829-6689
www.coastwalk.org/

Community Colleges
Some offer group hiking classes:

Skyline, San Mateo, Cañada
www.smccd.net

Foothill, De Anza
http://www.fhda.edu/

Environmental Museums
**California Academy
of Sciences**   415-750-7145
www.calacademy.org/

Coyote Point Museum   650-342-7755
www.coyoteptmuseum.org/

Filoli Center—Docent tours
of wildland area   650-364-2880
www.filoli.org/

**Golden Gate
National Parks Conservancy**   415-560-3000
www.parksconservancy.org/

Greenbelt Alliance   415-398-3730
www.greenbelt.org/

Hiking Clubs—e.g. Sierra Club
San Francisco Main Office   415-977-5500
http://www.sierraclub.org/

American Volkssport
San Francisco   415-334-4279
San Jose   408-376-0992
http://www.ava.org/

Horsemen's Associations—San Mateo County Volunteer Horse Patrol, San Mateo County
Horsemen's Assn.   650-368-8200
http://www.smcha.org

Marine Science Institute—Discovery Voyage, mostly for school groups
www.sfbaymsi.org/   650-364-2760

Mountain Parks Foundation   831-335-3174
www.mountainparks.org/

Peninsula Open Space Trust   650-854-7696
www.openspacetrust.org/

Pescadero Marsh
Natural Preserve   650-879-2170
www.bahiker.com/
southbayhikes/pescaderomarsh.html

Santa Cruz Mountains
Natural History Association   831-335-3174
                               or Dial-A-Hike
                               415-948-9198

Santa Cruz Mountains
Trail Association   415-968-2412
www.stanford.edu/~mhd/trails/

Sempervirens Fund   650-968-4509
www.sempervirens.org/

Senior Centers—Some offer group walks:
call cities

Sierra Club—Local chapters offer hiking,
bicycling, backpacking, climbing and kayaking
trips
Loma Prieta Chapter   415- 390-8411
http://lomaprieta.sierraclub.org/

The Nature Conservancy   415-281-0423
http://nature.org/

The Trail Center—A 4-county nonprofit, volunteer trail information and trail maintenance
clearinghouse   415-968-7065
www.trailcenter.org/

Women's Outdoor Network—
Recreation resource for active
Bay Area women   415-494-8583
www.pcbvi.org/services/recreation.htm

Youth Groups   Boy Scouts, Girl Scouts, and
Campfire units and YMCA, YWCA

Map List

Index

Numbers in **boldface** refer to primary entry for that area.

Wilderness Press covers the San Francisco Bay Area

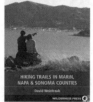

North Bay Trails
Hiking Trails in Marin, Napa & Sonoma Counties

Fifty-six routes in the coastal salt marshes, remote mountaintops, and shady redwood groves of the North Bay. Includes clear, easy-to-follow directions, photos, and maps.

ISBN 0-89997-378-7

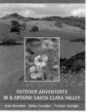

South Bay Trails
Outdoor Adventures in & around Santa Clara Valley

Explore Silicon Valley's 125,000 acres of public open space, from San Jose to the Santa Cruz Mountains. Over 100 routes and 568 miles of trails in the southern San Francisco Bay Area are described.

ISBN 0-89997-284-5

East Bay Trails
Outdoor Adventures in Alameda & Contra Costa Counties

Fifty-three hikes in 31 parks in the East Bay parklands offer respite and recreation, from the Carquinez Strait to the Ohlone Wilderness, San Francisco Bay to Mt. Diablo.

ISBN 0-89997-213-6

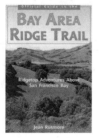

Bay Area Ridge Trail
Ridgetop Adventures Above San Francisco Bay

This official guide covers the 230 completed miles of the planned 425-mile recreation trail encircling the San Francisco Bay. Includes trailhead access, on-the-trail directions, side trips, facilities, and maps.

ISBN 0-89997-280-2

For ordering information, contact your local bookseller or Wilderness Press, www.wildernesspress.com.